Hysteroscopy, Resectoscopy and Endometrial Ablation

Hysteroscopy, Resectoscopy and Endometrial Ablation

Edited by

Eric J. Bieber, MD

Geisinger Medical Center, Danville, PA

and

Franklin D. Loffer, MD

Department of Obstetrics and Gynecology, University of Arizona, Phoenix, AZ

The Parthenon Publishing Group
International Publishers in Medicine, Science & Technology

A CRC PRESS COMPANY

BOCA RATON   LONDON   NEW YORK   WASHINGTON, D.C.

Notice to readers: The indication and dosages of all drugs in this book have been recommended in the medical literature and conform to the practice of the general medical community. The medications described do not necessarily have specific approval by the Food and Drug Administration (FDA) for use in the diseases and dosages for which they are recommended. The package insert for each drug should be consulted for use and dosage as approved by the FDA. Because standards of usage change, it is advisable to keep abreast of revised recommendations, particularly those concerning new drugs.

Published in the USA by
The Parthenon Publishing Group
345 Park Avenue South, 10th Floor
New York
NY 10010
USA

Published in the UK and Europe by
The Parthenon Publishing Group
23–25 Blades Court
Deodar Road
London SW15 2NU
UK

Library of Congress Cataloging in Publication Data
Data available on request

British Library Cataloguing-in-Publication Data
Data available on request

ISBN 1-84214-117-1

Typeset by AMA DataSet Ltd., Preston, UK
Printed and bound in the USA

Contents

List of contributors

J. A. Abbott, MD, PhD
University of New South Wales
Royal Hospital for Women
Randwick, NSW 2031
Australia

R. Barnes, MD
Department of Obstetrics and Gynecology
Northwestern University
Feinberg School of Medicine
Chicago, IL
USA

E. J. Bieber, MD
Geisinger Medical Center
Danville, PA
USA

P. G. Brooks, MD
UCLA School of Medicine
Cedar-Sinai Medical Center
Los Angeles, CA
USA

E. Confino, MD
Division of Reproductive Endocrinology and
    Infertility
Department of Obstetrics and Gynecology
Northwestern Feinberg School of Medicine
Chicago, IL
USA

J. Cooper, MD
Department of Obstetrics and Gynecology
University of Arizona School of Medicine
Phoenix, AZ
USA

J. R. Elliott, BSc, BASc, MESc
110–12051 Horseshoe Way
Richmond, BC
Canada V7A 4V4

R. J. Gimpelson, MD
Department of Obstetrics and Gynecology
St. Louis University School of Medicine
St. Louis, MI
USA

S. Levrant, MD
Partners in Reproductive Health
Tinley Park, IL
USA

F. D. Loffer, MD
Department of Obstetrics and Gynecology
University of Arizona
Phoenix, AZ
USA

K. R. Loughlin, MD
Department of Urology
Brigham and Womens' Hospital
Boston, MA
USA

A. Magos, BSc, MD, MRCOG
Minimally Invasive Therapy Unit and
    Endoscopy Training Centre
University Department of Obstetrics and
    Gynecology
The Royal Free Hospital
London NW3 2QG
UK

E. Skalnyi, MD
Novacept Inc.
1047 Elwell Court
Palo Alto, CA 94303
USA

R. M. Soderstrom, MD
Department of Obstetrics and Gynecology
University of Washington School of Medicine
Seattle, WA
USA

A. Taylor, MBBS, MRCOG
Minimally Invasive Therapy Unit and
    Endoscopy Training Centre
University Department of Obstetrics and
    Gynecology
The Royal Free Hospital
London NW3 2QG
UK

D. E. Townsend, MD, FACOG
Private Practice
Park City
Utah
USA

R. D. Tucker, PhD, MD
Department of Pathology
University of Iowa Hospitals and Clinics
Iowa City, IA
USA

R. F. Valle, MD
Department of Obstetrics and Gynecology
Northwestern University Medical School
680 N. Lake Shore Drive, Suite 1015
Chicago, IL 60611
USA

T. G. Vancaillie, MD
University of New South Wales
Royal Hospital for Women
Randwick, NSW 2031
Australia

D. B. Yackel, MD, FRCSC
MDMI Technologies Inc.
110–12051 Horseshoe Way
Richmond, BC
Canada V7A 4V4

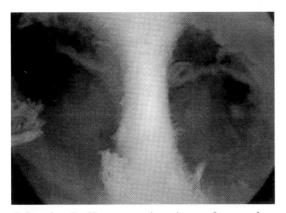

Color plate I Hysteroscopic view of complete uterine septum

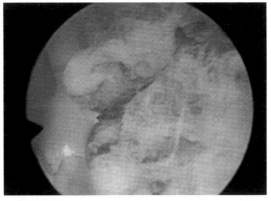

Color plate II Resectoscopic resection of uterine septum with electric knife: initial division

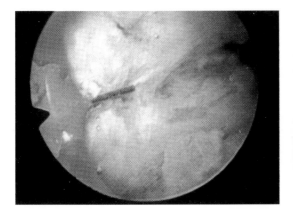

Color plate III Resectoscopic resection of uterine septum with electric knife: deeper cutting

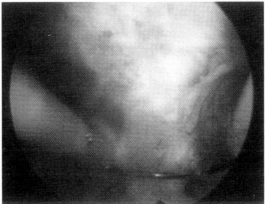

Color plate IV Resectoscopic resection of uterine septum with 180° loop

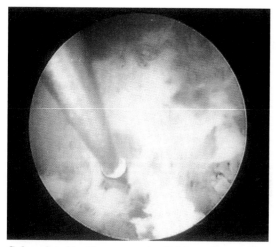

Color plate V Hysteroscopic division of extensive fundal intrauterine adhesions: initial division of adhesions

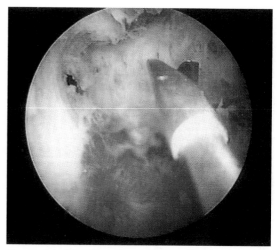

Color plate VI Hysteroscopic division of extensive fundal intrauterine adhesions: right uterotubal cone is visible

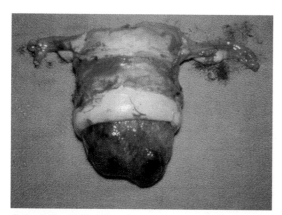

Color plate VII The size of submucous myomas is probably self-limiting – this fibroid measuring approximately 6 cm could no longer be contained in the uterine cavity

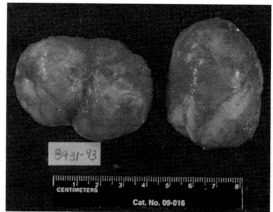

Color plate VIII These leiomyomas, which were removed intact through an abdominal incision, show that the shape of leiomyomas is not always round. More may lie intramurally than is apparent on hysteroscopic view. A grading scale would probably correctly have identified the degree of intramural extension for the leiomyoma on the right. However, the constricted area as soon on the specimen on the left could have given the impression that the intramural portion was smaller than that projecting into the uterine cavity

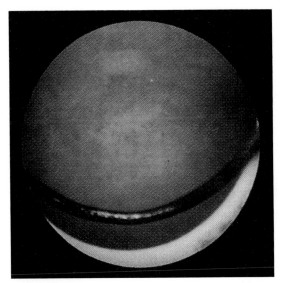

Color plate IX The appearance of the uterine cavity at the start of endometrial resection

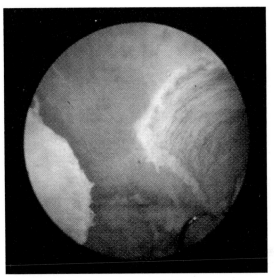

Color plate X The endometrial/myometrial interface during surgery

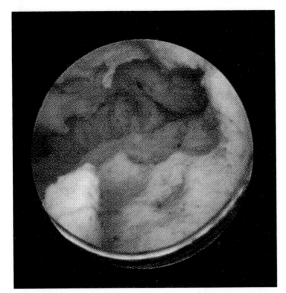

Color plate XI The appearance of the uterine cavity at the end of endometrial resection

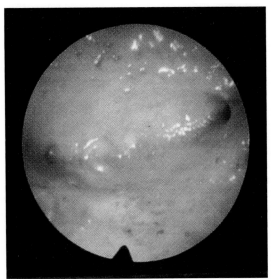

Color plate XII Photo of uterus – normal cavity

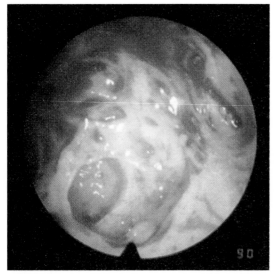

Color plate XIII Photo of uterus – postablation (synechiae)

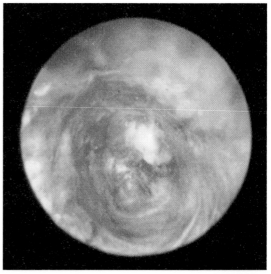

Color plate XIV Photo of uterus – postablation (narrowed and cylindrical)

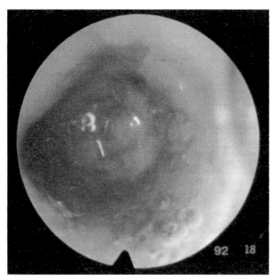

Color plate XV Uterine cavity before curettage

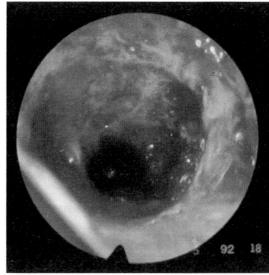

Color plate XVI Uterine cavity after curettage

Preface

Hysteroscopy first achieved limited interest among modern gynecologists in the early 1970s when it was thought that it might be suitable to replace laparoscopy as an effective method of female sterilization. The electrical techniques in use at that time had several disadvantages that resulted in its abandonment.

The second spurt of enthusiasm for learning hysteroscopy occurred in the early 1980s when the formed-in-place silicone plug was being investigated. Although a successful sterilization technique, it received no commercial support and is no longer available. About this same time, the ability to ablate the endometrial cavity for the control of menorrhagia using Nd:Yag laser energy was published. The enthusiasm that followed this technique further increased interest in hysteroscopy.

However, it was the introduction of the resectoscope and electrical energy to perform intrauterine surgery that has resulted in the most recent and widespread increased interest in diagnostic and operative hysteroscopy. The ready availability of electricity as an energy source in virtually all hospitals and the ability to apply this form of treatment based on the experience of urologists, has made this technique available to most experienced hysteroscopists.

Since the publication of our text, *Gynecologic Resectoscopy* (Blackwell Science, Inc., Cambridge, MA, USA, 1995), hysteroscopy has continued to be used by more gynecologists. In addition, simpler and equally effective methods of endometrial ablation have been developed which have allowed those gynecologists who had not developed traditional hysteroscopic operative skills to provide this procedure to their patients.

Hysteroscopic sterilization techniques have also been developed and are now available.

The division of the subject into the chapters we have selected is certainly arbitrary. There is inevitably a cross over between chapters on techniques, theoretical considerations and procedures. However, we selected contributing authors who could act as spokesmen for the techniques described. They were asked to provide not only a manual for accomplishing the procedure, but also the rationale and results based on the procedure. In this fashion it is hoped that the reader will be able to achieve a balanced view of the value and uses of the hysteroscope, resectoscope and other novel ablation technologies. Inevitably in a multi-authored text, there might initially appear to be conflicting opinions. Rather than confusing the reader, this should simply alert them to the fact that there are generally several ways of accomplishing the same goal.

Undoubtedly, some of the more difficult and complex intrauterine surgical procedures will eventually be carried out by a limited number of hysteroscopists. However, it is our belief that all gynecologists should be capable of evaluating the uterine cavity by hysteroscopy and of accomplishing the more common and simpler intrauterine surgical procedures.

We hope that this text will further encourage physicians to develop their hysteroscopic skills and allow those already experienced in diagnostic hysteroscopy to advance their skills in hysteroscopic intrauterine surgery.

Eric J. Bieber, MD
Franklin D. Loffer, MD

Acknowledgements

It was our hope when this book was conceived that it would provide a source for practicing gynecologic endoscopists who are using or wish to use the hysteroscope, resectoscope and ablation technologies. It is clear as one reviews the literature on intrauterine surgery that electrical energy has assumed increasing importance and is more versatile than either mechanical or laser energy.

Since it was first published, non-hysteroscopic methods of endometrial ablation have been developed and hysteroscopic sterilization has become available. Since these are important advances in operative hysteroscopy we have included numerous new chapters.

We intended that this text provide not only a manual of instruction in order to perform hysteroscopic surgery, but also to present the theoretical considerations that led to variation in techniques. It would have been impossible to accomplish this without the expertise, wisdom and skill of our contributors. We are indeed appreciative for the sharing of their experience with our readers.

Others have also made this text possible including publisher David Bloomer and Pam Lancaster, the production editor, who have allowed us a smooth interface with the publication of this material. In addition, we each must acknowledge our personal staff's contributions, including Marilyn Harter's help in researching material and Carole Jones' untiring efforts in preparation of the manuscripts.

Finally, I wish to express my appreciation and love to my wife, Trish Loffer, and family, who tolerated the months of clutter in the study and the hours of absence among that clutter (FDL). I would also like to thank my wife, Edie Bieber, for tolerating my dream chasing, my parents George and Audrey who taught me to reach and dream higher then I believed I could, and my children Brandon and Andrew who continue to help remind me that dream chasing keeps us young (EJB).

1

The origins of the resectoscope

K. R. Loughlin

There are several reasons why a knowledge and understanding of the origins of the resectoscope should be important to the modern surgeon. First, the resectoscope is one of the most common surgical instruments in use today. In 1989, over 400 000 transurethral resections of the prostate were performed[1]. Its use in gynecology has significantly increased over the last decade. Second, the same scepticism and uncertainty that surrounds many aspects of surgical innovation today were present during the development of the resectoscope. Perspective can be gained by recalling what was said in a textbook of urology over 35 years ago:

'Despite the extensive salesmanship with which transurethral resection was promoted in the early 1930s as a simple, successful operation without important danger, the procedure has suffered greatly at the hands of both trained and untrained blunderers with an overall mortality and morbidity in excess of open operation. Yet, today, in the hands of the competent, the mortality is not over two to four percent in all cases, hemorrhage and infection being the grave and relating frequent complications. Bleeding may occur weeks or even months postoperatively. Transurethral resection is decidedly an operation only for expert experienced hands[2].'

The resectoscope, like most significant surgical advances, cannot be credited to one individual.

The development of the resectoscope was the culmination of the independent as well as joint efforts of basic scientists and clinicians to solve a surgical problem. The genesis of the resectoscope can best be credited to the work of Bottini, who in 1877 described his galvanocautery incisor. His incisor was fitted with a platinum blade and connected to a source of electricity using insulated wires. However, Bottini's instrument did not permit the surgeon any visualization of the obstructive lesion. Modifications of Bottini's instrument were made by Freudenberg, Goldschmidt, Wishard and Chetwood, but none of their designs achieved widespread acceptance[3].

Nesbit credits the development of the resectoscope to three discoveries: the incandescent lamp, high-frequency current and the fenestrated sheath[3]. Thomas Edison invented the incandescent lamp in 1879 and within a decade duRocher had constructed a cystoscope that incorporated the incandescent lamp.

In 1900, the first American-made cystoscope was designed by Reinhold Wappler and William Otis in New York and was presented at the American Association for Genito-Urinary Surgeons in 1900[3]. Early contributions and continued modifications of the resectoscope were made by Hugh Young, William Braasch and Bransford Lewis. However, the next major advance in resectoscope design belongs to Maximilian Stern and Joseph McCarthy.

In 1926, Stern published an article describing his instrument for transurethral resection of the prostate[4]. Stern designed a cutting hoop that consisted of a small ring of tungsten about 0.5 cm in diameter placed at right angles to the end of an insulated shaft. The tungsten loop was positioned in front of the eye of the telescope and was moved backward toward the operator to cut tissue. Stern's original illustrations are reproduced in Figures 1 and 2. Stern is credited with first using the term 'resectoscope'.

During the time when the early resectoscopes were undergoing development, other technological advances were occurring in parallel. A young physicist in Boston, William T. Bovie, was working on the development of a new electrosurgical unit to cauterize tissue. The first time Bovie's unit was used clinically was October 1, 1926, at the Peter Bent Brigham Hospital[5]. Harvey Cushing was the operating surgeon and he used Bovie's electrocautery unit to remove a vascular myeloma. Bovie's work made the

application of diathermy possible to open surgical procedures. Also, Bovie's investigations into the applications of surgical electrocautery laid the foundation for further refinement of the resectoscope. However, early on, clinical surgeons were sceptical of the electrocautery unit and did not embrace its use.

Bovie ultimately sold his patent for the electrocautery unit to the Liebel–Florshelm Company for one dollar[5].

The early applications of electrical current for transurethral prostate resection were cumbersome. Edward L. Keyes Jr and Clyde W. Collings are credited with the first use of cutting electrical current for prostatic obstruction[3]. They employed a vacuum tube to supply the current and were unable to use the current underwater, so they distended the bladder with oil[3]. They reported their initial experience at the American Urological Association meeting in June, 1924. It was not until 1931, however, that the vacuum tube generator had sufficient power to enable the urologist to cut tissue underwater. A machine using a vacuum tube generator was developed by Frederick Wappler and was marketed by the ACMI company under the name of the Comprex Oscillator[3].

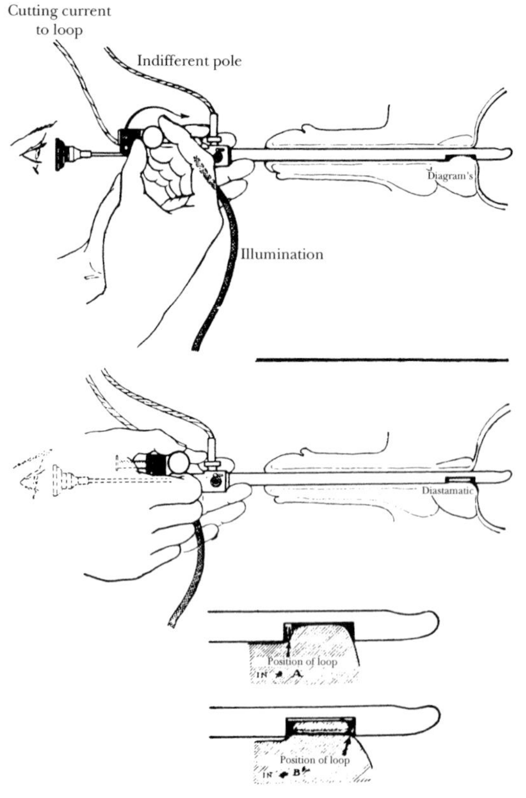

Figure 1 Stern's resectoscope as it appeared in the *Journal of the American Medical Association*, 1926. Reproduced from reference 4, with permission. ©1926, American Medical Association

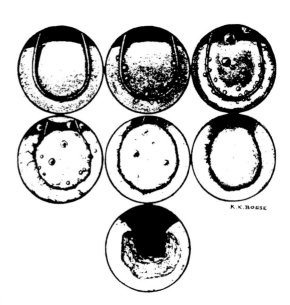

Figure 2 Stern's resectoscope loop, 1926. Reproduced from reference 4, with permission. ©1926, American Medical Association

In addition to improvements in optics and electrocautery, the introduction of the fenestrated tube facilitated the development of the resectoscope. Hugh Young first used a fenestrated tube for his cold punch instrument in 1909[3]. However, Young's original instrument did not permit visualization of the prostate by the surgeon. A few years later, Braasch developed a fenestrated sheath that incorporated direct visualization. In 1926, Bumpus, at the Mayo Clinic, further modified Braasch's instrument by using a tubular knife connected to high-frequency coagulatory current. Bumpus is credited with designing the first instrument for transurethral resection that incorporated the incandescent lamp, high-frequency electrical current and the fenestrated tube[3].

A North Carolina urologist, Theodore Davis, utilized the Bovie generation for transurethral resections. Perhaps his major contribution was the development of a magnetic foot switch that enabled the operating surgeon himself, rather than an assistant, to turn the electrical current off and on.

Joseph McCarthy first reported on his new modification of this resectoscope in a two-page report in the *Journal of Urology* in 1931[6]. In 1932, McCarthy further modified his resectoscope, which was in reality the forerunner of the modern instrument. His design included a foroblique lens system with magnification as well as a Bakelite sheath for insulation. That year, McCarthy wrote a classic article in the *New England Journal of Medicine* entitled 'The management of prostatic obstruction by endoscopic revision'[7]. A picture of McCarthy's instrument appears in Figure 3. Further refinement of the resectoscope continued, and Reed Nesbit persuaded Frederick Wappler, the President of American Cystoscope Makers, Inc., to design a resectoscope that could be used with one hand[3]. This would permit the surgeon's other hand to be placed into the O'Conor drape and to palpate the prostate transrectally during the resection.

Once the resectoscope became established as a viable surgical instrument, the choice of irrigation fluid became a subject of debate. The early experience with sterile water had resulted in red cell hemolysis and renal failure. Creevy and Webb[8] published some of the early work using an isotonic (4%) glucose solution as an irrigation fluid in order to prevent hemolysis. Subsequently, most endoscopic resectionists have used either mannitol, sorbitol or glycine as irrigating solutions. All these solutions are less hypotonic with plasma, and, therefore, do not

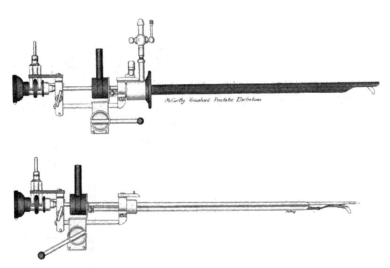

Figure 3 McCarthy's resectoscope as it appeared in the *New England Journal of Medicine*, 1932. Reproduced from reference 7, with permission. ©1932 Massachusetts Medical Society

carry the risk of intravascular hemolysis; however, they can cause hyponatremia.

In 1975, Iglesias and co-workers[9] published a report on their resectoscope, which has emerged as the 'modern' resectoscope and is presently used by most surgeons who perform transurethral resections of the prostate. The new Iglesias resectoscope permits simultaneous suction and continuous irrigation, which results in better visualization of the fluid and lower bladder pressure. The design for the Iglesias resectoscope appears in Figure 4.

The development of the resectoscope essentially took a century to complete. Multiple individuals, some known and some unknown, contributed to its development. The major events that led to the ultimate creation of the resectoscope appear on the 'time line' in Figure 5. It would be naive to assume that the refinement of the resectoscope is complete. Undoubtedly, as long as surgeons use a resectoscope to treat patients, they will continue to redesign, modify and perfect the instrument.

1870

– 1877 Bottini–galvanocautery incisor
– 1879 Edison–incandescent lamp

1880

1890

1900 – 1900 Wappler–first American cystoscope

– 1909 Young–fenestrated tube

1910

1920

– 1926 Bovie–electrosurgical unit
1926 Stern–resectoscope loop

1930

– 1932 McCarthy–foroblique lens

1940

– 1947 Creevy–research on irrigating solutions

1950

1960

1970

– 1975 Iglesias–continuous irrigation resectoscope

1980

Figure 5 Development of the resectoscope

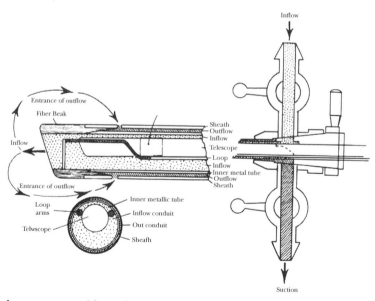

Figure 4 Iglesias' resectoscope with continuous irrigation and suction as described in the *Journal of Urology*, 1975. Reproduced from reference 9, with permission

References

1. Holtgrewe HL, Mebust WK, Dowd JB, *et al.* Trans-urethral prostatectomy: practice aspects of the dominant operation in American urology. *J Urol* 1989;141:248–53

2. Campbell MF. Tumors of the urogenital tract. In Campbell MF, ed. *Principles of Urology.* Philadelphia: WB Saunders, 1957:444–510

3. Nesbit RM. A history of transurethral prostatic resection. In Silber SJ, ed. *Transurethral Resection.* New York: Appleton-Century-Crofts, 1977:1–17

4. Stern M. Resection of obstructions at the vesical orifice. *J Am Med Assoc* 1926;87:1726–30

5. Goldwyn RM. Bovie: the man and the machine. *Ann Plast Surg* 1979;2:135–53

6. McCarthy JF. A new apparatus for endoscopic plastic surgery of the prostate, diathermia, and excision of vesical growths. *J Urol* 1931;26:695–6

7. McCarthy JF. The management of prostatic obstructions by endoscopic revision. *N Engl J Med* 1932;207:305–12

8. Creevy CD, Webb EA. A fatal hemolytic reaction following transurethral resection of the prostate gland: a discussion of its prevention and treatment. *Surgery* 1947;21:56–66

9. Iglesias JJ, Sporer A, Gellman AC, *et al.* New Iglesias resectoscope with continuous irrigation, simultaneous suction, and low intravesicle pressure. *J Urol* 1975;114:929–33

2

Hysteroscopic and resectoscopic instrumentation

S. Levrant

Hysteroscopy and resectoscopy require the use of specialized endoscopic instruments that differ from the endoscopic instruments used for laparoscopy, urology, gastroenterology, etc. Instruments that are common to hysteroscopy and resectoscopy include the endoscope (hysteroscope), light source, distention media and irrigation systems, electrosurgical devices and video camera systems. Unique to resectoscopy is the resectoscope and its electrodes. Knowledge of and experience with the basic techniques and instrumentation of diagnostic and operative hysteroscopy are prerequisite to safe and successful resectoscopy. Endometrial ablation can now be performed using not only the resectoscope, but also with hysteroscopy, or by specific devices that ablate the endometrial tissue by use of bipolar radiofrequency energy, heat or extreme cold.

HYSTEROSCOPES

Flexible hysteroscopes are slender endoscopes, similar in design to gastrointestinal endoscopes that can bend 120–160° at the tip, which is particularly helpful in visualizing an irregularly shaped uterus. Diagnostic flexible hysteroscopes have one channel for fluid; operative flexible hysteroscopes have a second channel, usually 2 mm in diameter for instrumentation. The outer diameter ranges from approximately 3.1 mm for diagnostic hysteroscopes to 5 mm for operative hysteroscopes. Advances over recent years have resulted in improved image size, resolution and brightness due to increases in the number of image fibers and improved optics. Some cameras have angles as wide as 100°. Flexible hysteroscopes have been particularly useful for office diagnostic hysteroscopy.

The rigid hysteroscope consists of a telescope and a sheath system. Diagnostic and operative sheaths are available as single- or continuous-flow systems with one, two or no operating channels that can accommodate scissors, biopsy forceps, grasper forceps and electrodes ranging in size from 3 to 7 Fr. The outer diameter of the hysteroscope sheath ranges from 3 to 8 mm. The size of the hysteroscope increases as the telescope size increases, if it has channels for a continuous-flow system (for low-viscosity fluids) and as the number of operating channels increase. There are a variety of different systems available from several manufacturers. One manufacturer makes a hysteroscope with an offset eyepiece that allows for a straight instrument channel. The offset eyepiece adds comfort to the surgeon operating without a camera, but when attached to the camera, the added length can impede rotation of the telescope to view the uterine cornua. The operative instruments are flexible or semirigid and come in several sizes as previously stated. The unipolar electrode for coagulation and the bipolar Versapoint™ system by Gynecare (a division of Ethicon Inc., Somerville, NJ, USA) are also available for use through the operating channels. Newer smaller hysteroscopes allow diagnostic hysteroscopy to be performed without the need of cervical dilatation and operative procedures to be undertaken with hysteroscopes the same size as the older diagnostic sheaths. A smaller telescope in a larger sheath allows for the use of a larger scissor or grasper. The decrease in instrument size with increased optics has expanded the range of hysteroscopy in both the office and operating room.

RESECTOSCOPES

The gynecological resectoscope is a modified urological resectoscope having a shorter, blunter insulating beak at its distal end (Figure 1). The first reports of gynecological applications of this technique utilized the urological resectoscope[1-4]. The gynecological resectoscope consists of a rigid 3- or 4-mm hysteroscope (telescope), the resectoscope working element, an inner sheath and an outer sheath (Figure 2). The electrodes and the electrosurgical device attach to the resectoscope working element, which contains a built-in finger-controlled spring system that moves the electrode forward and back. Gynecological resectoscopes utilize a passive spring mechanism. The electrode is

inside the sheath in the resting position, advances past the sheath against the spring, and then returns to the sheath (during cutting) by the force of the spring. The electrodes move about 3–4 cm within the visual field of the telescope. Electrical current should only be applied to the electrode when the operative site is completely visualized and the electrode is returning to the sheath.

The original resectoscope was a single-flow device with only an inflow sheath. This is still available for use with high-viscosity distention media. The continuous-flow resectoscope provides continuous flushing of low-viscosity

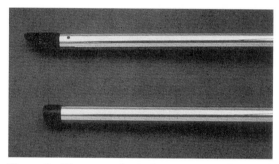

Figure 1 The gynecological resectoscope (bottom) has a shorter, blunter insulating beak than the urological resectoscope (top). Photograph courtesy of Richard Wolf Medical Instruments Corp.

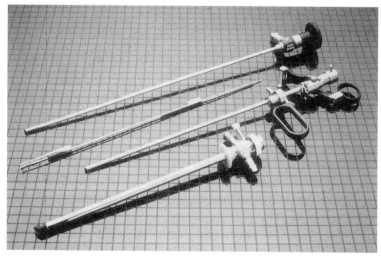

Figure 2 Telescope, electrode, resectoscope working element and assembled inner and outer sheaths. Photograph courtesy of Karl Storz Endoscopy

distention media, resulting in better visualization and safer surgery. The distention media inflow is through the inner sheath and the outflow is through the outer sheath (Figures 3 and 4). The double-channelled sheaths are designed for minimal inflow resistance and have a slightly higher outflow resistance. This resulting continuous flow increases visibility while maintaining intrauterine pressure and distention. The pattern of holes at the distal end of the outer sheath varies according to manufacturer (Table 1, Figures 4 and 5).

Resectoscopes come in a variety of sizes (Table 1). The 24 (8-mm), 25, 26, 27 (9-mm) and 28 Fr resectoscopes utilize the 4-mm telescope. They have separate inflow and outflow sheaths and open (U-shaped) wire-loop electrodes. These resectoscopes are used for all aspects of resectoscopic surgery, but are particularly well suited for the resection of submucosal myomas and large polyps. The 21 and 22 Fr (7-mm) resectoscopes utilize the 3-mm telescope. They have one sheath that contains both the inflow and outflow channels and closed wire-loop electrodes. These smaller resectoscopes are the same size as operative hysteroscopes and are both well suited for removal of small polyps, lysis of intrauterine adhesions and lysis of uterine septa. The smaller resectoscopes are particularly useful in women with cervical stenosis. Resectoscopes are 30–35 cm in total length and have working distances of 18–22 cm (Table 1).

Continuous-flow resectoscopes are listed by manufacturer and size (maximum outer sheath diameter). The four basic electrode designs (see Figure 7), plus several variations on these designs, are available with 25 Fr and larger resectoscopes. Electrode selection/variety tends to be limited with the smaller resectoscopes; however, this varies with manufacturer and is expected to improve.

The light cable and distention medium inflow attach on the top, and the distention medium outflow attaches on the bottom. Reversal of the distention medium inflow and outflow attachments will hinder effective intrauterine distention and visibility (Figure 3).

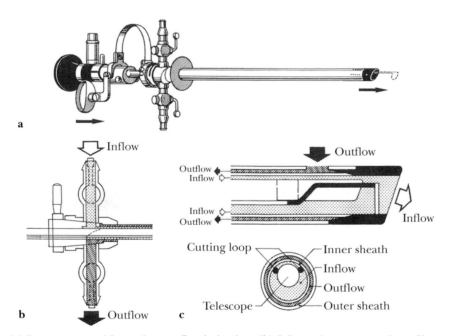

Figure 3 (a) Resectoscope with continuous-flow irrigation. (b) Schematic representation of in- and outflow channels. (c) Longitudinal section of the instrument tip. Cross-section shows the fluid outflow, which lies between the inner and outer sheaths, the inner tube with telescope, cutting loop connectors and lumen for inflow irrigating solution. Reproduced from reference 5, with permission from Elsevier

The electric cable attachment site varies with manufacturer. There are two basic designs for how the instruments lock in place. One is a rotary or twisting lock mechanism, and the other is a snap-in connection (Figures 2 and 6). The rotary design can untwist while rotating the resectoscope during surgery, if one is not careful. The snap-in system will not unlock while rotating the instrument; however, if not held correctly, the resectoscope may unlock when

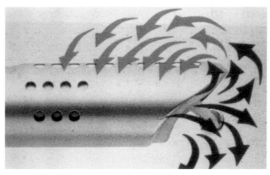

Figure 4 Distal tip of Olympus 9-mm outer sheath. Note top and side hole pattern with schematic of intrauterine irrigation flow. Photograph courtesy of Olympus Corp.

moved within the uterine cavity or removed from the uterine cavity.

ELECTRODES

There are four basic designs of resectoscopic electrodes: the loop, bar/barrel, ball and point or knife-like tip (Figure 7). The loop electrodes are used primarily to shave or remove myomas and polyps. The 90°, 45° and 120° loops are well suited for this purpose. The 0° loop and point or knife-like tips can be used for resection of septa or lysis of intrauterine adhesions. Endometrial ablation is performed using the 90° loop, the ball, the bar/barrel electrode, or some combination of the three. Electrode surface area is inversely proportional to energy density. Thin, loop, electrodes produce high energy densities that cut or vaporize tissue. The ball and bar/barrel electrodes increase the electrode surface area, thereby decreasing current density and heating. The depth of coagulation achieved is dependent on the electrode surface area, time of exposure, and the electrical source and power (see Chapter 3)[6]. Most resectoscopes use monopolar electrodes. Gynecare makes a

Table 1 Continuous-flow resectoscopes

Manufacturer	Size	Telescope size (mm)	Viewing angle°	Outer sheath outflow holes	Connector	Features
Circon ACMI (Southborough, MA, USA)	25.6 Fr	4	12, 30	top and bottom	snap-in	rotatable working element
Gynecare (a division of Ethicon Inc., Somerville, NJ, USA)	27 Fr	4	30	top and bottom	snap-in	bipolar energy
Karl Storz Endoscopy-America Inc., (Culver City, CA, USA)	22 Fr	2.9	12	encircle (single row)	rotary/twist	rotatable
	26 Fr, 28 Fr	4	0, 12, 30	top and bottom		
Olympus America Inc. (Melville, NY, USA)	8 mm	3	12	top and side	snap-in	rotatable
	9 mm	4	12, 30	top and side		optical obturator rotatable sheath
	25 Fr	4	12, 25	top and side	rotary/twist	rotatable ports
Richard Wolf Medical Instruments Corp. (Vernon Hills, IL, USA)	27 Fr, 28.9 Fr	4	12, 25	top and side	and snap-in	

7 mm = 21 Fr (French); 8 mm = 24 Fr; and 9 mm = 27 Fr

bipolar resectoscopic system and Conceptus Inc. (San Carlos, CA, USA) make the ERA sleeve accessory that consists of an outer sheath which incorporates a dispersive electrode that converts a resectoscope from monopolar to bipolar energy.

TELESCOPES

The same telescopes used for diagnostic and operative hysteroscopy are used with the resectoscope. These are panoramic telescopes with a rod lens optical system and range from 1.9 to 4 mm outer diameter. The telescope is focused at infinity; therefore, the image is smaller than actual size when it is positioned away from the

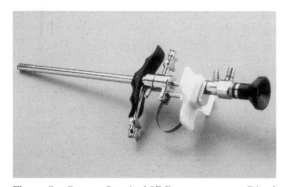

Figure 5 Cooper Surgical 27 Fr resectoscope. Distal tip of outer sheath has hole pattern that encircles the sheath. Photograph courtesy of CooperSurgical, Inc.

object[7]. Magnification is inversely proportional to the distance of the object from the lens[7]. The working distance is 30–35 mm, and because hysteroscopes are monocular, there is little depth perception. The panoramic field varies from approximately 70° to 120°, depending on model and manufacturer. Telescopes are available with a viewing angle of 0°, 5°, 12°, 15°, 25° or 30° (Figure 8). The optic systems have improved over the years to produce brighter sharper images with smaller diameter telescopes. The acute angle telescopes (25° and 30° foroblique) are better suited for visualizing the uterine cornua and lateral walls. For operative hysteroscopy and resectoscopic surgery, there is no single angle of vision that is best for all situations. The fully extended electrode or operative instrument may go beyond the field of view when using a 30° telescope, or partially beyond the view using a 0° telescope. Which angle telescope is used for hysteroscopy and resectoscopy is based on surgeon preference. Prior to purchasing a hysteroscope or resectoscope system, one should operate with the different angles of vision to determine which is best. Ideally, operating with each of the different telescopes within the same uterine cavities should be tried. Having both 0–12° and 25–30° telescopes available for hysteroscopic and resectoscopic systems gives the surgeon greater flexibility.

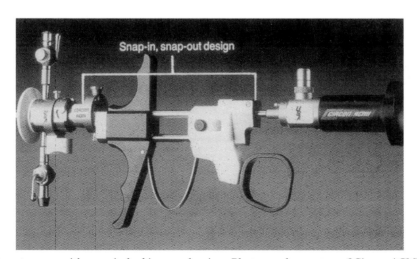

Figure 6 Resectoscope with snap-in locking mechanism. Photograph courtesy of Circon ACMI

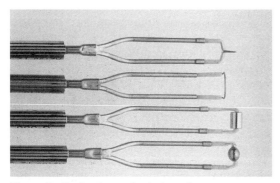

Figure 7 Basic electrode designs for resectoscopy: point, loop, bar/barrel and ball. Photograph courtesy of Olympus Corp.

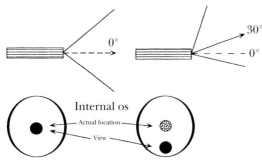

Figure 8 Field of view between 0° (on left) and 30° foroblique telescope. As the 30° telescope passes through the cervical canal with the telescope's axis of symmetry aimed ventrally (at the symphysis pubis), the internal os appears lower in the field of view than where it actually lies

DISTENTION DEVICES

Intrauterine distention during hysteroscopy can be achieved using a variety of distention media. Common to all methods is the goal of using the lowest possible intrauterine pressure and medium flow rate to achieve adequate visualization of the uterine cavity. Adequate distention and visualization of the uterine cavity is usually achieved with intrauterine pressures in the range of 40–80 mmHg. As the intrauterine pressure exceeds the mean arterial pressure within the uterus, the risk of medium absorption rises.

Carbon dioxide insufflators for hysteroscopy are low-flow, low-pressure devices that are not interchangeable with the high-flow laparoscopic insufflators. Flow rates are usually 40–60 ml/min and should not exceed 100 ml/min. Pressure settings should not exceed 100 mmHg and usually 40–80 mmHg is sufficient. Some hysteroscopic insufflators have the operator set the intrauterine pressure and the CO_2 is instilled until that pressure is achieved. Other insufflators allow the operator to preset for the flow rate which then decreases as the intrauterine pressure rises.

Hyskon® (CooperSurgical, Trumbull, CT, USA) is a highly viscous fluid medium that is usually administered by an assistant pushing a 20–50 cc syringe filled with the Hyskon. A pump designed for Hyskon uses CO_2 from a high-pressure source and a reducing valve to limit flow rate to deliver a preset amount of Hyskon. The Hyskon is released at intervals by the surgeon by use of a foot pedal.

Low-viscosity liquid media can be delivered by gravity or by pump. Hanging low-viscosity distention media approximately 8 feet above the floor (a few feet above the patient) and using wide-bore urological tubing (transurethral prostatic resection (TUR) tubing) has been successfully employed by many surgeons. A bag of fluid 3–4 feet above the patient can result in intrauterine pressures of 70–100 mmHg[8]. Standard intravenous (IV) tubing, because of its narrow diameter and high resistance to flow, does not allow a satisfactory distention medium flow rate. Standard IV tubing should not be used for resectoscopic surgery. The use of pressure cuffs on 1- or 3-liter bags of fluid is discouraged, since the intrauterine pressure and flow rate cannot be measured and may exceed safe limits resulting in excessive fluid absorption[9].

A number of hysteroscopic pumps or fluid management systems are available for hysteroscopic and resectoscopic surgery. These systems integrate a pump, usually with preset intrauterine pressure and/or fluid flow rates, and a means of determining the fluid loss or deficit. The pump may be either mechanical using a peristaltic roller, a bladder compression or centrifugal. The pumps maintain constant intrauterine pressures by varying the distention fluid flow rates. Fluid deficits are calculated either by computing the input/output deficit of the measured volume or measured weight of the fluid medium utilized. Inaccuracies may result from the up to 5% volume error of commercially available fluid containers and/or the leakage of fluid on the operating room floor or surgical drapes[10]. The accuracy of intra-uterine pressure measurements may be influenced by leakage around the instruments, resistance of the hysteroscope/resectoscope input or output port or stopcock, and by the amount of suction applied to the outflow port. Dirt or differences in the instruments of differing manufacturers may alter the resistance of input and output ports. In general, flow rates are between 50 and 200 ml/min, but may be set as high as 450 ml/min to 1 liter/min with some machines. Intrauterine pressures can be set between 0 and 150 mmHg on most machines, but usually should not exceed 80 mmHg. The minimal pressure needed to provide adequate distention and visualization should be used at all times. Newer machines have visual and audible alarms to alert the surgeon of difficulty. Manufacturers of hysteroscopic pumps include Circon ACMI (Southborough, MA, USA), Davol Inc. (subsidiary of C.R. Bard Inc., Cranston, RI, USA), Gynecare, Karl Storz Endoscopy-America Inc. (Culver City, CA, USA), Olympus America Inc. (Melville, NY, USA) and Richard Wolf Medical Instruments Corp. (Vernon Hills, IL, USA).

ELECTROSURGICAL DEVICES

A high-frequency electrosurgical unit with a digital wattage indicator is preferable to one with arbitrary dial settings. For safer electro-surgery, the electrosurgical unit should be isolated electrically and advantage taken of developments in the return electrode, i.e. the Valleylab (a division of Tyco Healthcare Group LP, Boulder, CO, USA) return electrode monitoring circuit (REM), or equivalent. The Gynecare Versapoint bipolar system requires the use of the Gynecare Versapoint bipolar generator that is used for both the bipolar hysteroscopic electrodes and the bipolar resectoscope. The Gynecare Versapoint generator unit has diagnostic circuits that not only monitor system performance but also automati-

cally adjust power settings to the attached electrode. The ERA sheath by Conceptus fits over most manufacturer's resectoscopes and is compatible with most electrosurgical units[11].

VIDEO EQUIPMENT

Attaching the video camera to the telescope and performing the surgery while viewing the images on a video monitor magnifies the surgical field, dramatically improves the surgeon's comfort and allows for greater participation and interest of the operating-room staff. The equipment requirements for resectoscopy are the same as those for hysteroscopy and essentially the same as those for laparoscopy.

The basic components include a video camera, high-resolution medical video monitor, video recorder and color video printer.

Camera

Video camera technology has advanced rapidly with increased resolution, increased light sensitivity and, most importantly, enhanced digital processing of the video image. Cameras currently used for endoscopy consist of a lens and either one or three solid-state integrated-circuit image sensors referred to as charge coupled devices (CCDs) or chips. In single-chip cameras, the picture element contains thousands of photosensitive cells, or pixels, that detect the colors red, green or blue. In a camera in which one-third of the pixels are devoted to each color, only one-third of the image falls on any given color. The camera circuitry, then, has to generate colors electronically for the areas that fall on the other pixel colors. Three-chip cameras have three picture elements, each devoted to a single color (red, blue and green), and each sees the entire image. Single-chip cameras have a 20% reduction in pixel resolution as a result of color filtration, but require approximately 15% less light than three-chip cameras. This is changing with increased technology; new three-chip cameras require less light than older single-chip cameras.

Video noise and background graininess, or snow, are measured by the signal-to-noise (S/N) ratio on a logarithmic scale. The higher the S/N ratio, the better the picture. The better single-chip cameras have S/N ratios of around 47 dB compared to S/N ratios of 60+ dB for three-chip cameras.

Differences in single-chip camera systems include the camera head and telescopic optics; the color reproduction, tone and tints are essentially the same. Single-chip cameras come in two sizes, the half-inch chip and the two-thirds-inch chip. The latter has increased resolution (450–550 lines) compared to the former (300–450 lines); 600–800 lines of resolution are generated by three-chip cameras. Three-chip cameras have increased color separation and resolution, and decreased noise, compared to single-chip camera systems.

Features to look for with any camera include a small, lightweight camera head with focusing ring and zoom feature (usually 25–40 mm) and a camera system that has automatic adjustments for its various features and no more than three buttons. Some of these features include gain control (compensates for reflections of bright images), brightness (shutter) control (regulates light through the light source), color adjustment and white balance.

Additional advances in camera technology include the 'Hyper HAD™' CCD (Sony Corp., Tokyo, Japan) which improves light sensitivity by capturing the light that falls between pixels and by digital technology. Camera image transmission and processing have traditionally utilized analog technology. Digital processing involves converting the analog waveform to the binary language utilized by computers. Digital signal processing has improved the image quality of the analog camera systems on the market. This is why today's cameras are better than those of just a few years ago. The other advantage of digital processing is that it allows direct communication with other digital technology, i.e. computers and telecommunications, as well as digital image storage. Surgical images can be stored digitally on any computer storage device such as a CD or DVD, enhanced using computer software, and then printed or used to produce slides. The stored image files can be incorporated into the operative report or electronic medical system, or transmitted via the Internet. Integrated digital systems include the camera, monitor, printer and digital image storage device (computer, CD or DVD burner) or VCR. Advances to look for include digital cameras, which could have the camera chip at the tip of the endoscope, bypassing the traditional optics system entirely.

Monitor

The medical monitors found in many operating rooms have about 450–600 lines of resolution. This is all that is needed for the single-chip camera. To take full advantage of the increasing resolution of three-chip cameras, it is necessary to have a high-resolution medical monitor or high-definition TV that has 700+ lines of resolution.

Light source

There are a number of options when it comes to light sources. The 150 W lamp with or without flash generator is certainly sufficient for hysteroscopy and resectoscopy. However, the xenon or metal halide light sources are better suited for videotaping and still photography. Xenon light sources can give a bluish color distortion, while metal halides can give a reddish color distortion. However, these color distortions are corrected by most camera systems.

Video recorder

Video recorders also come in a variety of formats and sizes. The standard VHS recorder has approximately 250 lines of resolution, and the super VHS (S-VHS) recorder has approximately 400 lines of resolution. Both utilize half-inch tape as does the Betacam or Betacam SP system. While the 0.75-inch U-matic SP high-band recording, referred to as BVU, is considered professional quality, the 0.75-inch U-matic low band is considered semi-professional. When editing is required, either 0.75-inch U-matic format is superior to the 0.5-inch VHS tape systems. However, for routine documentation of endoscopic surgery, a professional-grade VHS recorder is sufficient. The 8-mm format (V8) is also available for documentation of hysteroscopic surgery.

Video standards

There are three major video standards used in the world. The NTSC (National Television Standard Committee) standard is used in North America, Japan and parts of South America and Asia. The PAL (phase-alternating line) standard is used in Western Europe, Australia, New Zealand and parts of Africa and the Far East. The SECAM (Séquentiel Couleur a Mémoire) standard is used in France, Eastern Europe and parts of Africa and Asia. The standards differ in how color is encoded and the number of image lines. PAL and SECAM have 625 image lines compared to 525 lines with NTSC. PAL is more expensive than NTSC but has increased color stability and reproduction. Improved image quality with the NTSC system is achieved with the 'Y/C' (luminance–chrominance) output. In the NTSC system, the RGB (red, green, blue) signal is encoded into a single composite. Camera systems with the Y/C output encode the RGB signal electronically into separate luminance (black and white) and chrominance (color) signals, but do not encode these two signals into the final composite NTSC signal[12]. The resulting image has decreased bleeding of colors and superior quality. The entire video system, from video camera to recorder and then to monitor, must maintain the signal in the Y/C form throughout.

ANCILLARY INSTRUMENTS

Accessory instruments required for diagnostic, operative hysteroscopy and resectoscopy include a weighted speculum and vaginal wall retractors or a single-hinged (open-side) speculum, conventional double-tooth tenaculum and cervical dilators. Operative instruments include scissors, grasping forceps and biopsy forceps. It is important to ensure the proper size of accessory instrument for the hysteroscope to be used. These instruments are small and delicate, so it wise to have a back-up set available. To remove myoma chips during resectoscopy, myoma-grasping forceps are very useful; however, polyp forceps, pituitary rongeur, ring forceps, or curette can be used instead. When using low-viscosity liquid distention media, larger diameter urology tubing should be used. Standard IV tubing has a smaller diameter and a much higher resistance to flow. Use of special surgical drapes, which funnel fluids into a drain pouch, is exceedingly important in monitoring input and output during resectoscopy. Special drapes and tubing sets are part of the various fluid irrigation systems described above that are very helpful with resectoscopy and operative hysteroscopy. Special fluid management tubing systems, like the Brooks' Disten-U-Flo™ fluid management system (ACMI, Southborough, MA, USA) are designed for use with diagnostic hysteroscopy. Because there can be drainage from around the cervix, even when attaching the outflow port directly to the fluid management system, surgical drapes that funnel fluid into a pouch should be used. Urological and neurosurgical drapes were used prior to the design and marketing of gynecological resectoscopic surgical drapes.

OPERATING ROOM SET-UP

The operating room should be arranged to minimize clutter and maximize efficiency for the surgeon and nursing staff. Diagnostic hysteroscopy can be performed in an office procedure room or the operating room. Minimal equipment requirements, in addition to the hysteroscope, are a light source, accessory instruments and CO_2 insufflator or tubing for high- or low-viscosity fluids. The operating room set-up for operative hysteroscopy and resectoscopy are similar adding an electrosurgical device, irrigation pump or fluid management system, camera, monitor and some means of image documentation. Arrangement of equipment should be part of the planning before procedures begin. Placement of the video camera cable, light source cable, electrosurgical cable and distention-medium input and output tubing need to be considered. In addition, there is the Foley catheter and foot pedal to the electrosurgical unit. If the bottom drape pouch has a valve at the bottom, this and the output tubing may both be connected to suction. If a distention-medium irrigation system is used, this is an additional piece of equipment the displays of which should be clearly visible. A clear and unobstructed view of the video monitor that does not cause the surgeon's neck to strain is essential. This is accomplished with either a monitor near the head of the table or a video cart with a swivel arm for the monitor, or by placing the monitor near the patient's hip with the monitor high on the cart and the patient's hip slightly flexed. Urological or Allen stirrups are better than the traditional candy cane stirrups for these purposes. Generally, the light source, video monitor and video camera are on one cart; therefore, these three cables will go together in one direction. Placing the irrigation tubing (and device) and electrosurgical unit on the opposite side of the patient usually works best. The surgical assistant or scrub nurse may stand to the side of the surgeon, or on the patient's side, depending on operating room size and personal preference. Either the circulating nurse or anesthesiologist should be assigned to monitor input/output prior to starting the surgery.

The surgeon should have a working knowledge of the camera equipment. This should include start-up, basic troubleshooting and the ability to explain how to record the surgery on the VHS or print pictures using the video printer to someone who has never laid eyes on the equipment. A complete understanding of how to put together the hysteroscope or resectoscope and connect the electrodes and cables is essential for hassle-free surgery.

If you do not understand your equipment, you will one day have to explain to your patient that you had to cancel or could not complete her surgery because of technical difficulties (your usual operating-room staff called in sick!).

ENDOMETRIAL ABLATION DEVICES

There are now several alternatives to resectoscopic endometrial ablation. Four alternative techniques have been approved by the US Food and Drug Administration (FDA), one hysteroscopic and three non-hysteroscopic, and several other techniques are in development. Non-hysteroscopic techniques approved by the FDA include a device using a balloon heated with fluids, a cryoablation device and a bipolar electrode.

The first non-surgical device approved by the FDA (1997) is the ThermaChoice® Uterine Balloon Therapy System by Gynecare, a division of Ethicon Inc. The ThermaChoice system consists of a silicone balloon that is inserted into the uterus, inflated with a heated solution of dextrose and water to 87°C (188°F) for 8 min. The HER Option™ Uterine Cryoblation Therapy™ System by CryoGen Inc. (San Diego, CA, USA) was approved by the FDA in April 2001. The HER Option Uterine Cryoblation Therapy System uses a cryoprobe that produces temperatures of −100°C (−148°F). These cold temperatures are produced at the tip of the probe creating an ice ball that advances through tissue destroying the uterine lining in approximately 10 min. Ultrasound is used to guide and monitor the procedure. Also approved by the FDA in April 2001 is the NovaSure™ Impedence Controlled Endometrial Ablation System by Novacept (Palo Alto, CA, USA). A metallic-mesh triangular bipolar electrode is expanded out of a slender tube into the uterus and brought into contact with the endometrial tissue by means of gentle suction. The bipolar electrode delivers radiofrequency energy by means of a radiofrequency controller that desiccates and coagulates the endometrium and underlying superficial myometrium in approximately 90 s. No hysteroscope or ultrasound is used to view the uterus during this procedure. The Hydro ThermAblator® Endometrial Ablation System (HTA) by Boston Scientific (Natick, MA, USA) was approved by the FDA in April 2001. This device circulates heated saline, 90°C (194°F), inside the uterus for 10 min by means of a sheath and tubing attached to a hysteroscope. The surgeon uses the hysteroscope to view the uterus during the procedure. Devices utilizing microwave energy, diode laser, unipolar electrodes and photodynamic therapy are currently under investigation. One of these devices is the GyneLase™ by Karl Storz that uses their ELITT™ (endometrial laser intrauterine thermal therapy) procedure. ELITT consists of a diode laser to deliver 830-nm wavelength laser light to the endometrial cavity by means of a transcervical applicator. The absorbed light is transformed into heat thereby destroying the endometrium.

References

1. Neuwirth RS. A new technique for and additional experience with hysteroscopic resection of submucous fibroids. *Am J Obstet Gynecol* 1978;131:91–4

2. Haning RV, Harkins, PG, Uehling DT. Preservation of fertility by transcervical resection of a benign mesodermal uterine tumor with a resectoscope and glycine distending medium. *Fertil Steril* 1980;33:209–10

3. DeCherney AH, Polan ML. Hysteroscopic management of intrauterine lesion and intractable uterine bleeding. *Obstet Gynecol* 1983;61:392–7

4. DeCherney AH, Russell JB, Graebe RA, *et al.* Resectoscopic management of mullerian fusion defects. *Fertil Steril* 1986;45:726–8

5. Matouschek E. *Urologic Endoscopic Surgery.* Toronto: B.C. Decker Inc., 1989

6. Soderstrom RM. Electricity inside the uterus. *Clin Obstet Gynecol* 1992;35:262–9

7. Siegler AM, Valle RF, Lindemann HJ, Mencaglia L. *Therapeutic Hysteroscopy Indications and Techniques.* St Louis: CV Mosby, 1990:10–35

8. Indman PD, Brooks PG, Cooper JM, *et al.* Complications of fluid overload from resectoscopic surgery. *J Am Assoc Gynecol Laparosc* 1988;5:63–7

9. Loffer FD. Laser ablation of the endometrium. *Obstet Gynecol Clin N Am* 1988;15:77–89

10. Isaacson KB. Complications of operative hysteroscopy. *Obstet Gynecol Clin N Am* 1999;26:39–51

11. Isaacson K, Nardella P. Development and use of a bipolar resectoscope in endometrial electrosurgery. *J Am Assoc Gynecol Laparosc* 1997;4:385–90

12. Indman PD. Instruments and video cameras for operative hysteroscopy. *Clin Obstet Gynecol* 1992;35:211–24

3

Tissue effects of radiofrequency electrosurgical currents

R. D. Tucker

Electrosurgery utilizes alternating radio-frequency (RF) currents to cut and coagulate tissue. In monopolar electrosurgery, current flows from the electrosurgery generator to the active electrode, to the surgical site tissue, and through the patient's body until it is collected at the return electrode or 'ground pad'; the circuit is then complete as the current is returned to the generator. Electrosurgery can also be bipolar in which the current flows from the generator to one electrode, to the surgical site tissue, then to a second electrode in close proximity to the first electrode at the surgical site, and finally it is returned to the generator to complete the circuit. The electrode(s) does not heat, but, rather, the tissue heats as it resists the flow of the RF alternating current. Thus, electrosurgical currents accomplish the surgical action of cutting and coagulating by heat. This effect is different from true electrocautery, in which electrical currents are used to heat a wire and the hot wire coagulates tissue. Unlike electrosurgery, electrocautery cannot cut tissue or be used in a fluid medium.

Electrosurgery began in 1891, when French physicist d'Arsonval discovered that alternating currents at frequencies of 2000 to 2 million cycles/s (2 kHz to 2 MHz, where Hertz or Hz equals cycles/s) when applied to living tissue caused heating without muscle or nerve stimulation[1]. By 1910, the American surgeon, William Clark, routinely used electrosurgical coagulation to remove benign and malignant tumors of the head, neck, breast and cervix[2]. In

the same year, Edwin Beer utilized RF alternating current to remove endoscopically bladder tumors and growths at the bladder neck[3]. In the mid-1920s, many different electrosurgical machines became commercially available in Europe and the United States. However, it was not until William Bovie, a Harvard physicist, collaborated with Harvey Cushing, the Chief of Surgery at Peter Brent Brigham Hospital, that a machine capable of cutting and coagulating tissue became generally accepted by surgeons[4,5].

Updating this chapter is difficult as the histological tissue effects have not changed from those mentioned in the first edition; in fact, the tissue effects are the same as have occurred since the technology was first used at the turn of the 20th century. Although there have been a few notable early studies on electrosurgical tissue effects[6], the study has been a more recent development as physicians have tried to evaluate the efficacy and safety of new techniques and procedures, notably in laparoscopy and endoscopy. This chapter will describe the various histological effects of electrosurgical current and will conclude with some of the new technologies that are available to allow physicians to control better the tissue effects.

TISSUE EFFECTS OF ELECTROSURGERY

The goal of this section is not to turn gyne-cologists into experts on surgical pathology but rather to provide examples of the effect of RF current on tissue and to guide the gynecologists to aid in the histological evaluation of tissue samples. Most pathologists are unfamiliar with the examination of electrosurgical damage and are reluctant to provide a cause and effect diagnosis. Subtle effects of low temperature (40–80°C) are often missed. Therefore, in order to obtain valid information, the gynecologist must be sufficiently familiar with the tissue effects of RF current to provide the necessary clinical input to the pathologist evaluating the samples; this becomes especially important for the evaluation of potential complications.

Figures 1–8 are of sections obtained by contact desiccation on the mucosal surface of pig bladder at 30 W in coagulation mode for 3 s using a Valleylab Force 2™ generator (Valleylab, Boulder, CO, USA). The samples were then excised immediately and prepared for histological analysis. Figures 9 and 10 were obtained utilizing the same procedure on dog stomach mucosa and rabbit uterus, respectively.

Figures 11 and 12 are sections from a human laparoscopic procedure in which the small bowel was desiccated unintentionally; the burn was not excised until 1 week postsurgery. Figures 13 and 14 are from a human endoscopic procedure, a polypectomy in the colon; the sample was excised 4 days post-procedure.

Tissue stains

Unfortunately, there is no one histological stain that is diagnostic of electrosurgical damage or will allow demarcation of cells that will ultimately undergo necrosis. Therefore, in analyzing electrosurgical damage, it may be necessary to employ multiple stains to determine the extent of damage.

The most commonly and routinely used stain is hematoxylin and eosin (H & E). The stain consists of two parts: hematoxylin, a nuclear stain, and eosin, a negative-charged plasma stain. The hematoxylin stains nuclei blue, while the eosin stains erythrocytes, collagen and

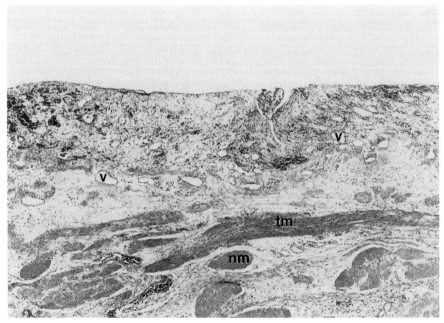

Figure 1 Mucosal surface of a pig bladder contact desiccated for 3 s at 30 W from a Valleylab Force 2 electrosurgical generator. The entire surface is necrotic with the total loss of normal architecture. Vacuoles (v) are scattered throughout the surface. Thermally damaged muscle (tm) underlies the necrotic surface and stretches across the entire figure. Underlying the thermally damaged muscle are several normal muscle fibers (nm). Magnification × 10

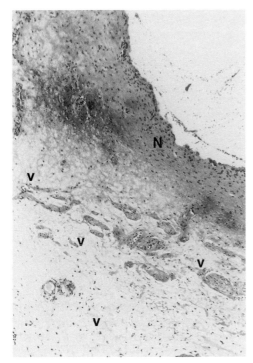

Figure 2 Section of the mucosal surface of another pig bladder contact desiccated similar to Figure 1. The entire surface shows necrotic tissue (N). Underlying the necrotic tissue throughout the section is a fine lacework of small vacuoles (v) created by the vaporization of cellular and extracellular fluids and shrinkage of tissue. Magnification × 20

As trichrome stains contain a connective tissue stain, they are particularly useful in examining tissues rich in collagen.

Another stain useful in examining electrosurgical thermal damage is picrosirius red. This stain colors collagen and reticulum a deep red, nuclei are colored black, and all other tissue elements are colored bright yellow. As collagen and reticular fibers are strongly anisotropic in longitudinal section, upon viewing with polarized light, the collagen and reticulum fibers show strong birefringence. Denatured collagen and reticulum fibers show little birefringence; this effect is demonstrated in Figure 10. The area of rabbit uterus with the electrosurgical thermal damage is shown as a dark red tissue with no birefringence while the overlying normal muscle shows strong birefringence at the right of the section, which fades towards the left of the figure. The stain is extremely useful at demonstrating thermal damage immediately postelectrosurgical cutting or coagulation. However, damage viewed several days postsurgery may be equivocal. During evaluation, it must be remembered that collagen and reticular fibers are isotropic in cross-section and, therefore, produce little birefringence if cut in that plane.

Histological view of electrosurgical damage

As stated above, electrosurgical damage is caused by heat. Heating that is rapid and intense, more than 100°C, will cause the vaporization of intra- and extracellular fluids, thereby producing a cutting action. Temperatures less than 100°C cause a desiccating or coagulation action. Intra- and extracellular proteins are irreversibly denatured at temperatures between 80 and 100°C. Temperatures between 60 and 80°C will cause reversible damage to some proteins, e.g. the unfolding of collagen chains without destroying the collagen triple helixes. At temperatures of less than 60°C, changes to tissues are more subtle and may be confined to specific cells or specific cellular components.

In electrosurgical coagulation, the tissue temperature immediately surrounding the

cytoplasm of muscle or epithelial cells varying shades or intensities of pink. Figure 11 shows a section of small bowel damaged by electrosurgery and stained with H & E. The stain is readily available in all pathology laboratories. H & E stained slides are excellent for viewing morphology, and most pathologists are comfortable reading H & E stained tissue.

A trichrome stain combines a plasma stain and a connective fiber stain; various trichrome stains are available, including Gomori, Mallory and Masson. These stains color cell cytoplasm and muscle fibers red, collagen, green or blue, depending upon the specific chemical solution, and nuclei, blue to black. Figure 12 shows the same section as Figure 11, but stained with trichrome. These three-colored stains give added contrast and, therefore, may make areas of electrosurgical damage easier to demarcate.

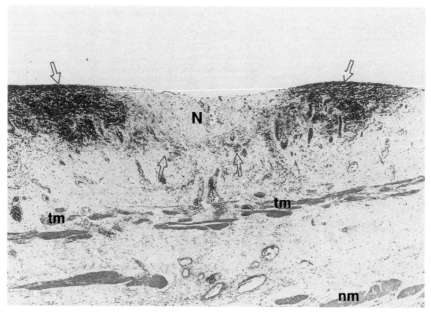

Figure 3 Section of pig bladder contact desiccated in a similar manner to Figure 1. There is a large necrotic area (N) in the center of the figure. Laterally and beneath the necrotic area, there is considerable hemorrhage (open arrows). The muscle cells (tm) spanning the entire figure are elongated and shrunken by thermal damage. Normal muscle (nm) is seen in the bottom right-hand corner. Magnification × 10

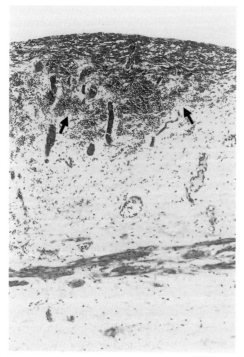

Figure 4 High magnification of Figure 3 showing hemorrhage (open arrows) and underlying thermally damaged muscle. Magnification × 20

active electrode will be the highest; there is a thermal gradient created in which the tissue temperature varies from high temperature to normal body temperature over a given distance. Figure 15 is a diagrammatic representation of the variation of temperature in tissue over distance for an electrosurgical coagulation. As RF current follows the paths of least resistance and these paths vary from millisecond to millisecond according to the state of desiccation (or the resistance of the desiccated tissue), the isothermal gradients will not be uniform and will vary dynamically. The thermal gradients may be large as tissue temperatures vary from 100°C to body temperature in a few millimeters. Hot spots distant to the surgical site can be created by the RF current following a low-resistance path, such as a blood vessel.

The unpredictable flow of current through low-resistance paths is only one uncertainty in the histological evaluation of electrosurgical damage. The plane through which the tissue section is taken also creates variation. Consider the diagrammatic electrosurgical burn in Figure 15; if sections are obtained in planes A, B

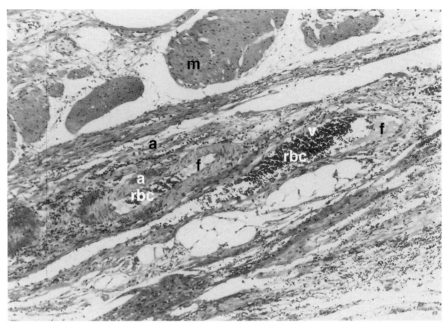

Figure 5 Section from a pig bladder contact desiccated in a similar manner to Figure 1; the section is from a low-temperature area removed from mucosal contact desiccation. Muscle cells (m) at the top of the figure are normal. However, beneath the muscle cells, there are two vessels both showing thermal damage. The artery (a) shows nuclear changes in the endothelial cells and a fibrin clot (f) with red blood cells (rbc) occluding the entire lumen. The adjoining vein (v) shows a longitudinal cut with a partially occluding clot with fibrin and red blood cells. Magnification × 25

and C, the histological analysis will vary greatly. The damage will be easily visible in sections taken through planes A and B, as these sections are through high-temperature areas in which protein denaturation would have occurred, while a section taken in plane C will show significantly less thermal effect. However, a systematic analysis would yield deep thermal damage to the tissue in the circled area; this 'hot spot' would be surrounded by tissue that is close to body temperature and displays little damage.

The variation of histology depending on the section location can become a problem when evaluating electrosurgical injuries as demonstrated in Figures 13 and 14. These slides were taken from a patient who underwent polypectomy; the patient presented 4 days post-procedure with peritonitis and free air in the abdomen. The microscopic description of the pathology report from the apparent site of perforation noted the acute inflammation on the serosal surface that extended into the

muscularis propria layer with intact mucosa. This is represented in the low-power photomicrograph on the left of Figure 13. The damage is obvious on the serosal surface of the bowel and extends into the muscle. From this single slide one cannot tell if the damage originated from the serosa or the mucosa. A closer examination of the mucosa, the area marked by a box on the left of Figure 13, is shown at higher power on the right of the figure. The glands in the mucosa at the left do not appear to be the same compared with the normal glands at the right. The cells do not exhibit nuclei and the normal architecture has been disrupted. These cells demonstrate electrosurgical heat damage. Serial cuts were made in the block; after 88 3-μm steps into the block the perforation became obvious (Figure 14). Notice that the muscle layer shows necrosis and shortening that is more pronounced at the mucosal surface; this demonstrates that the current originated from inside the bowel.

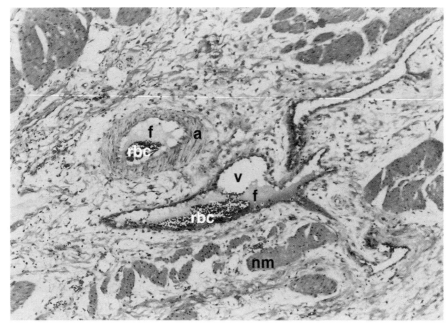

Figure 6   Section from pig bladder with a contact desiccation on the mucosa created in a manner similar to Figure 1. The section shows an artery (a) and vein (v) surrounded by completely normal muscle cells (nm). The artery is occluded by a fibrin clot (f) with embedded red blood cells (rbc). The endothelial cells demonstrate nuclear shape changes from thermal damage. The adjoining vein is also occluded with a large clot. Magnification × 25

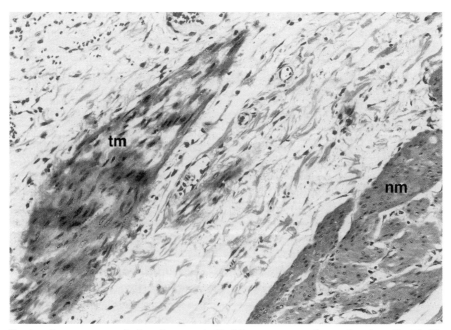

Figure 7   Section from a contact desiccation on pig bladder mucosa performed as described in Figure 1. The figure shows two muscle bundles. The lower bundle is normal muscle (nm). The other bundle demonstrates thermally damaged muscle (tm). A comparison of nuclei between bundles shows that the thermally damaged muscle has pyknotic hyperchromic nuclei and few normal nuclei. Magnification × 50

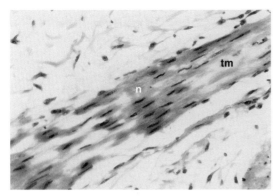

Figure 8 Section from a contact desiccation performed on pig bladder mucosa in a similar manner to Figure 1. The figure shows a high magnification of a thermally damaged muscle fiber (tm). The muscle bundle shows the predominance of hyperchromic pyknotic nuclei (n). Magnification × 60

The effect of variations in temperatures and the differences between stains in analyzing the damage is illustrated in Figures 11 and 12. These samples were taken from the same tissue block and are adjacent sections. Both sections show the same full-thickness bowel burn without perforation. The mucosal surfaces are toward the bottom of the sections; the mucosa at the far left of the figures is normal and progresses toward the right with increasing damage and total loss of normal mucosal architecture by the center of the images. Both the H & E and trichrome stains show extensive damage in the right half of the figures; these are areas of high temperature in which the normal architecture is replaced by homogeneous-appearing necrotic tissue. Also in the necrotic area, vacuolization is seen throughout the bowel wall. In lower-temperature zones, large amounts of hemorrhage are seen on the serosal surfaces. Thrombi are seen in vessels. At higher-power magnification, these vessels show not only red cells but organized clots with fibrin. In the H & E slide, damage to the muscle layer is difficult to assess; however, the normal muscle architecture is disrupted from the center of Figure 11 to the right-hand side of the section. Analysis of the muscle damage in the trichrome section (Figure 12) is significantly easier to assess. In

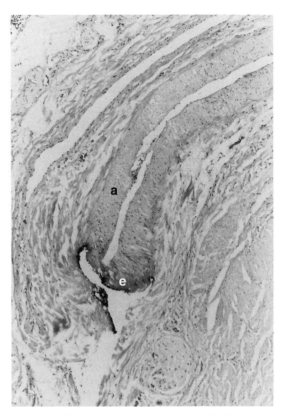

Figure 9 Section of a dog stomach in which contact desiccation was performed for 3 s at 30 W with a Valleylab Force 2 electrosurgical generator. The section shows a longitudinal cut of a small artery (a) distant to the mucosal coagulation. The top of the vessel is essentially normal; however, at the center, there is a necrotic area and endothelial damage (e). Magnification × 9

this figure, the muscle fibers adjacent to the serosal surface have been disrupted and large numbers of vacuoles are seen while the muscle nearest to the mucosal surface appears more normal. The fact that the damage on the serosal surface extends further than the mucosal surface and the muscle damage is more extensive on the cells facing the serosal surface confirms that the RF flow originated on the serosa.

During contact desiccation (i.e. the electrode touching the tissue during activation), temperatures can be quite high and, therefore, tissue destruction considerable. The histological picture under lying the electrode is

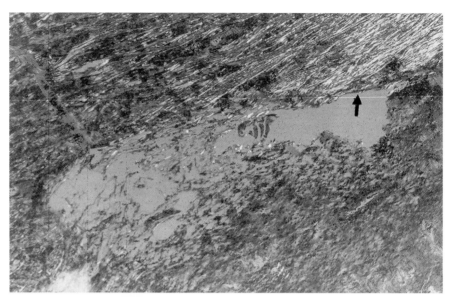

Figure 10 Section of rabbit Fallopian tube contact desiccated for 3 s at 30 W from a Valleylab Force 2 electrosurgical generator. The section is stained with picrosirius red and viewed with polarized light. The tissue in the lower right-hand area is thermally damaged and shows very little birefringence. The tissue overlying the damaged part shows birefringence (open arrow), which fades toward the left of the figure

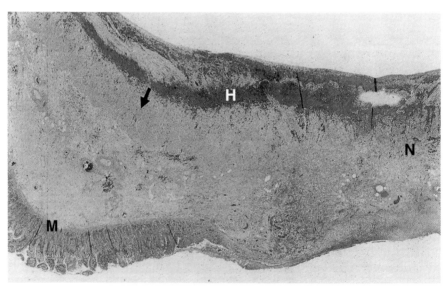

Figure 11 Section of human ileum that was burned inadvertently on the serosal surface (top of picture). The burn is a full thickness with the necrotic tissue (N) on the right side of the figure. The mucosa (M) on the far left of the figure is normal, but by the middle of the figure, all normal architecture is lost. A large amount of hemorrhage (H) is seen on the entire serosal surface. The muscle fibers facing the mucosa (open arrow) are normal while the muscle near the serosa show thermal damage, including vacuolization

simple; it consists of complete disruption of the normal tissue architecture and the replacement with homogeneous necrotic tissue. Also seen in areas of intense thermal heat are vacuoles created by the vaporization of fluid and the shrinkage of desiccated tissue. Figure 1 shows this effect in pig bladder. Vacuoles are seen not only near the surface but also deep in the

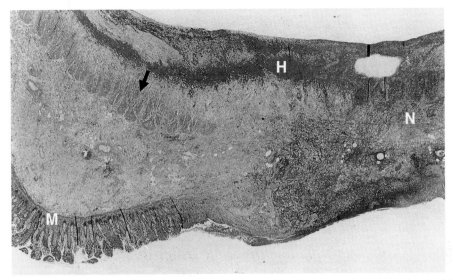

Figure 12 The adjacent section of tissue as shown in Figure 11. This section was stained with Masson trichrome and shows the same histological changes as in Figure 11

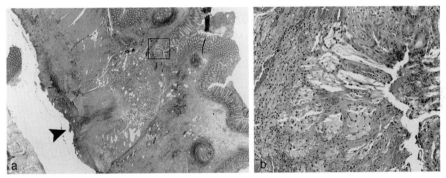

Figure 13 (a) Low-power photomicrograph (magnification × 2.5) of the colon, 4 days after a polypectomy. The inflammation and necrosis at the serosal surface, indicated by the arrow head, is obvious. The mucosa, while intact, does not appear normal. (b) Higher magnification (× 25) of the area indicated by the box in the low-power view. The left of this view shows necrotic ghost cells and abnormal glands, while normal mucosa is on the right

underlying tissue. The entire surface of the section is necrotic, and most of the underlying muscle cells are thermally damaged. Figure 2 shows a section from another bladder that demonstrates extensive small vacuoles underlying the necrotic surface. Electrosurgical burn sections, such as this, are easy to diagnose as a result of the large necrotic area and the more subtle tissue changes occurring at the margin of the necrotic area.

High-temperature areas denature most proteins and, therefore, produce uniform-appearing necrosis; lower temperatures produce activation of the coagulation cascade, vascular endothelial damage and thrombi. Even lower temperatures produce thermal damage to vessel walls and bleeding rather than clotting. As a result, slides taken at the periphery of an electrosurgical burn may show considerable hemorrhage. Figure 3 demonstrates this effect. At the center, there is a necrotic zone showing little normal architecture. At the periphery of the high-temperature zone, there is considerable hemorrhage laterally and some

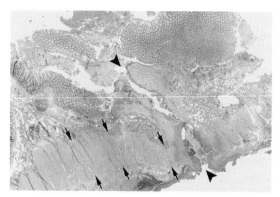

Figure 14 Section from the same tissue block as in Figure 13, but taken deeper into the block. The perforation is indicated with arrowheads. The muscle layer shows more necrosis on the mucosal side; the arrows indicate the normal muscle layer

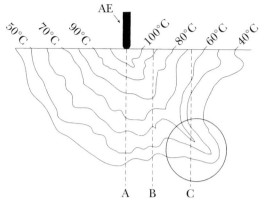

Figure 15 Diagrammatic representation of the thermal gradients underlying an active electrode (AE). The temperatures vary from 100°C immediately under the electrode to 40°C at the outer margin. The isothermal lines will vary dynamically depending upon changes in tissue resistance that effect the heat produced within the tissue. The dotted lines perpendicular to the tissue marked A, B and C show hypothetical histology sections through the tissue. If a histological section is taken at section C, the circled area will show a hot spot of over 60°C, which would be surrounded entirely by tissue of much lower temperature and displaying few thermal effects

hemorrhage in underlying tissue. Hemorrhage in this section demarcates the necrotic tissue. Much of the underlying muscle layer shows thermal damage. It is impossible to determine if these underlying tissues, which are not overtly necrotic, are viable; however, these areas have sustained sufficient thermal damage that these cells would probably undergo necrosis over time. Only the muscle in the bottom right corner of the figure shows minimal thermal effect. Figure 4 shows a higher magnification of the hemorrhage demonstrated in Figure 3. The muscle cells underlying the hemorrhage demonstrate considerable thermal damage, including muscle cell elongation and nuclear shape changes. Nuclear changes include elongation, shrinkage and hyperchromasia.

As discussed earlier, sections taken through low-temperature areas may show only subtle electrosurgical damage. As current follows the path of least resistance, blood vessels are particularly susceptible to damage; the damage can occur far from necrotic areas and may be surrounded by totally normal tissue. Figure 5, from a pig bladder, shows an artery and vein surrounded by normal muscle. Within the artery, a clump of red cells is embedded in a fibrin clot; this thrombus has occluded the vessel. This artery endothelium also demonstrates typical nuclear thermal damage. In close approximation is a large vein partially occluded with a fibrin clot. Figure 6 shows another pig bladder artery and vein with electrosurgically caused thrombi. Although connective tissue surrounding the vessels shows heat damage, the muscle immediately adjacent to the vessels demonstrates little thermal effect. Figure 9 is a section from a dog stomach taken immediately after the electrocoagulation on the mucosal surface. The figure shows a large vessel in longitudinal section completely surrounded by normal tissue. The great majority of the vessel is totally normal except for a very small area of heat damage to the endothelium at the center of the figure. Such an effect may have been caused by the narrowing of the vessel, creating an increased resistance and, therefore, a larger power with resulting necrosis.

Another subtle effect often overlooked in assessing electrosurgical damage is cellular nuclear change. As nuclei are particularly susceptible to thermal damage, it is important in assessing the extent of the electrosurgical burn to pay close attention to nuclear changes. Figure 7 was taken from an electrosurgical coagulation on the mucosa of a pig bladder. The figure demonstrates two muscle bundles, the lower bundle being normal and the upper bundle showing considerable cellular changes. Comparing the nuclei between bundles, the thermally damaged nuclei are hyperchromic and elongated with many showing a twisting confirmation (i.e. pyknotic). Figure 8 shows a higher magnification of a muscle bundle; hyperchromic pyknotic nuclei predominate and few normal undamaged nuclei are seen.

INFLUENCE OF TECHNOLOGY ON ELECTROSURGICAL TISSUE EFFECTS

Electrosurgical generators typically provide little control of the effects of the RF currents. Generators usually provide the operator with several monopolar options: a pure cut waveform (a sine wave with little coagulation effect), a coagulation waveform (a low duty cycle waveform with high voltage capable of producing deep coagulation), and a series of blend waveforms that cut and provide varying degrees of coagulation. Bipolar outputs that are intended for coagulation are also provided.

The typical generator gives the operator control of the monopolar and bipolar power output. While the operator can control the power setting and the generator voltage (by waveform selection), these values can vary dramatically with the tissue impedance (AC resistance) during cutting and coagulating. Such variations led to the lack of reproducibility in the tissue effects.

Microprocessor technology in new generators has enabled control of the waveforms, generator voltage and power output that has not been previously possible. This new generation of generators has given the surgeon more reproducible tissue effects. It has also enabled manufacturers to optimize generator output to specific electrodes or specific procedures. Different operating characteristics, i.e. constant voltage or constant power and

electrode variations, make it imperative that surgeons are familiar with each generator that they employ.

With respect to endometrial ablation several new devices warrant specific mention. New bipolar resectoscopes are available that work in a similar fashion to monopolar systems, except that the current is confined to flow in a small volume of tissue about the surgical site and they work in a saline environment. They provide cutting and coagulation with less collateral damage than corresponding monopolar systems. Another technology also involves bipolar electrodes but works by an entirely different mechanism. The instruments consist of an electrode at the tip and a cylindrical return electrode on the shaft, only a few millimeters away from the tip. When the instrument is activated in saline away from tissue, current flows between the electrodes in the saline, the saline is heated and a vapor pocket is created around the tip. This pocket consists of ionized saline. As the instrument is brought close to the tissue, arcs travel through the vapor pocket to the tissue at the surgical site, then exit the tissue and travel through the saline to the return electrode. The vapor pocket has a high impedance which limits the amount of surgical current. The generator has feedback systems to initiate and sustain the vapor pocket about the active electrode. Operated in this fashion the instrument can reproducibly vaporize a layer of tissue with little damage to underlying structures. If the active electrode comes into contact with the tissue, thus eliminating the vapor pocket, the instrument would behave as a bipolar coagulator and be capable of deep coagulation, an unintended effect; however, the generator has current-limiting capabilities to prevent this unintended operation.

CONCLUSIONS

Electrosurgical damage is caused by tissue resisting the flow of RF current, creating heat, and thus, the surgical effect of cutting or coagulation. Electrosurgical tissue damage is a continuum of effects ranging from high-temperature denaturing of proteins to low-temperature changes. The areas of tissue in high-temperature zones undergo necrosis and the complete loss of normal architecture with vacuolization. Tissue in lower-temperature zones displays varied changes, such as hemorrhage, thrombosis, perivascular damage and pyknotic hyperchromic nuclei. Unfortunately, it is histologically difficult to determine if tissue in low-temperature areas would, with time, undergo necrosis. No single histological stain is diagnostic of electrosurgical damage, and in difficult cases, multiple stains may need to be employed to determine cause and effect and to demarcate damaged areas.

References

1. d'Arsonval A. Action physiologique des courants alternatifs a grand frequence. *Arch Physiol Norm Path* 1893;5:401–8, 789–90
2. Clark WL. Oscillatory desiccation in the treatment of accessible malignant growths and minor surgical conditions: a new electrical effect. *J Adv Ther* 1911;29:169–83
3. Beer E. Removal of neoplasms of the urinary bladder. A new method employing high frequency (Oudin) currents through a catheterizing cystoscope. *J Am Med Assoc* 1910;54:1768–9
4. McLean AJ. The Bovie electrosurgical current generator: some underlying principles and results. *Arch Surg* 1929;18:1863–73
5. Cushing H. Electrosurgery as an aid to the removal of intracranial tumors. With a preliminary note on a new surgical-current generator by WT Bovie. *Surg Gynecol Obstet* 1928;47:751–84
6. McLean AJ. Characteristics of adequate electrosurgical current. *Am J Surg* 1932;18:417–41

4

Preoperative evaluation for resectoscopic surgery

R. Barnes

It is a well-accepted axiom in surgery that a successful outcome depends on appropriate preoperative evaluation to establish the correct diagnosis and to determine the appropriate surgical therapy. A successful surgical outcome also depends on proper preoperative patient preparation. This chapter will consider the preoperative evaluation of patients presenting for resectoscopic surgery, appropriate preoperative preparation with regard to prophylactic antibiotics, preparation of the cervix for dilatation and anesthesia.

PREOPERATIVE EVALUATION

Uses of the gynecological resectoscope include removal of intrauterine growths, endometrial ablation or excision, incision of a uterine septum and lysis of intrauterine adhesions. Of these indications the resectoscope is ideally suited for excision of intrauterine growths such as leiomyomata and polyps. Recently, the thermal balloon has gained popularity for endometrial ablation because of its ease of use and outcomes similar to those following resectoscopic ablation. Although there are successful reports of the use of the resectoscope for incision of a uterine septum and for lysis of intrauterine adhesions, these procedures are more commonly performed with the operative hysteroscope and scissors.

Evaluation of recurrent spontaneous abortion and infertility

Evaluation of the uterine cavity by hysterosalpingogram or hysteroscopy is an essential step in the work-up of recurrent spontaneous abortion. A congenital uterine anomaly is present in about 10% of women with three or more consecutive first-trimester spontaneous abortions[1]. The most common finding is a septate, followed by a bicornuate, uterus. If a septum is present, transvaginal ultrasound can often distinguish between a septate and bicornuate uterus. In doubtful cases, magnetic resonance imaging (MRI) should be performed preoperatively or laparoscopy should be performed at the time of a septal lysis to confirm a septate uterus. Postoperatively, a hysterosalpingogram is useful to verify that the uterine cavity is normal. Occasionally, septal lysis is incomplete and a second surgical procedure is necessary.

Hysteroscopic lysis of a uterine septum has become standard therapy in patients with recurrent spontaneous abortion. A retrospective study found a successful pregnancy rate of 87% in patients who had 95% pregnancy wastage prior to treatment[2]. There are no prospective randomized trials verifying these retrospective studies. A uterine septum does not always result in recurrent spontaneous abortion. About 3% of fertile women undergoing tubal ligation were found to have a septate or bicornuate uterus based on operative findings and postoperative hysterosalpingogram[3]. There was no increase in pregnancy wastage in the affected women. Thus, it is not clear that an incidental finding of a uterine septum requires surgical therapy.

Patients requiring treatment of intrauterine adhesions or Asherman's syndrome usually present with recurrent pregnancy wastage or infertility. In the USA, the great majority of patients acquire intrauterine adhesions as a result of curettage of a pregnant or recently pregnant uterus. A less common cause is uterine surgery, such as myomectomy. Genital tuberculosis is a common cause of intrauterine adhesions in Third World countries. About half of patients with intrauterine adhesions present with a history of infertility and about half with a history of recurrent pregnancy loss[4]. Menstrual history is not particularly useful in establishing the diagnosis, as patients with extensive adhesions can present with eumenorrhea, hypomenorrhea or amenorrhea. Thus a hysterosalpingogram is useful to diagnose and to determine the extent of adhesions preoperatively and, postoperatively, to confirm the success of the procedure. The effects on pregnancy after lysis of intrauterine adhesions depend on the severity of the adhesions. Successful term pregnancy occurred in 81% of women with mild adhesions, in 66% with moderate adhesions, but in only 32% with severe adhesions[4].

Evaluation of abnormal uterine bleeding

Abnormal uterine bleeding is an extremely common problem. In England, about 30 per 1000 female patients a year consult with their general practitioners for evaluation of abnormal uterine bleeding. About 20% of referrals from general practitioners to gynecologists are for abnormal uterine bleeding, and of those referred, about half undergo hysterectomy[5]. Because of the high incidence of abnormal bleeding and likelihood of hysterectomy, proper evaluation and consideration of non-surgical therapies are essential to the management of abnormal uterine bleeding.

The critical distinction to be made in the evaluation of abnormal uterine bleeding is whether it is associated with ovulation or anovulation. For the purposes of this chapter, abnormal uterine bleeding associated with anovulation will be referred to as dysfunctional uterine bleeding (DUB). Menorrhagia is defined as heavy menses in ovulatory women, while metrorrhagia is irregular bleeding during an ovulatory cycle (Table 1). The distinction between ovulatory and anovulatory bleeding is critical because causes and therapies are distinct.

Menometrorrhagia

The diagnosis of menorrhagia, or heavy menstrual bleeding, is usually made by the

Table 1 Causes of abnormal uterine bleeding

Menometrorrhagia
Anatomical
  leiomyomata
  endometrial polyp
  adenomyosis
Intrauterine device
Bleeding disorders
  von Willebrand's disease
  platelet disorders
Hypothyroidism or hyperthyroidism
Essential menorrhagia

Dysfunctional uterine bleeding
Physiological
  perimenarcheal and perimenopausal anovulation
Hypothalamic dysfunction
  stress
  exercise
  weight loss
Hyperprolactinemia
Premature ovarian failure
Androgen excess
  polycystic ovary syndrome
  late onset 21-hydroxylase deficiency
Hypothyroidism or hyperthyroidism
Consequences of chronic anovulation
  endometrial hyperplasia
  endometrial cancer

patient. Menstrual bleeding lasting longer than 7 days or associated with clotting is common in menorrhagia. The average menstrual blood loss is about 40 ml per cycle; any loss > 80 ml is associated with an increase risk of anemia and is considered menorrhagia[6,7]. Because accurate measurement of menstrual blood loss is inconvenient and cumbersome, the diagnosis of menorrhagia is subjective, and often the only objective indicator available to the physician is an abnormally low hemoglobin.

Metrorrhagia may be physiological when it presents as midcycle spotting, which is probably the result of falling estradiol levels during the time of luteinizing hormone surge. Any other metrorrhagia is abnormal and deserves investigation.

Menometrorrhagia is often difficult to distinguish from DUB. Ovulation should be confirmed in uncertain cases by a serum progesterone > 3 ng/ml or the finding of secretory endometrium on biopsy. Basal body temperature charting is useful to time the above tests (Table 2).

Table 2 Evaluation of abnormal uterine bleeding

All patients
Pregnancy test if sexually active
Complete blood count
Thyroid stimulating hormone
Platelet count, prothrombin time, partial
  thromboplastin time and platelet function
  analysis if coagulation disorder suspected

Ovulatory versus anovulatory
Endometrial biopsy
Serum progesterone
Basal body temperature

Ovulatory bleeding (menometrorrhagia)
Saline infusion sonography
Endometrial biopsy (if over 40 years old)

Anovulatory bleeding (dysfunctional uterine bleeding)
Prolactin, follide stimulating hormone
If androgen excess present: testosterone, free
  testosterone, 17-hydroxyprogesterone
If anovulatory for > 1 year: endometrial biopsy
If unresponsive to medical therapy: rule out
  anatomical defect

Causes of menometrorrhagia

Uterine leiomyomata, particularly those that distort the uterine cavity, endometrial polyps and adenomyosis are common anatomical abnormalities causing menometrorrhagia. Of women undergoing hysteroscopy for menorrhagia, 10–15% had submucosal fibroids and 15–30% had endometrial polyps[8]. Adenomyosis was found in hysteroscopic biopsy specimens in 37% of 90 menorrhagic women. If the uterine cavity was normal, 66% had significant adenomyosis[8]. Adenomyosis was found in 46% of 43 women with an enlarged uterus without evidence of leiomyomata on ultrasound who had hysterectomy for recurrent menorrhagia[9]. All intrauterine devices (IUDs), with the exception of those containing progestins, increase the prevalence of menorrhagia. Depending on the type used, menorrhagia occurs in 25–50% of IUD users after 1 year[7].

Hyperthyroidism rarely causes menometrorrhagia. Polymenorrhea or hypermenorrhea was noted in only 8% of 214 reproductive-aged women with hyperthyroidism[10]. Hypothyroidism causes a range of menstrual abnormalities from amenorrhea to menometrorrhagia[11]. In a recent study of 171 reproductive-aged women with hypothyrodism, 23% had menstrual abnormalities. Menorrhagia accounted for about one-third of the abnormalities[12]. Early hypothyroidism has been found in 22% of women with menorrhagia[13]. Overt hypothyroidism was found in 2% of women with menorrhagia evaluated for endometrial ablation[8].

Although it is uncommon for bleeding disorders to present to the gynecologist with abnormal uterine bleeding, the possibility should always be considered. Von Willebrand's disease has been found in patients considered for endometrial ablation[8]. In particular, bleeding disorders should be considered in adolescents admitted to hospital with acute menorrhagia. A primary coagulation disorder has been reported in almost 20% of such patients, with 50% of patients hospitalized with excessive bleeding at menarche having clotting disorders. Von Willebrand's disease and platelet abnormalities, such as idiopathic thrombocytopenia, were the most commonly found disorders[14].

There is some debate as to whether tubal sterilization increases a woman's risk of increased menstrual and intermenstrual bleeding, often referred to as the post-tubal-sterilization syndrome. A recent study of over 9500 women who underwent tubal sterilization and 573 whose partners underwent vasectomy found no increased risk of abnormal bleeding in the tubal sterilization group. The women who underwent sterilization had significantly fewer days of bleeding and significantly lesser amounts of bleeding and dysmenorrhea[15]. Essential menorrhagia is the final cause of menorrhagia. It has been reported to occur in about 10% of Western European women[7]. Since it is a diagnosis of exclusion, it may be difficult to distinguish from adenomyosis.

Evaluation of menometrorrhagia

The patient presenting with menometrorrhagia should be evaluated for the presence of an anatomical abnormality (Table 2). Often, this is easily accomplished by palpating a fibroid uterus on physical examination. However, symptomatic submucosal fibroids or endometrial polyps can be present in a normal-size

uterus (Figure 1). Therefore, all patients should undergo transvaginal ultrasound with saline infusion of the uterine cavity (saline infusion sonography (SIS)). When compared to findings at hysterectomy or hysteroscopy, SIS is superior to either transvaginal ultrasound or hysterosalpingography for detecting intracavitary lesions and is equal to diagnostic hysteroscopy[16,17]. SIS is equivalent to hysteroscopy and more reliable than either transvaginal ultrasound or MRI in detecting endometrial polyps[17,18]. SIS is equivalent to MRI in detecting submucosal fibroids and can give information regarding intramural extension[18]. SIS is easier to perform and better accepted by patients than hysteroscopy, hysterosalpingography or MRI[19]. MRI is more effective than SIS in determining intramural extension of submucous myomas and in the diagnosis of adenomyosis[18,19].

The preoperative diagnosis of adenomyosis may be difficult to make. The physical finding of a diffusely enlarged, tender uterus is not always present. Transvaginal ultrasound has been found to be about 80% sensitive in detecting adenomyosis with a 26% false-positive rate[9]. The most reliable preoperative method for detecting adenomyosis is MRI[19,20]. Based on histopathological diagnosis, MRI correctly diagnosed adenomyosis in 88% of cases versus 53% of cases for transvaginal ultrasonography. MRI correctly distinguished between leiomyomata and adenomyosis in 92 of 93 patients with an enlarged uterus.

Thyroid stimulating hormone (TSH) should be measured in all patients with menorrhagia as a screening test for both hypo- and hyperthyroidism. If there is suspicion of a clotting disorder, a prothrombin time, partial thromboplastin time, platelet count and platelet function analysis should be performed. Endometrial biopsy should be considered, particularly in women over 40, to rule out endometrial hyperplasia or cancer.

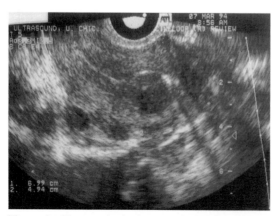

Figure 1 Transvaginal ultrasound demonstrates a 3-cm intracavity fibroid in a patient with normal uterine size who presented with menometrorrhagia

Medical therapy of menometrorrhagia

Resectoscopic removal of a submucosal fibroid or polyp in patients with menometrorrhagia who have not completed childbearing or otherwise wish to keep their uterus has rapidly become standard practice. In patients with menorrhagia, no anatomical abnormality and no desire for fertility, ablation of the endometrium is a possible therapy. However, it must be emphasized that these patients require proper evaluation as outlined above. If hypothyroidism is present, patients respond very quickly to thyroid hormone replacement therapy with a rapid decline in menstrual blood loss[11,21]. If deep adenomyosis is felt to be present, most authors believe that a hysterectomy, and not ablation, is a more appropriate therapy. Adenomyosis is a frequent finding in hysterectomy specimens from patients failing ablation[22,23].

Medical therapy is often effective for treating essential menorrhagia and should be attempted before an ablation. The oral contraceptive pill decreases menstrual blood loss by 50%[24]. The progesterone-containing IUD reduces blood loss by 65% after 1 year[25]. The levonorgestrel-releasing IUD reduces menstrual blood loss by 96% after 12 months in patients with essential menorrhagia[26]. In a randomized trial in women with menorrhagia, the levonorgestrel IUD was as effective as endometrial resection, as determined by hemoglobin concentrations after 6 months of therapy[27]. Danazol 200 mg daily for 3 months has been reported to reduce menstrual blood loss by 80%[28].

Antiprostaglandins reduce menstrual blood loss by 20–50%[7,26,29,30]. Systemic antifibrinolytic agents like tranexamic acid and ε-aminocaproic acid have been used in Europe and reduce menstrual blood loss by 50%[7,24]. However, side-effects of these agents, such as nausea, diarrhea and dizziness, limit their usefulness. In addition, at least three cases of intracranial arterial thrombosis have been described in women using antithrombolytics for menorrhagia[7]. In the author's view, they should not be considered as an alternative to endometrial ablation.

Gonadotropin releasing hormone (GnRH) agonists have been investigated in patients with essential menorrhagia or adenomyosis. There are reports of pregnancy following agonist therapy of severe adenomyosis[31,32]. A GnRH agonist together with hormone replacement therapy has also been reported to treat essential menorrhagia effectively[33]. Because of their expense, GnRH agonists should be reserved for use in women with essential menorrhagia or adenomyosis who are unresponsive to any other medical therapy and who wish to preserve childbearing.

Dysfunctional uterine bleeding

In the author's experience, any cause of anovulation with normal estrogen levels can present as DUB (Table 1). Anovulatory cycles are considered to be physiological in the first year after menarche and in the perimenopause and do not require extensive hormonal evaluation[34]. However, the cause of anovulatory cycles at other times in a woman's reproductive life should be investigated (Table 2). Prolactin and TSH should be measured in all patients with anovulation, whether they present with amenorrhea, oligomenorrhea or DUB, to rule out hyperprolactinemia and hypothyroidism. Follicle stimulating hormone (FSH) should also be measured, as dysfunctional bleeding may occur during the transition to premature ovarian failure, just as it does at the time of physiological menopause.

DUB is a common symptom of androgen excess. In women with dysfunctional bleeding and evidence of hirsutism or acne, the diagnosis of polycystic ovary syndrome can be made by finding elevated total or free testosterone. Late-onset or non-classic 21-hydroxylase deficiency is an uncommon cause of androgen excess, occurring in < 5% of hyperandrogenic women. It can be reliably ruled out by a 17-hydroxyprogesterone of < 2 ng/ml[35].

If there is no evidence of hyperprolactinemia, hypothyroidism, premature ovarian failure or androgen excess, patients with DUB fit into the category of hypothalamic dysfunction. They may be anovulatory due to stress, weight loss, exercise, or the cause may be idiopathic. These patients can be reassured that, as long as they continue to withdraw to a progestin challenge, there is no serious cause for their anovulation.

The long-term consequence of chronic anovulation is endometrial hyperplasia and carcinoma. Chronically anovulatory women have a three-fold increased risk of endometrial cancer[36]. An endometrial biopsy should be considered in all patients with anovulatory bleeding, particularly those over 40 years old. Some authors recommend that an endometrial biopsy be performed in a patient of any age with a history of anovulatory bleeding of > 1 year duration because there have been reports of endometrial cancer in patients as young as 15 years of age[34,37].

Treatment of dysfunctional uterine bleeding

When DUB is due to hyperprolactinemia, a dopamine agonist, such as bromocriptine, is effective in restoring ovulatory function. Some hyperprolactinemic patients may be treated with periodic progestin withdrawal. Patients with DUB and hypothyroidism respond quickly to thyroid hormone replacement therapy, as noted above.

In other patients with hypothalamic dysfunction and DUB, periodic progestin administration is effective in restoring a normal bleeding pattern (Table 3). A progestin, such as medroxyprogesterone acetate, is given by mouth 5 mg daily for the first 13 days of each month. There is evidence that at least 13 days of

Table 3 Medical therapy of abnormal uterine bleeding

Ovulatory bleeding (essential menorrhagia)
Birth control pill
Antiprostaglandins
Antithrombolytics
Danazol
Progesterone IUD

Dysfunctional uterine bleeding
Acute episode
  birth control pill
  IV conjugated equine estrogen
Chronic control
  monthly progestin
  birth control pill

IUD, intrauterine device; IV, intravenous

progestin therapy is necessary to eliminate the risk of endometrial hyperplasia[38]. The birth control pill is also effective in patients with DUB. It is particularly useful in patients with polycystic ovary syndrome as it helps control symptoms of androgen excess.

Occasionally, patients with DUB present with acute episodes of extremely heavy bleeding that require immediate therapy. In these patients, progestins alone are not effective, and estrogen must also be given. An effective outpatient therapy is to give any low-dose oral contraceptive pill, one pill twice daily for 5–7 days. Patients usually stop bleeding within 12–24 h, but therapy should be continued for the full 7 days. Upon completion of therapy, the patient will have a self-limited episode of bleeding, which may be heavy. Five days after discontinuing the dosage, the birth control pill can be restarted, one tablet daily as for contraception[39]. In patients with significant anemia, the withdrawal bleed may be postponed by continuing the oral contraceptive until the hemoglobin level is adequate to allow a withdrawal bleed. In women requiring in-patient observation and therapy, intravenous Premarin® has been shown to be effective in the treatment of DUB; 25 mg is given every 3–4 h for up to three doses[40]. After treating the acute episode of bleeding, it is important to put patients on chronic intermittent progestin therapy or the birth control pill to prevent further episodes.

Endometrial ablation may not be the ideal therapy in patients with DUB, because chronic anovulation and unopposed ovarian estrogen production will continue despite ablation. Since the endometrium is not completely destroyed in all endometrial ablations, there is a continued need of progestin therapy to prevent endometrial carcinoma in the residual islands. Endometrial carcinoma has been reported in a variety of circumstances following endometrial ablation including two perimenopausal patients 3 and 5 years after an endometrial ablation for DUB[41,42]. Endometrial carcinoma has also been found at the time of initial endometrial resection in women with normal preoperative diagnostic hysteroscopy and endometrial sampling[42,43]. Hysterectomy may be a more appropriate surgical choice for patients who cannot tolerate or do not respond to medical therapy for DUB.

PREOPERATIVE CONSIDERATIONS IN RESECTOSCOPIC SURGERY

Preoperative considerations in patients undergoing resectoscopic surgery include the use of agents to cause endometrial atrophy, cervical preparation, prophylactic antibiotics and consideration of appropriate anesthesia during surgery. The question of preoperative endometrial preparation will be considered in Chapter 5.

A review of hysteroscopic surgery for removal of intrauterine growths or for endometrial ablation revealed a number of preoperative strategies[22,23,44–52]. Prophylactic antibiotics were used in about one-half of the series. The most commonly used prophylactic antibiotic was doxycycline. Postoperative infections were rare. In a series of 575 endometrial resections receiving prophylactic amoxicillin and clavulanate, there were nine cases (1.6%) of endometritis[52]. The author is not aware of any randomized trial of prophylactic antibiotics in resectoscopic surgery. It would not be unreasonable to use prophylactic antibiotics in cases that are prolonged or require multiple transcervical insertions of the resectoscope.

Some authors recommend the insertion of laminaria the day before surgery because use of the resectoscope requires dilatation of the cervix up to a 31 Hegar dilator[44,50]. However, as with prophylactic antibiotics, evidence from randomized trials is lacking. Randomized trials have shown the synthetic prostaglandin misoprostol to be effective for cervical preparation. Oral misoprostol 400 µg 12 h prior to diagnostic hysteroscopy increased baseline cervical dilatation and decreased cumulative force required for dilatation in premenopausal women[53], but not in postmenopausal women[54]. Vaginal misoprostol 200 µg 9–10 h before operative hysteroscopy resulted in significantly increased baseline cervical dilatation, decreased operative time and decreased cervical tears compared to placebo[55].

The majority of patients in these series received general anesthetic. Regional anesthesia, such as an epidural block, has been used with equal success[22,46,49,50]. However, a randomized trial of general versus epidural anesthesia for hysteroscopic endometrial resection found significantly greater absorption of the glycine distention fluid in women randomized to epidural anesthesia[56]. One paper reported the use of intravenous sedation and paracervical block in 40 patients undergoing endometrial ablation[46]. Only two of the 40 required additional anesthesia. Thus, conduction anesthesia as well as intravenous analgesia and pericervical block are effective for pain control for patients undergoing resectoscopic surgery.

CLINICAL PEARLS

(1) Menstrual history is a poor predictor of extent of intrauterine adhesions.

(2) Patients presenting for septal lysis with a history of miscarriage should be worked up for other causes prior to surgery.

(3) Uterine fibroids, endometrial polyps and adenomyosis are common anatomical abnormalities causing menometrorrhagia.

(4) Preoperative diagnosis of adenomyosis is difficult.

(5) Evaluation of the uterine cavity, TSH and possibly coagulation studies and endometrial biopsy are the core work-up in patients with menorrhagia.

(6) Medical therapy is very effective in many patients with menorrhagia.

(7) In anovulatory patients, prolactin, TSH and FSH should be evaluated. In patients with signs of hyperandrogenism, androgens should be evaluated.

(8) In anovulatory patients, endometrial biopsy should also be considered to rule out hyperplasia.

(9) In patients with acute heavy bleeds, estrogen must be given. Progestins are ineffective.

(10) It is unclear if prophylactic antibiotics are effective in decreasing infectious morbidity for hysteroscopy.

(11) Preoperative laminaria use has not yet been shown to be effective prior to hysteroscopy.

(12) General, regional and paracervical blocks have all been effectively utilized as anesthetic regimens.

References

1. Li TC. Recurrent miscarriage: principles of management. *Hum Reprod* 1998;13:478–82

2. March CM, Israel R. Hysteroscopic management of recurrent abortion caused by septate uterus. *Am J Obstet Gynecol* 1987;156:834–42

3. Simon C, Martinez L, Pardo F, *et al.* Mullerian defects in women with normal reproductive outcome. *Fertil Steril* 1991;56:1192–3

4. Valle RF, Sciarra JJ. Intrauterine adhesions: hysteroscopic diagnosis, classification, treatment, and reproductive outcome. *Am J Obstet Gynecol* 1988;158:1459–70

5. Coulter A, Bradlow J, Agass M, *et al.* Outcomes of referrals to gynaecology outpatient clinics for menstrual problems: an audit of general practice records. *Br J Obstet Gynaecol* 1991;98:789–96

6. Hallberg L, Hogdahl AM, Nilson L, *et al.* Menstrual blood loss – a population study. *Acta Obstet Gynecol Scand* 1966;45:320–51

7. Eijkeren Van MA, Christiaens GCML, Sixma JJ, *et al.* Menorrhagia: a review. *Obstet Gynecol Surv* 1989; 44:421–9

8. McCausland AM. Hysteroscopic myometrial biopsy: its use in diagnosing adenomyosis and its clinical application. *Am J Obstet Gynecol* 1992; 166:1619–28

9. Fedele L, Bianchi ST, Dorta M, *et al.* Transvaginal ultrasonography in the diagnosis of diffuse adenomyosis. *Fertil Steril* 1992;58:94–7

10. Krassas GE, Pontikides N, Kalstas Th, *et al.* Menstrual disturbances in thyrotoxicosis. *Clin Endocrinol* 1994;40:641–4

11. Scott JC Jr, Mussey EL. Menstrual patterns in myxedema. *Am J Obstet Gynecol* 1964;90:161–5

12. Krassas GE, Pontikides N, Kaltsas Th, *et al.* Disturbances of menstruation in hypothyroidism. *Clin Endocrinol* 1999;50:655–9

13. Wilansky DL, Greisman B. Early hypothyroidism in patients with menorrhagia. *Am J Obstet Gynecol* 1989;160:673–7

14. Classens AE, Cowell CA. Acute adolescent menorrhagia. *Am J Obstet Gynecol* 1981;139:277–9

15. Peterson HB, Jeng G, Folger SG, *et al.* The risk of menstrual abnormalities after tubal sterilization. *N Engl J Med* 2000;343:1681–7

16. Soares SR, Reis MM, Camargos AF. Diagnostic accuracy of sonohysterography, transvaginal sonography, and hysterosalpingography in patients with uterine cavity diseases. *Fertil Steril* 2000;70:406–11

17. Dueholm M, Forman A, Jensen ML, *et al.* Transvaginal sonography combined with saline contrast sonohysterography in evaluating the uterine cavity in premenopausal patients with abnormal uterine bleeding. *Ultrasound Obstet Gynecol* 2001;18:54–61

18. Dueholm M, Lundorf E, Hansen ES, *et al.* Evaluation of the uterine cavity with magnetic resonance imaging, transvaginal sonography, hysterosonographic examination, and diagnostic hysteroscopy. *Fertil Steril* 2001;76:350–7

19. Bradley LD, Falcone T, Magen AB. Contemporary management of abnormal uterine bleeding. *Obstet Gynecol Clin* 2000;27:1–28

20. Togashi K, Ozasa HI, Konishi I, *et al.* Enlarged uterus: differentiation between adenomyosis and leiomyoma with MRI imaging. *Radiology* 1989;171:531–4

21. Higham JM, Shaw RW. The effect of thyroxine replacement on menstrual blood loss in a hypothyroid patient. *Br J Obstet Gynaecol* 1992;99:695–6

22. Derman SG, Rehnstrom J, Neuwirth RS. The long-term effectiveness of hysteroscopic treatment of menorrhagia and leiomyomas. *Obstet Gynecol* 1991;77:591–4

23. Daniell JF, Kurtz BR, Ke RW. Hysteroscopic endometrial ablation using the rollerball electrode. *Obstet Gynecol* 1992;80:329–32

24. Nilsson L, Rybo G. Treatment of menorrhagia. *Am J Obstet Gynecol* 1971;110:713–20

25. Bergqvist A, Sjukhuset A, Malmo RG. Treatment of menorrhagia with intrauterine release of progesterone. *Br J Obstet Gynaecol* 1983;90:255–8

26. Milson L, Anderson K, Andersch B, *et al.* A comparison of flurbiprofen, tranexamic acid, and a levonorgestrel-releasing intrauterine contraceptive device in the treatment of idiopathic menorrhagia. *Am J Obstet Gynecol* 1991;164:879–83

27. Crosignani PG, Vercellini P, Mosconi P, *et al.* Levonorgestrel-releasing intrauterine device versus hysteroscopic endometrial resection in the treatment of dysfunctional uterine bleeding. *Obstet Gynecol* 1997;90:257–63

28. Chimbira TH, Anderson ABM, Naish C, *et al.* Reduction of menstrual blood loss by danazol in unexplained menorrhagia: lack of effect of placebo. *Br J Obstet Gynaecol* 1980;87:1152–8

29. Hall P, Maclachalan N, Thorn N, *et al.* Control of menorrhagia by the cyclo-oxygenase inhibitors naproxen sodium and mefenamic acid. *Br J Obstet Gynaecol* 1987;94:554–8

30. van Eijkeren MA, Christiaens G, Geuze HJ, *et al.* Effects of mefenamic acid on menstrual hemostasis in essential menorrhagia. *Am J Obstet Gynecol* 1992;166:1419–28

31. Nelson JR, Corson SL. Long-term management of adenomyosis with a gonadotropin-releasing hormone agonist: a case report. *Fertil Steril* 1993;59:441–3

32. Hirata JD, Moghissi KS, Ginsburg KA. Pregnancy after medical therapy of adenomyosis with a gonadotropin-releasing hormone agonist. *Fertil Steril* 1993;59:444–5

33. Thomas EJ, Okuda KJ, Thomas NM. The combination of a depot gonadotropin-releasing hormone agonist and cyclical hormone replacement therapy for dysfunctional uterine bleeding. *Br J Obstet Gynaecol* 1991;98:1155–9

34. Bayer SR, DeCherney AH. Clinical manifestations and treatment of dysfunctional uterine bleeding. *J Am Med Assoc* 1993;269:1823–8

35. Azziz R, Hincapie LA, Knochenhauer ES, *et al.* Screening for 21-hydroxylase-deficient non-classic adrenal hyperplasia among hyperandrogenic women: a prospective study. *Fertil Steril* 1999;72:915–25

36. Coulam CB, Annegers JF, Kranz JS. Chronic anovulation syndrome and associated neoplasia. *Obstet Gynecol* 1983;61:403–7

37. Farhi DC, Nosanchuk J, Silverberg SG. Endometrial adenocarcinoma in women under 25 years of age. *Obstet Gynecol* 1986;68:741–5

38. Mishell DR. Abnormal uterine bleeding. In Herbst AR, Mishell DR, Stenchever MA, *et al.* eds. *Comprehensive Gynecology.* St Louis: Mosby Year Book, 1992:1079–99

39. Dysfunctional uterine bleeding. In Speroff L, Glass RH, Kase NG, eds. *Clinical Gynecologic Endocrinology and Infertility,* 6th edn. Baltimore: Lippincott Williams & Wilkins, 1999:575–93

40. DeVore GR, Owens O, Kase N. Use of intravenous premarin in the treatment of dysfunctional uterine bleeding – a double-blind randomized control study. *Obstet Gynecol* 1982;59:285–91

41. Copperman AB, DeCherney AH, Olive DL. A case of endometrial cancer following endometrial ablation for dysfunctional uterine bleeding. *Obstet Gynecol* 1993;82:640–2

42. Valle RF, Baggish MS. Endometrial carcinoma after endometrial ablation: high risk factors predicting its occurrence. *Am J Obstet Gynecol* 1998;179:569–72

43. Colafranceschi M, Bettocchi S, Mencaglia K, *et al.* Missed hysteroscopic detection of uterine carcinoma before endometrial resection: report of three cases. *Gynecol Oncol* 1996;62:298–300

44. Townsend DE, Richart RM, Paskowitz RA, *et al.* Instruments and methods. *Obstet Gynecol* 1990;76:310–13

45. Loffer FD. Removal of large symptomatic intrauterine growths by the hysteroscopic resectoscope. *Obstet Gynecol* 1990;76:836–40

46. Garry R, Erian J, Grochmal SA. A multi-centre collaborative study into the treatment of menorrhagia by Nd-YAG laser ablation of the endometrium. *Br J Obstet Gynaecol* 1991;98:357–62

47. Corson SL, Brooks PG. Resectoscopic myomectomy. *Fertil Steril* 1991;55:1041–4

48. Pyper RJD, Haeri AD. A review of 80 endometrial resections for menorrhagia. *Br J Obstet Gynaecol* 1991;98:1049–54

49. VanDamme JP. One-stage endometrial ablation: results in 200 cases. *Eur J Obstet Gynecol Reprod Biol* 1992;43:209–14

50. Indman PD. Hysteroscopic treatment of menorrhagia associated with uterine leiomyomas. *Obstet Gynecol* 1993;81:716–20

51. Dwyer N, Hutton J, Stirrat GM. Randomised controlled trial comparing endometrial resection with abdominal hysterectomy for the surgical treatment of menorrhagia. *Br J Obstet Gynaecol* 1993;100:237–43

52. O'Connor H, Magos A. Endometrial resection for the treatment of menorrhagia. *N Engl J Med* 1996;335:151–6

53. Ngai SW, Chan YM, Liu KL, *et al.* Oral misoprostol for cervical priming in non-pregnant women. *Hum Reprod* 1997;12:2373–5

54. Ngai SW, Chan YM, Ho PC. The use of misoprostol prior to hysteroscopy in postmenopausal women. *Hum Reprod* 2001;16:1486–8

55. Preutthipan S, Herabutya Y. Vaginal misoprostol for cervical priming before operative hysteroscopy: a randomized controlled trial. *Obstet Gynecol* 2000;96:890–4

56. Goldenberg M, Cohen SB, Etchin A, *et al.* A randomized prospective comparative study of general versus epidural anesthesia for transcervical hysteroscopic endometrial resection. *Am J Obstet Gynecol* 2001;184:273–6

5

Uterine preparation prior to surgery

E. J. Bieber

The concept of preparation of the uterus prior to surgery has received increasing attention as we strive to achieve higher success rates and facilitate our procedures. When DeCherney and Polan first reported on resectoscopic endometrial ablations, most of their patients were chronically sick with acute bleeding, and although there was no time for medical pretreatment, they achieved good results[1]. As the applications and indications of hysteroscopic and resectoscopic procedures have broadened, we see far fewer acute patients.

For the novice hysteroscopist, visualization is critical. There is nothing more frustrating to the beginning hysteroscopist than setting up the necessary equipment, only to insert the hysteroscope into a sea of blood and excess tissue that cannot be cleared. There are several preoperative and operative measures that will keep this experience to a minimum and potentially facilitate operative procedures.

The primary goals of pretreatment are to:

(1) Decrease the endometrial thickness and/or myoma size;

(2) Decrease vascularity of the endometrium or myomata;

(3) Decrease blood loss at the time of surgery;

(4) Decrease operative time;

(5) Increase hemoglobin prior to surgery in anemic patients;

(6) Improve visualization and ease of surgery;

(7) Possibly improve overall success and feasibility rates.

More recently, there has been interest in treating patients after surgery to enhance the results. Interestingly, in the case of fertility patients, this may be the opposite treatment to that of a patient undergoing endometrial ablation.

Currently, many different methods are used in attempting to achieve these goals, ranging from appropriate timing during the cycle to medical or mechanical methods. Like many other applications in obstetrics and gynecology, none of the medical treatments discussed are approved as hysteroscopy endometrial pretreatments by the Food and Drug Administration (FDA). Once the FDA has approved a drug, physicians are not limited in their ability to use these agents for unlabelled applications. Such is the case with all medical agents discussed herein.

PRETREATMENT REGIMENS

Hysteroscopy during the proliferative phase

The simplest form of uterine preparation might be considered to be performance of a procedure during the early proliferative phase. Review of the endometrial height at various times during the menstrual cycle demonstrates the lowest or most basal endometrium following menses (Figure 1). An impressive increase in endometrial height occurs as a response to

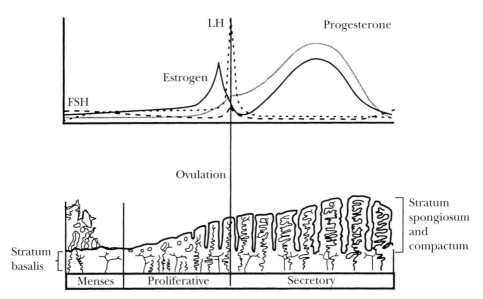

Figure 1 Demonstration of the change in endometrial height during the menstrual cycle. LH, luteinizing hormone; FSH, follicle stimulating hormone

the endometrial mitogen estrogen. Diagnostic hysteroscopy is most easily performed after menses, prior to the excessive endometrial build-up, which occurs as early as the mid- to late proliferative phase. Performance of hysteroscopy during the luteal phase is more difficult, because disruption of endometrial tissue often occurs during hysteroscope insertion or manipulation. Excessive tissue may obscure intracavitary abnormalities and subtle lesions. In addition, luteal phase hysteroscopy carries the risk of disrupting a chemically undetectable pregnancy. In some cases, we have been forced to perform hysteroscopies during the menstrual cycle. With modern continuous-flow hysteroscopes (see Chapter 2), even in cases of heavy bleeding, good visualization is almost always achievable.

While we find the early proliferative phase an excellent time for diagnostic and simple operative procedures, on occasion, a surprising amount of tissue is present.

Progestational agents

Progestins are commonly used in clinical practice to antagonize the effects of estrogen and initiate programmed endometrial changes, which allow a timed withdrawal bleed. These effects have been used to treat patients prior to hysteroscopic procedures. Progestins limit the growth of endometrium by multiple actions. When used over extended time periods, progestins induce pseudodecidual changes and eventual atrophy.

Multiple regimens have been used for this purpose, including depo-medroxyprogesterone acetate (DMPA), oral medroxyprogesterone acetate and (MPA) norethindrone. In the depot formulation, DMPA is administered as a 150-mg intramuscular injection. Studies evaluating DMPA have found depo-injections to cause pharmacological and contraceptive effects for at least 3 months[2]. With the regimen of 150 mg every 3 months, approximately 50% of patients will become amenorrheic after 1 year and 60–70% amenorrheic after 2 years[3]. This demonstrates the atrophy that ultimately takes place. Unfortunately, the effect is somewhat unpredictable, and approximately 10% of women have menorrhagia at 12 months[3].

Alternative regimens have used norethindrone 5 mg twice a day or oral MPA 10 mg three times a day for periods of 45–60 days.

Common progestational side-effects are listed in Table 1[3,4].

Progestins may also have a role in stabilizing the endometrium of patients who have required estrogen to decrease significant blood loss. Stabilization of the endometrium with cessation of bleeding allows an increase in hematocrit in anemic patients as well as creating an even endometrium that will be appropriately shed once the progestin is withdrawn. This type of initial regimen may then be followed by other medical pretreatment regimens, i.e. gonado-tropin-releasing hormone (GnRH) agonists, danazol, or further progestins.

Oral contraceptives

Like progestins, oral contraceptives are often used clinically to regulate and decrease the amount of menstrual flow. Previous studies have documented decreases of greater than 40% of pretreatment loss using reliable methods for quantification of menstrual blood loss[5]. Current combined oral contraceptives contain pro-gestins in all active hormonal days, and, thus, there is a continual antagonism to the estrogen component. It is for this reason that oral contra-ceptives were considered a reasonable pre-treatment option.

Table 1 Common progestational side-effects

GnRHa
Hot flushes/sweats (80%)
Headaches (30%)
Vaginitis (20–30%)
Emotion/lability (20%)

Danazol
Hot flushes/sweats (50–60%)
Androgen-like effects (30%)
Weight change (20–30%)
Headaches (20%)

Progestins
Menstrual abnormalities (25%)
Headache (15%)
Abdominal discomfort (13%)
Nervousness (10%)
Decreased libido (5%)

GnRHa, gonadotropin releasing hormone agonist

Unfortunately, the estrogenic stimulus is not completely suppressed, even on very low-dose preparations. Because of this, there are relatively few patients who become amenorrheic from atrophy, and most patients have some level of endometrial proliferation. Although the endometrium is decreased compared with that of the ovulatory patient, there may be enough endometrium to interfere with visualization.

In the case of patients being pretreated prior to endometrial ablation, there may be difficulty in achieving destruction of the endometrium to the basal level. Previous publications have documented the ability of continuous oral con-traceptives to cause a decidual-like effect and amenorrhea, thus the term pseudo-pregnancy. As with progestins, there is a variable response of the endometrium, and many months of treat-ment may be required to achieve the desired effect. It is for these reasons that the authors have found limited utility for oral contraceptives in preoperative endometrial preparation for hysteroscopy.

Danazol

Danazol has been used extensively in Europe for preoperative endometrial preparation. Danazol is a 2,3-isoxazol derivative of 17α-ethinyl testosterone. The medication was intro-duced over two decades ago and has been stud-ied as a treatment in numerous gynecological disorders.

Pharmacodynamic studies have shown that the drug is almost completely absorbed from the gastrointestinal tract with peak serum levels 2 h later and almost no drug seen after 8 h[6]. It is from these data and efficacy data that the recommended regimen is 200 mg every 6–8 h.

Danazol has multiple mechanisms of action. Baseline levels of gonadotropins are unchanged, but there is a decrease in mid-cycle gonadotropin surge. Estradiol levels are decreased to a low follicular phase level. Sex hormone-binding globulin levels are markedly decreased with a subsequent elevation in free testosterone levels. This explains the increased prevalence of androgenic symptoms in patients taking danazol.

While some studies have suggested comparable efficacy of lower doses and decreased side-effects with the diminished dose, this is in disagreement with other trials[7,8]. In addition, there is concern that decreased doses may not cause full suppression because of the metabolism of the drug, and this may, in turn, cause less endometrial suppression in the pretreatment patient. Unfortunately, as the clinician increases the dose, significant side-effects are seen (Table 1).

In general, patients should be placed on medication for 6 weeks prior to undergoing surgery. In addition, an effort should be made to rule out pregnancy as the potential for virilization exists should pregnancy occur[9].

Gonadotropin releasing hormone agonists

Gonadotropin releasing hormone agonists (GnRHa) were originally introduced as a medical treatment for patients with prostate cancer. In recent years, many applications for these agents to gynecological disease have been evaluated. During initial animal trials, it was noted that acute administration of GnRHa caused a stimulatory effect, as would be expected for an agent with an agonist effect[10]. Chronic administration, to the surprise of the investigators, caused pituitary downregulation and desensitization, acting in an almost antagonist fashion. Reversal of administration caused a return to the original stimulatory effect. This may be seen graphically in Figure 2. When given chronically, there is a variable period of agonist stimulation for 6–10 (± 2) days. A period of decreased hypothalamic–pituitary–ovarian axis function follows with an eventual reversible senescence. Investigations have suggested several mechanisms by which this type of phenomenon might occur. It is hypothesized that the receptor site–agonist complex causes downregulation and an uncoupling of the receptor–agonist occurs to cause a desensitization effect. The end result is a pseudomenopausal state with very low levels of circulating estradiol. It is this effect that is most clinically useful in the preoperative preparation of patients.

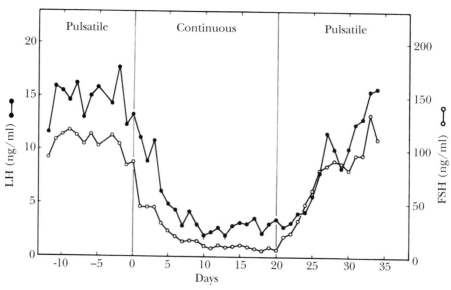

Figure 2 Pulsatile administration of gonadotropin releasing hormone (GnRH) in an ovariectomized monkey demonstrates normal gonadotropin (LH, luteinizing hormone; FSH, follicle stimulating hormone) release. Continuous infusion induces an incremental decrease over 7–10 days. Reinstitution of the intermittent or pulsatile release reverses the suppression with a return to baseline gonadotropin levels. Reproduced with permission from reference 10

GnRHa are synthesized by modifying the native GnRH molecule at the N-terminal end and near the sixth amino acid. These chemical changes impart greater potency and inhibit degradation enzymes, thereby extending the half-life. Three GnRHa are presently approved in the USA for the treatment of endometriosis: nafarelin acetate, leuprolide acetate and goserelin acetate. Table 2 summarizes the administration and dosage for the various GnRHa available. All three have different delivery systems. Nafarelin is available as a 400-µg intranasal spray. Leuprolide is available in either a depoformulation of microspheres or as a subcutaneous daily injection and goserelin is available as a long-acting subcutaneous implant.

GnRHa have been shown to decrease the size of a significant percentage of all fibroids, decrease uterine volume and elevate hemoglobin levels during treatment. In a European multicenter study, Serra and colleagues reported that treatment with 4 months of GnRHa resulted in 53% of individual myomas decreasing in size more than 50% of the inital pretreatment volume, while 18% of myomas were unchanged or increased in size[11]. Friedman and colleagues found similar results in their randomized, prospective, double-blind multicenter study[12]. They demonstrated a mean uterine volume reduction of 36% at 12 weeks and 45% at 24 weeks in patients treated with leuprolide acetate. It is from these data that most clinicians consider 3 months of pretreatment adequate to reduce myoma size. Shorter treatment regimens have also been evaluated.

In one study, a short course GnRHa treatment regimen found a volume reduction of 35% at 1 month and 44% at 2 months[13].

Golan and co-workers evaluated the GnRHa D-Trp 6-luteinizing hormone releasing hormone (LHRH) and found a decrease in operative times and the amount of intra-operative blood loss when performing surgery on leiomyomas[14].

In patients presenting with menorrhagia and anemia, immediate surgery may have a higher incidence of blood transfusion. Vercellini and colleagues demonstrated a mean hemoglobin rise from 8.5 to 13.3 g/dl in patients treated for 6 months with the GnRHa goserelin[15]. Interestingly, 51% of their control group required blood transfusion whereas no medical treatment patient was transfused intra- or post-operatively.

Suction curettage prior to hysteroscopy

Several reports have discussed the use of a suction curette mechanically to denude the endometrium prior to operative hysteroscopy. In these cases, preoperative medication is not required. Interestingly, one author felt performance of the procedure during the late luteal or menstrual phase of the cycle allowed the clearest visualization[16]. He hypothesized that late luteal or menstrual endometrium may be more loosely attached and, thus, more easily separated from the basalis during suction. Performance of a procedure during these time periods does risk interruption of a chemically non-detectable pregnancy. In a second report,

Table 2 Three gonadotropin releasing hormone agonists (GnRHa) available in the USA and two agonists commonly used outside the USA are compared for route of administration and dosing

Generic name	Trade name	Available in USA	Route of administration	Dose
Leuprolide	Lupron®	yes	intramuscular	3.75–7.5 mg/monthly
			intramuscular	11.25 mg (3-month dose)
			subcutaneous	0.5–1.0 mg/daily
Nafarelin	Synarel®	yes	intranasal	400–800 µg/daily
Goserelin	Zoladex®	yes	subcutaneous implant	3.6 mg/monthly
Tryptorelin	Decapeptyl®	no	intramuscular	3.75 mg/monthly
			subcutaneous	0.25–0.5 mg/daily
Buserelin	Suprefact®	no	intramuscular	900–1200 µg/daily

the procedure was performed during the early follicular phase without difficulty[17]. Both groups felt that the advantages of this type of preparation were cost savings, no wait for medication to cause endometrial atrophy, and obtaining tissue for histological evaluation. In one patient, preoperative endometrial biopsy demonstrated anovulatory endometrium without atypia. At the time of endometrial ablation, suction curettage demonstrated atypical hyperplasia. Concern was raised regarding the possible suppressive effect of a preoperative medication. The clinical relevance of abnormal endometrium that suppresses to normal is debatable. In addition, endometrial biopsies have demonstrated an impressive ability to rule out endometrial disease[18]. However, regardless of the technique used for ablation and preparation, suspicious or unusual areas seen during procedures should be biopsied or resected for histological analysis, regardless of previous histology.

EFFICACY OF PRETREATMENT REGIMENS

In the original publication by DeCherney and Polan on the use of the urologic resectoscope to manage patients with septa, polyps, myomas, and abnormal uterine bleeding, no specific pretreatment regimen was utilized[1]. Septum patients had surgery during the proliferative phase. Patients with intractable uterine bleeding had all been initially treated with 25 mg of intravenous conjugated estrogens and failed. They then underwent endometrial cauterization using the wire loop.

In 1989, Vancaillie reported on the use of a ball-end resectoscope to ablate the endometrium in 15 patients[19]. He suggested that menstruation might be the ideal period in which to perform ablation, but dismissed this as 'technically difficult'. His regimen of pretreatment was daily oral MPA, 5 mg/75 lb, beginning on day 2 of the cycle with performance of the procedure 3–4 weeks later. In short-term follow-up, 14 of 15 patients had amenorrhea or hypomenorrhea.

Goldrath reported on the use of danazol for treatment prior to laser endometrial ablation[20]. He recommended 800 mg/day for 25 days prior to surgery and described a 'very thin atrophic endometrium in which telangiectasia is present'. Using this protocol, he had excellent or good results in 299 of 321 women.

In contrast to Goldrath, Lefler and colleagues reported about patients undergoing endometrial coagulation: '. . . Danazol resulted in inconsistent thinning of the endometrium which often shredded off, obscuring vision during the procedure, and which may have left thicker areas of the endometrium uncoagulated'[17]. They reported a non-statistically significant increase in amenorrhea rates in patients who underwent coagulation ablation using vasopressin and suction curettage versus patients undergoing laser ablation and a pretreatment regimen of 200 mg of danazol twice daily.

In a study of patients undergoing transcervical resection of the endometrium (TCRE), the authors found that 800 mg/day of danazol for 6 weeks prior to surgery decreased fluid deficit and procedure duration. In this non-randomized trial they noted three patients in the untreated group who had fluid deficits over 1000 ml versus none in the danazol-treated arm[26].

Gimpelson and Kaigh compared results obtained with a heterogeneous group of medical preparations (danazol, leuprolide and nafarelin) to patients who underwent suction curettage prior to endometrial ablation[16]. Their study was neither prospective nor randomized but offered interesting conclusions. No statistical differences were noted between the study groups when evaluating for reduction of bleeding or amenorrhea. Non-statistically significant decreases in operative times and the amount of fluids used or absorbed were seen in the suction curettage group. Because the suction curettage patients were later in the series, influence of operator experience and equipment evolution make comparisons difficult. This form of pretreatment offers the theoretic advantages of decreased cost and an additional histological specimen. Some surgeons have suggested the addition of a procedure (suction curettage) might lead to increased operative times and, thus, the question of increasing operating room cost. In addition, there are concerns regarding the ability of suction curettage completely to denude the endometrium to the level of the basalis to allow the most effective destruction when performing endometrial coagulation. Such issues may be less important when performing endometrial resection (see Chapter 14). It is also difficult to understand how suction curettage, which causes endometrial trauma and bleeding, would lead to decreased intravasation from these open vessels. In a study from Taiwan, Yin and colleagues evaluated use of a 'thorough' suction curettage prior to hysteroscopic resection. While their patient satisfaction with the surgery was only 60% and 10% of patients required a second procedure (either repeat ablation or hysterectomy), they concluded that curettage was cheap, effective and acceptable[27].

While additional tissue may be sent for further histological evaluation, it is the editor's recommendation that all patients being considered for ablative procedures be adequately evaluated prior to ablation with office sampling, hysteroscopy, or previous dilatation and curettage. Minassian and Mira recently reported on a patient who had refractory menorrhagia and underwent thermal balloon ablation[28]. Dilatation and curettage, and subsequent pathology at the time of ablation, found complex hyperplasia with atypia. While we have also seen patients with documented abnormal histology at the time of ablation (which was normal at previous sampling), it is unclear how such abnormalities might respond to medical pretreatment or if this abnormal pathology would have been missed without sampling. Randomized, prospective evaluations may help in answering these critical questions.

Brooks and Serden reported on the use of a single dose of the GnRHa leuprolide acetate depot prior to resectoscopic endometrial ablation[21]. When administered during the luteal phase, the agonist effect is generally inconsequential. Following menses, pituitary downregulation and desensitization will have occurred. At this point, endogenous estradiol levels should be close to castration levels, and little proliferation should occur in the postmenstrual basal endometrium. Interestingly, anecdotal reports have described increased bleeding in either preablation or myomectomy patients following GnRHa administration. Although relatively uncommon, expectant hormonal management with estrogen is appropriate in these cases, and rarely is surgical treatment necessary. In patients treated with a single dose of GnRHa, the endometrium was described as being '... thinned in all patients, with inactive glands, reduced vascularity, and atrophic stroma'.

Serden and Brooks compared amenorrhea rates achieved following ablation with either no preparation, danazol, progestins, or leuprolide acetate[22]. Progesterones were dropped from the protocol because of difficulties with tissue from the decidualized endometrium interfering with surgery. Amenorrhea rates were 41% for danazol, 43% with no preparation, and 67% for leuprolide acetate during the short follow-up. In another study, various preoperative treatment strategies were compared by analyzing the endometrial histology from the resected tissue[23]. Progestins (DMPA or norethindrone)

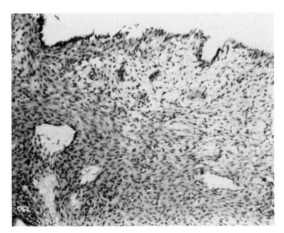

Figure 3 Photomicrograph of endometrium after progestin therapy. Edema, angiectasia and decidual reaction are notable. Reproduced from reference 23 with permission

were noted to induce endometrial thickening secondary to tissue edema. Vascular proliferation and angiectasia were noted with this preparation (Figure 3). In patients who were untreated but had their surgery performed during the proliferative phase, the endometrium was described as thin and hypovascular but histologically dysfunctional. Patients treated with depo-leuprolide acetate had reproducible results, with the endometrium noted to be thin, mostly atrophic, and without tissue edema (Figure 4). In contrast, danazol demonstrated a variable effect, which was reported to be independent of dose or duration of treatment. The endometrium was found to be dysynchronous with variable vascularity and tissue thickness (Figure 5).

In another study evaluating efficiency of GnRHa, Perino and colleagues prospectively compared leuprolide acetate with no treatment in patients undergoing septal incision, endometrial ablation and submucous myomectomy[24]. They documented no difference in the septum group but found statistically significant reductions in operative time, intraoperative bleeding, volume of media infused and failure rates (continued abnormal bleeding after 1 year or persistence of fibroid after 2 months) in the group of patients undergoing submucous myomectomy and pretreated

with a GnRHa. In the endometrial ablation pretreatment group, decreases were seen in operative time, intraoperative bleeding and media used, but similar failure rates were recorded.

In contrast, Fedele and co-workers in comparing GnRHa versus danazol in pretreatment of patients undergoing hysteroscopic metroplasty found that danazol allowed faster introduction of the resectoscope through the cervix and that overall the metroplasty was simpler[30].

In an interesting small study, Taskin and associates evaluated use of two doses of GnRHa versus placebo in patients undergoing rollerball ablation[31]. They used glycine mixed with a tracer of 2% alcohol to access intravasation of the media. Statistically significantly lower levels of blood ethanol as well as a decrease in sodium were noted in the GnRHa-treated patients. This is consistent with the premise of GnRHa decreasing vascularity and possibly fluid intravasation.

Multiple recent studies have also attempted to elucidate the impact of pretreatment on procedure success. In a large retrospective series of 1000 consecutive laser ablations, Phillips and colleagues reported that type of endometrial preparation was not correlated to success or increased risk of hysterectomy[32].

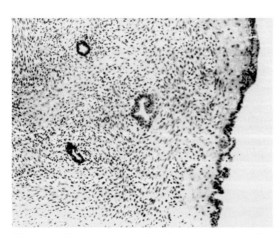

Figure 4 Photomicrograph of endometrium after leuprolide therapy, showing atrophy, sparse glands and dense stroma. Reproduced from reference 23 with permission

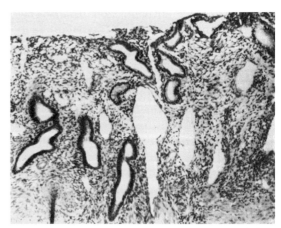

Figure 5 Photomicrograph of endometrium after danazol therapy. Angiectasia is extensive and thickness is less than with progestins. Reproduced from reference 23 with permission

Brolmann and co-workers had prospectively evaluated patients pretreated with GnRHa prior to endometrial resection[33]. In 24/32 cases endometrium was reduced in thickness, in one patient there was no change and in 7/32 the endometrium was slightly increased. This may represent the variable response some patients have to GnRHa.

Additional comparative trials include that of Fraser and colleagues who randomized patients to GnRHa or danazol 200 mg twice a day for 2 months prior to rollerball ablation[34]. At 6 months 74% of GnRHa and 62% of danazol patients were amenorrheic. Blood loss was markedly decreased in the GnRHa group from 94.8 to 1.0 ml and in the danazol group from 97.9 to 7.4 ml. Alford and Hopkins evaluated the use of GnRHa, danazol, tamoxifen or Depo-Provera® prior to rollerball ablation[35]. In this non-randomized trial, the surgeon rated the degree of endometrial atrophy as completely atrophic, intermediate atrophy or no response. Amenorrhea postablation was improved when complete atrophy was noted, whereas no patients were amenorrheic when 'no response' was seen. Twenty-four of the 30 patients treated with GnRHa or Danocrine® had complete atrophy versus 0/10 patients treated with Depo-Provera or tamoxifen.

Sorensen and co-workers evaluated the weight of endomyometrial strips in patients undergoing endometrial resection who were randomly assigned to no treatment, GnRHa 4–6 weeks preoperatively or GnRHa 4–6 weeks preoperatively and one injection on the day of surgery[36]. Surgical duration as well as the weight of resected strips was statistically lower for both GnRHa groups versus no treatment, and amenorrhea or scanty bleeding rates were higher for the GnRHa groups at 12 months' follow-up. It was unclear if the addition of the GnRHa injection on the day of surgery (postoperative treatment) had any clinically significant effect.

In a more recent and larger prospective randomized study, Shawki and associates pretreated patients prior to endometrial ablation with dilatation and curettage, GnRHa for 1 month, GnRHa for 3 months, danazol for 3 months, or oral MPA[37]. Table 3 shows the results from this trial. Unfortunately, a limiting factor was the use of both rollerball ablation and resection for treatment as well as the limited number of patients in each arm. None the less, as demonstrated by the improvement in all arms of the study, endometrial ablation, regardless of pretreatment regimen chosen, is a very effective technique.

Sowter and colleagues also recently evaluated endometrial pretreatment for endometrial ablation[38]. They found 12 studies that met the criteria for inclusion in the evaluation. After using their rigorous evaluation techniques they concluded that: 'Endometrial thinning prior to hysteroscopic surgery in the early proliferative phase of the menstrual cycle for menorrhagia improves both the operating conditions for the surgeon and short term post-operative outcome'. They also noted that GnRHa produced a more consistent result than danazol.

The choice of a pretreatment regimen depends on physician preference and skill, type of procedure to be performed, and preoperative status, i.e. hemoglobin. Many

Table 3 Data comparing pretreatment regimens prior to endometrial ablation. Adapted from reference 37

Preoperative preparation (n)	Operative time (min)	Improvement (%)	Amenorrhea (%)
Dilatation and curettage (39)	68	100	18
GnRHa 1 month before procedure (23)	39	91	39
GnRHa for 3 months before procedure (26)	37	92	38
Danazol 400–600 mg/day for 3 months before procedure (26)	43	92	35
MPA 15 mg orally (17)	54	85	26

GnRHa, gonadotropin releasing hormone agonist; MPA, medroxyprogesterone acetate

authors have 'favorite' protocols; the editor's standard pretreatment regimens are presented in Table 4.

POSTOPERATIVE TREATMENT

Postoperative endometrial suppression has gained increasing interest as clinicians strive to achieve higher amenorrhea rates after endometrial ablation. The idea of postoperative suppression is based on the premise that many women will have islands of non-coagulated or partially coagulated endometrium that will ultimately regenerate and lead to menstrual bleeding. In many cases, there is likely to be residual endometrium as 50% of women continue to have some level of bleeding following ablation. Some clinicians believe that postoperative hormonal inhibition will decrease the stimulus for regeneration of such tissues, possibly improving the overall success rate. Townsend and colleagues used such a regimen when they first reported on rollerball coagulation[25]. Twenty-five of 50 patients treated received 400 mg of MPA in the recovery room. None of these patients had bleeding in a

Table 4 Editor's most commonly used pretreatment protocols for endometrial and myoma preparation

Surgical procedure	Pretreatment regimen
Rollerball endometrial ablation	GnRHa – 2 months (if begun follicular phase) GnRHa – 1 month (if begun luteal phase) no pretreatment suction curettage
Septum resection	surgery during proliferative phase
Endometrial resection	surgery during proliferative phase or GnRHa agonist – 1–2 months
Thermal ablation	suction curettage
Myomectomy	GnRHa – 3 months (depending on size)
Polypectomy	no pretreatment

GnRHa, gonadotropin releasing hormone agonist

follow-up period of 6–12 months. Unfortunately, their long-term follow-up was not published.

In one of the few published reports addressing this issue, Goldrath found a significant improvement in amenorrhea rates after Nd:YAG laser ablation and a postoperative injection of 150 mg of MPA[20]. The group of patients treated with ablation alone without postoperative treatment had an amenorrhea rate of 37.3%, whereas those treated with both ablation and postoperative DMPA had a 69.3% rate of amenorrhea. The overall success rate (non-persistence of menorrhagia) was similar in both groups, but the increase in amenorrhea in the treatment group was impressive. Unfortunately, the groups are not compared as to length of time from surgery to re-evaluation, nor is comment made as to when cases were performed relative to the author's experience. Goldrath additionally alludes to the use of Danocrine postoperatively but dismisses this as impractical because of the extended healing period (up to 6 months) for the endometrium. Maia and co-workers also used 20 mg/day of oral MPA for 2 months after endometrial resection and concomitant rollerball ablation[29]. They gave no endometrial preparation prior to surgery. Patients were followed for 12 months and noted 98% success (amenorrhea to light menstrual flow). It is unclear if the success was secondary to the use of post-procedure hormonal suppression, use of the double procedure of resection rather than ablation or other factors.

GnRHa have also been suggested as post-treatment adjuvants. It is felt that the significant hypoestrogenism these agents produce may also retard or prevent regeneration of damaged tissue. Although studies are currently evaluating these agents, no published studies are available.

Caustic agents, such as tetracyline, have also been considered for postoperative treatment (T. G. Vancaillie, personal communication). It is proposed that intrauterine installation of these compounds may also serve to inhibit further tissue regeneration or proliferation. Concerns include the risk of transtubal leakage into the peritoneal cavity, intravasation of the material, and vaginal irritation following installation.

As with the other proposed medical regimens, significant data are lacking regarding efficacy and incidence of potential complications.

Because of our clinical desire to achieve higher amenorrhea rates, we have become increasingly interested in managing the post-operative period. Unfortunately, the paucity of data does not aid in choosing a regimen. Consideration must be given to the side-effects, cost and potential risks of any medication used postoperatively.

CONCLUSIONS

Success of any ablative or resection procedure is likely multifactorial. This is the difficulty in designing and performing any clinical trial but is especially problematic in the area of preoperative endometrial treatment. There are many ways a surgeon can perform a TCRE or endometrial ablation ranging from depth of resection, approach to the cornua regions, power settings, type of current, etc. All of these may in minor or major ways have an impact on the ultimate success or failure of the procedure. The thermal balloon may offer one opportunity as a standardized procedure to further investigate which type of preparation (if any) is preferential. Until further information is available, we as surgeons must rely on the published literature as presented within this chapter as well as our personal experience with the various pretreatment methodologies and our preferred surgical approach.

CLINICAL PEARLS

(1) Diagnostic hysteroscopy is best performed during the early proliferative phase.

(2) Progestational agents are useful in antagonizing the effects of estrogen and in limiting endometrial growth.

(3) Danazol is a testosterone derivative that has many effects, including decreasing the mid-cycle gonadotropin surge and reducing estradiol levels to low follicular phase.

(4) GnRHa initially cause a gonadotropin surge with estrogen release but, with chronic administration, reduce gonadotropins and decrease estradiol to menopausal levels.

(5) GnRHa have been extensively used to decrease myoma size and vascularity and elevate hemoglobin prior to surgery.

(6) Few good large studies exist comparing the efficacy of different regimens.

(7) Preliminary data suggest thinner endometrium allows better visualization and may have higher success rates with decreased intravasation because of decreased vascularity.

(8) Progestins cause a decidual-like effect that may interfere with operative hysteroscopy.

(9) Post-treatment regimens are being evaluated in an attempt to increase amenorrhea and overall success rates.

References

1. DeCherney A, Polan ML. Hysteroscopic management of intrauterine lesions and intractable uterine bleeding. *Obstet Gynecol* 1983;61:392–6

2. Ortiz A, Hiroi M, Stanczyk F, *et al.* Serum medroxyprogesterone acetate (MPA) concentrations and ovarian function following intramuscular injection of depo-MPA. *J Clin Endocrinol Metab* 1977;44:32–8

3. Schwallie PC, Assenzo JR. Contraceptive use efficacy study utilizing medroxyprogesterone acetate administered as an intramuscular injection once every 90 days. *Fertil Steril* 1993; 24:331–9

4. *Physicians Desk Reference*, 48th edn. Oradell, NJ: Medical Economic Co., 1994:2442–3

5. Nilsson L, Rybo G. Treatment of menorrhagia. *Am J Obstet Gynecol* 1971;110:713–20

6. Israel R. Pelvic endometriosis. In Mishell DR, Davajan V, Lobo RA, eds. *Infertility, Contraception, and Reproductive Endocrinology*. Boston: Blackwell Scientific Publications, 1991:734–5

7. Biberoglu KO, Behrman SJ. Dosage aspects of danazol therapy in endometriosis: short-term and long-term effectiveness. *Am J Obstet Gynecol* 1981;139:645–54

8. Dmowski WP, Kapetanakis E, Scommegna A. Variable effects of danazol on endometriosis at 4 low-dose levels. *Obstet Gynecol* 1982;59:408–15

9. Quagliarello J, Greco MA. Danazol and urogenital sinus formation in pregnancy. *Fertil Steril* 1985;43:939–42

10. Belchetz PE, Plant TM, Nakai Y, *et al.* Hypophysial responses to continuous and intermittent delivery of hypothalamic gonadotropin-releasing hormone. *Science* 1978; 202:631–3

11. Serra GB, Panetta V, Colosimo M, *et al.* Efficacy of leuprolide acetate depot in symptomatic fibromatous uteri: the Italian multicentre trial. *Clin Ther* 1992;14:57–73

12. Friedman AJ, Hoffman DI, Comite F, *et al.* Treatment of leiomyomata uteri with leuprolide acetate depot – a double-blind, placebo controlled multicenter study. *Obstet Gynecol* 1991;77:720–5

13. Coddington CC, Brzyski R, Hansen KA, *et al.* Short-term treatment with leuprolide acetate is a successful adjunct to surgical therapy of leiomyomas of the uterus. *Surg Gynecol Obstet* 1992;175:57–63

14. Golan A, Bukovsky I, Pansky M, *et al.* Preoperative gonadotropin-releasing hormone agonist treatment in surgery for uterine leiomyomata. *Hum Reprod* 1993;8:450–2

15. Vercellini P, Bocciolone L, Columbo A, *et al.* Gonadotropin-releasing hormone agonist treatment before hyperectomy for menorrhagia and uterine leiomyomas. *Acta Obstet Gynecol Scand* 1993;72:369–73

16. Gimpelson RJ, Kaigh J. Mechanical preparation of the endometrium prior to endometrial ablation. *J Reprod Med* 1992;37:691–4

17. Lefler HT, Sullivan GH, Hulka JF. Modified endometrial ablation: electrocoagulation with vasopressin and suction curettage preparation. *Obstet Gynecol* 1991;77:949–53

18. Goldschmit R, Katz Z, Blickstein I, *et al.* The accuracy of endometrial pipette sampling with and without sonographic measurement of endometrium. *Obstet Gynecol* 1993;82:727–30

19. Vancaillie TG. Electrocoagulation of the endometrium with the ballend resectoscope. *Obstet Gynecol* 1989;74:425–7

20. Goldrath MH. Use of danazol in hysteroscopic surgery for menorrhagia. *J Reprod Med* 1990; 35:91–5

21. Brooks PG, Serden SP. Preparation of the endometrium for ablation with a single dose of leuprolide acetate depot. *J Reprod Med* 1991; 36:477–8

22. Serden SP, Brooks PG. Preoperative therapy in preparation for endometrial ablation. *J Reprod Med* 1992;37:679–81

23. Brooks PG, Serden SP, Davos I. Hormonal inhibition of the endometrium for resectoscopic endometrial ablation. *Am J Obstet Gynecol* 1991; 164:1601–6

24. Perino A, Chianchiano N, Petronio M, *et al.* Role of leuprolide acetate depot in hysteroscopic surgery: a controlled study. *Fertil Steril* 1993; 59:507–10

25. Townsend DE, Richart RM, Paskowith RA, *et al.* 'Rollerball' coagulation of the endometrium. *Obstet Gynecol* 1990;76:310–13

26. Kriplani A, Nath J, Takkar D, *et al.* Biochemical hemodynamic and hematological changes during transcervical resections of the endometrium using 1.5% glycine as the irrigating solution. *Eur J Obstet Gynecol Reprod Biol* 1998;80:99–104

27. Yin CS, Wei RY, Chao TC, *et al.* Hysteroscopic endometrial ablation without endometrial preparation. *Int J Gynecol Obstet* 1998;62:167–72

28. Minassian VA, Mira JL. Balloon thermoablation in a woman with complex endometrial hyperplasia with atypia. *J Reprod Med* 2001;46:933–6

29. Maia H Jr, Calmon LC, Marques D, *et al.* Administration of medroxyprogesterone acetate after endomyometrial resection. *J Am Assoc Gynecol Laparosc* 1997;4:195–200

30. Fedele L, Bianchi S, Gruft L, *et al.* Danazol versus a gonadotropin-releasing hormone agonist as preoperative preparation for hysteroscopic metroplasty. *Fertil Steril* 1996;65:186–8

31. Taskin O, Yalcinoglu A, Kucuk S, *et al.* The degree of fluid absorption during hysteroscopic surgery in patients retreated with goserelin. *J Am Assoc Gynecol Laparosc* 1996;3:555–9

32. Phillips G, Chien PF, Garry R. Risk of hysterectomy after 1000 consecutive endometrial laser ablations. *Br J Obstet Gynecol* 1998;105: 897–903

33. Brolmann HA, Koks CA, Bongers MY. Endometrial electrosurgical resection by hysteroscopy in 32 menorrhagic patients: endometrial preparation with a GnRH agonist may have some effect on results. *J Gynecol Surg* 1995;11:65–70

34. Fraser IS, Healy DL, Torode H, *et al.* Depot goserelin and danazol pre-treatment before rollerball endometrial ablation for menorrhagia. *Obstet Gynecol* 1996;87:544–50

35. Alford WS, Hopkins MP. Endometrial rollerball ablation. *J Reprod Med* 1996;41:251–4

36. Sorensen SS, Colov NP, Vejerslev LO. Pre and postoperative therapy with GnRH agonist for endometrial resection. A prospective, randomized study. *Acta Obstet Gynecol Scand* 1997;76: 340–4

37. Shawki O, Peters A, Abraham-Hebert S. Hysteroscopic endometrial destruction, optimum method for preoperative endometrial preparation: a prospective, randomized, multicenter evaluation. *J Soc Laproendosc Surg* 2002;6:23–7

38. Sowter MC, Lethaby A, Singla AA. Pre-operative endometrial thinning agents before endometrial destruction for heavy menstrual bleeding. *Cochrane Database Syst Rev* 2002;3:CD001124

6

Distention media

E. J. Bieber

The effective use of distending media is one of the most important aspects for improving visualization and decreasing hysteroscopic complications. While urologists have contended with the difficulties of distention and media choice for resectoscopy over the last five or six decades, gynecologists have only recently retraced their steps. This chapter describes all of the media commonly used for hysteroscopic surgery and focuses on those solutions that have the greatest utility in diagnostic, operative and electrosurgical hysteroscopy.

THE DIFFICULTY WITH DISTENTION

While many parallels exist between urological cystourethroscopy/resectoscopy and gynecological hysteroscopy, significant differences are present. The cervix is not easily dilated and represents a barrier to surgery. The uterus is significantly more muscular, and, thus, greater pressure (as compared to the bladder) is necessary to allow separation of the endometrial walls. This separation allows the potential space of the uterus to become a true space in which surgery may be effectively performed. Unfortunately, because of the vascular nature of the uterus, overdistention may not improve visualization past a certain threshold but may predispose the patient to a greater risk of fluid intravasation (Figure 1). Depending on the indication for surgery and type of instrumentation to be used, one medium may be more appropriate than another. A list of media commonly used in hysteroscopy is found in Table 1. Several factors are important in selecting a medium, including the type of surgery to be performed, the amount of bleeding anticipated at the time of surgery, and the need for electrosurgery. The optimal medium would have clear visibility with a refractive index of 1.00, be isotonic, allow easy cleaning of instruments used during surgery, and have minimal impact on plasma, extracellular and intracellular fluid volumes (Table 2). In addition, cost per liter of solution differs markedly between each fluid (Table 3). Unfortunately, this perfect medium does not exist, and as surgeons, we must know the benefits, risks and limitations of multiple media to choose the most appropriate for a given surgery.

TYPES OF DISTENTION MEDIA

Carbon dioxide

Carbon dioxide (CO_2) is a gas medium with excellent optical properties, and it is relatively easy to use. Its refractive index is 1.00, or essentially equivalent to air. CO_2 has found the greatest utility in diagnostic hysteroscopy, but has limited applicability to operative hysteroscopy or resectoscopy because of the bleeding encountered during these procedures. The low viscosity of CO_2 allows easy flow through the relatively small inflow portals of most hysteroscopes. Unfortunately, this characteristic allows CO_2 to migrate around the hysteroscope and out of the cervical os if overdilatation has occurred.

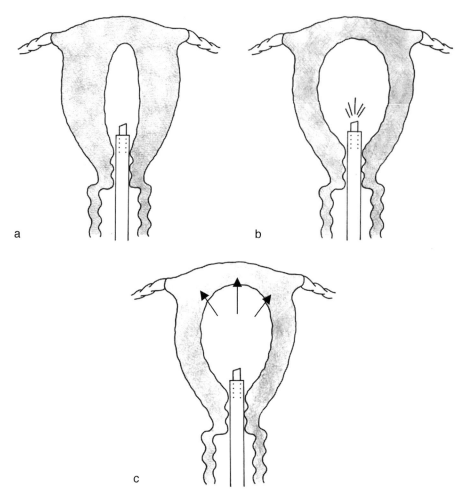

Figure 1 (a) Underdistention of the uterine cavity resulting in inadequate separation of the walls and decreased visualization; (b) adequate distention with excellent visualization; (c) increased intrauterine pressures giving no visual improvement but causing an increase in media intravasation

Rubin first reported on the use of CO_2 to distend and view the endometrium in patients with infertility[1]. He used a modified cystoscope and performed most of these procedures in the office setting. He later reported on the safety of using CO_2 to evaluate tubal patency in over 80 000 patients[2].

While excellent for diagnostic studies, the inability of CO_2 and blood to mix limits its application. The bubbles formed from this interaction can obscure the view and limit what can be successfully performed hysteroscopically.

Although a long safety history exists for CO_2 used hysteroscopically, there are concerns regarding potential problems if inappropriate insufflators are used. Dedicated hysteroscopic CO_2 insufflators have been manufactured for several decades. These insufflators are preset to limit either flow to below 100 ml/min or pressure to below 200 mmHg. Generally, excellent visualization is possible at pressure settings of 60–80 mmHg with an average flow rate of 50 ml/min. Laparoscopic insufflators (even older models) should never be used for hysteroscopy. The flow rates of > 1000 ml/min could

Table 1 Media commonly used for hysteroscopy

Low-viscosity media
Electrolyte containing
   lactated Ringer's
   0.45/0.9% normal saline
Non-electrolyte containing
   glycine (1.5%)
   sorbitol (3%)
   mannitol (5%)
   Cytal (sorbitol/mannitol) (3.2%)
   D_5W

High-viscosity media
   Hyskon

Gas media
Carbon dioxide

D_5W, dextrose 5% in water

Table 2 Characteristics of an 'ideal' medium

Isotonic
Clear visibility
Ease of instrument cleaning
Minimal impact on body fluid volumes
Ease of hysteroscopic delivery
Non-hemolytic
Non-conductive

Table 3 Cost comparison of various media, 1994

Solution	Size of bag (l)	Cost per unit* (US dollars)
1.5% Glycine	5	19.70
1.5% Glycine	3	12.20
3.0% Sorbitol	5	19.70
3.0% Sorbitol	3	12.20
0.9% Normal saline	1	3.66
0.9% Normal saline	2	6.66
0.9% Normal saline	3	9.75
Lactated Ringer's	3	10.50
Lactated Ringer's	5	17.00
D_5W	1	6.58

*List prices from Baxter
D_5W, dextrose 5% in water

cause a CO_2 pulmonary embolus. Baggish and Daniel reported on significant complications, including mortalities, from CO_2-cooled Nd:YAG laser tips being used for hysteroscopic ablation[3]. These cases demonstrate, *in vivo*, the risk of CO_2 emboli in high-flow systems where tissue disruption allows subsequent emboli formation.

Carbon dioxide remains an excellent medium for diagnostic evaluation. Its value for operative work is limited to simple operative procedures, such as intrauterine device (IUD) removal, polypectomy, or directed endometrial sampling. There is no role for CO_2 as a medium when using the resectoscope.

Normal saline, lactated Ringer's

Normal saline may be the optimal medium for performance of hysteroscopy using the Nd:YAG laser but has no utility when performing electrosurgery with standard instrumentation with the operative hysteroscope or resectoscope. However, recently a bipolar electrode has been introduced which is able to function with electrolyte-containing media. Like other low-viscosity fluids, saline readily mixes with blood. This is an advantage when using a continuous-flow instrument or an operative sheath with multiple ports. With these apparatus, the blood and saline mixture may be suctioned until a clear field is obtained. Optical characteristics for saline show a refractive index of 1.37. Although this is slightly different from CO_2, little difference may be appreciated clinically.

The greatest advantage of normal saline is its isotonicity. Attention must still be paid to the amount of intravasation as fluid overload may still occur. However, there is little concern regarding the possibility of hyponatremia should there be excess intravasation.

Lactated Ringer's is also an isotonic solution, and like normal saline, it contains electrolytes and is an unsatisfactory medium for electrosurgery.

Several manufacturers of electrosurgical generators are evaluating systems that would allow concurrent use of electrodes and saline as a distention medium. Presently, if standard electrosurgical generators are used with saline as a distending medium, no significant effect is achieved and the current diffuses in all directions. During a recent endometrial ablation, midway through the case, there was no tissue effect by the ball electrode. The problem was traced to the hanging of a 3-liter bag of normal saline instead of 1.5% glycine. On changing back to glycine, the desired electrosurgical effect was reinstated. Fortunately, it is unlikely that significant current density could be achieved to cause remote thermal injury in this type of situation.

Dextrose 5% in water or water

Dextrose 5% in water (D_5W) or water solutions are effective low-viscosity solutions. However, they have even greater limitations than normal saline or lactated Ringer's. Although electrolytically non-conductive, both have the disadvantage of causing dilutional hyponatremia. This is especially true for D_5W, which may markedly increase plasma volume, further exacerbating the hyponatremic nature of the solution. Like normal saline, both solutions mix well with blood and, theoretically, may be used in high-flow situations.

Water has optical properties that provide excellent visualization. This medium is severely limited in its operative indications by virtue of its ability to cause intravascular hemolysis and subsequent potential for renal damage[4]. It is for these reasons that water is not appropriate as a medium choice for hysteroscopy.

Glycine

Glycine is a distention medium commonly used by both gynecologists and urologists. The solution is a low-viscosity fluid, composed of a 1.5% mixture of the amino acid and commonly supplied in convenient 3-liter bags (Figure 2). This decreases the need for inconvenient nursing changes of distending media containers. Glycine has been the choice of urologists for decades in performing transurethral resections of the prostate (TURP) because of its excellent optical properties and lack of electrolytes[5].

Although some authors have referred to glycine as an isotonic fluid, it has an osmolality of only 200 mosmol/l and is a hypotonic fluid[6]. While posing little risk of intravascular hemolysis, there is a significant risk of volume overload and concurrent hyponatremia should this occur[7].

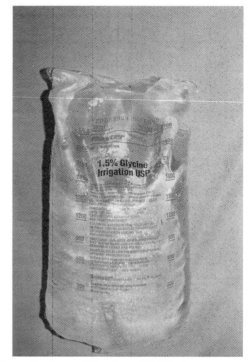

Figure 2 Large 3-liter bag of 1.5% glycine

Glycine metabolism is demonstrated in Figure 3. Once glycine has been intravasated, the intravascular half-life is 85 min. Following this, the amino acid is broken down to ammonia and glyoxylic acid via oxidative deamination in the liver and kidney. Ammonia is subsequently excreted as urea, and glyoxylic acid may be further reduced to oxalate.

It is unclear whether patients with underlying renal or hepatic abnormalities may be predisposed to elevated levels of the by-products of glycine metabolism. One report suggested hyperammonemia from excessive glycine metabolism during a TURP caused clinical toxicity, whereas other reports suggested there is no correlation in these levels even in patients with underlying liver abnormalities[4,8]. Oral L-arginine has been suggested as a protective agent, as it promotes ammonia breakdown through the urea cycle[9].

Glycine has been associated with acute, but transient, visual changes. In a small study, four of 18 patients experienced some level of visual alteration[10]. It is believed that glycine acts as a

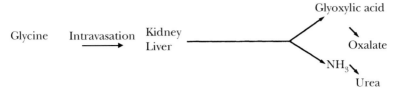

Figure 3 Glycine metabolism

neuroinhibitory substance at the retina, causing these reversible changes. Although cases of temporary postsurgical blindness have occurred, we know of no report of persistence.

Duffy and colleagues compared electrical parameters of 1.5% glycine, D_5W, distilled water and deionized water using a resectoscope in an *in vitro* experiment[11]. They found little difference in electrical properties between the four media. Interestingly, they found the addition of blood in varying concentrations resulted in current limiting and eventual electrosurgical generator shutdown[11]. They suggest that this situation may occur clinically when the surgeon is operating an electrode in a cavity with excess bleeding, demonstrating the importance of a functioning continuous-flow system.

Sorbitol and mannitol

Sorbitol and sorbitol/mannitol (Cytal; Abbott Laboratories, North Chicago, IL, USA) solutions have also been utilized for years by urologists and are available in large 3-liter bags. These solutions have similar problems to glycine in that they are hypotonic and may induce volume overload and hyponatremia if extensive intravasation were to occur. Cytal contains both 2.7% sorbitol and 0.54% mannitol. The mannitol was added to induce diuresis should fluid overload occur. Although anecdotal reports exist regarding the use of these agents during hysteroscopic surgery, there is little information regarding risk and benefit versus other distention agents.

Mannitol and sorbitol have similar structures in that they are both six-carbon molecules (Figure 4). However, they are metabolized and act very differently. Sorbitol is broken down to glucose and fructose, whereas little mannitol is

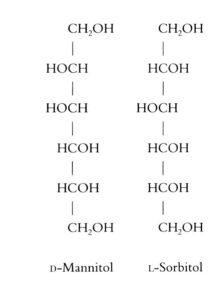

Figure 4 Chemical structure of mannitol and sorbitol, demonstrating marked similarity

metabolized. Because of its short half-life and subsequent renal excretion, mannitol acts effectively as an osmotic diuretic.

Increasing concern has been voiced as the literature becomes replete with reports of fluid overload and hyponatremia. This has focused attention on finding the 'best' medium possible. Because of its short half-life and the osmotic diuresis it induces, mannitol may come closest. While low-percentage mannitol solutions have an inadequate osmolar concentration, 5% mannitol has been suggested as an ideal medium[6]. At this concentration, the solution has an osmolarity of 274 mosmol/l, closely approximating the osmolarity of serum (280 mosmol/l).

Some writers have voiced concern regarding the 'stickiness' of the solution and a potential for carmelization at the electrode. Further evaluations may need to be performed clinically to substantiate mannitol as the preferential medium.

Hyskon®

Hyskon (CooperSurgical, Trumbull, CA, USA) is a high-viscosity solution composed of dextran 70 (32% W/V) in 10% dextrose (W/V). It contains glucose manufactured into high molecular weight (70 kDa) polymers. This solution has been effectively used for hysteroscopy and has also been used as a postsurgical adjuvant to attempt to decrease adhesions. Such a solution was first introduced for endoscopy in 1970 by Edstrom and Fernstrom[12]. The solution is highly viscous, clear and non-conductive since it contains no electrolytes[13]. In addition, the solution is poorly miscible with blood and is thus an excellent medium for performing operative hysteroscopy. Similar concerns have been expressed about the use of Hyskon, to those about mannitol for resectoscopy, in that both solutions may allow for carmelization around the active electrode. A more salient concern may be the inability to have adequate continuous flow given current hysteroscope design. Although the viscous nature of Hyskon reduces the large fluid volumes needed when using low-viscosity fluids, it is critical in operative hysteroscopy to have the ability intermittently to remove blood and/or debris from the operative field. It is likely that future instrument modifications will allow the use of resectoscopic electrodes and have multiple ancillary ports for accessory instrumentation or suction devices.

Because of the viscous nature of Hyskon, instruments must be specially cared for following a procedure. I have personally had a hysteroscope ruined because the instrument was not adequately cleaned on procedure completion. The solution will adhere to optical surfaces, valves, and intake and outflow portals. Use of hot water and cleansing solutions obviates these problems.

Another difficulty with Hyskon is the mechanism of delivery. The viscous nature of the solution makes delivery through the relatively small inflow channels of the hysteroscope somewhat difficult. Several devices for delivery have been created to decrease these difficulties and are further discussed in Chapter 2. A simple hand-held device using Archimedes principle allows easy, effective distention when using Hyskon (Figure 5).

A relatively recent addition to the hysteroscopic armamentarium has been the development of a bipolar electrode system that will function in a saline environment (Gynecare Inc., Menlo Park, CA, USA). Multiple bipolar electrodes (twizzle, ball, spring) are able to coagulate or vaporize in saline depending on the power setting (i.e. desiccation is 50 W whereas vaporcut is 200 W) (Figure 6). Early results from multiple investigators suggested the ability to treat a wide range of intrauterine lesions and disease[14–16]. A recent observational study by Marwah and Bhandari evaluated 151 cases of microhysteroscopy of which 50 patients underwent operative intervention with this 5-Fr bipolar electrode system and only one patient required additional use of the 27-Fr resectoscope[17]. In a larger study, Bettochi and colleagues treated 501 women with interuterine disease in the office with this small bipolar instrumentation[18]. He found that in spite of using no anesthesia or analgesia, 48–79% of patients were able to undergo their procedures without discomfort. This use of liquid media such as 0.9% normal saline with small hysteroscopes and small operative electrodes may allow performance of a significant number of hysteroscopies in the outpatient or office setting.

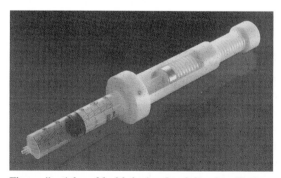

Figure 5 A hand-held device for delivering Hyskon through hysteroscope channels. Courtesy of Cook Ob/Gyn, Spencer, IN, USA

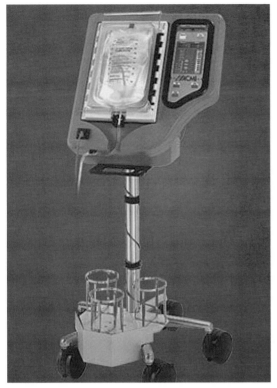

Figure 6 Bipolar electrode system. Courtesy of ACMI Corporation, Southborough, MA, USA

During the process of tissue vaporization gases will be released as tissue emplodes. In an interesting experiment, Munro and colleagues evaluated the composition of gas released *in vitro* from a monopolar vaporizing electrode in 1.5% of glycine and a bipolar electrode in normal saline[19]. Both types of electrodes released hydrogen, carbon monoxide and carbon dioxide – gases which are all highly soluble in serum.

COMPARATIVE STUDIES

In the early 1990s, we were early adopters of fluid media for diagnostic hysteroscopy instead of CO_2. Using a small hysteroscope with discrete inflow/outflow channels such as is seen in Figure 7, our group noted ease of surgery with excellent patient tolerance and improved visualization. This change was met with scepticism by many seasoned hysteroscopists who had used CO_2 successfully for many years.

It is only recently that multiple well done studies have been published comparing various media. Pellicano and associates performed a randomized prospective comparison of CO_2 versus normal saline in patients having outpatient hysteroscopy[20]. They found that use of normal saline decreased abdominal and shoulder pain, vasovagal reactions, operative time and had a higher satisfaction rate while requiring less analgesia post-procedure. This was consistent with earlier data from a similar prospective randomized trial from the Royal Free Hospital in London[21]. They similarly found an increase in abdominal and shoulder pain in the CO_2 group but also noted increased duration of procedures, need for cervical dilatation and had eight cases, which had to be converted from CO_2 to normal saline for technical problems. In a very large but non-randomized report, Perez-Medina and co-workers analyzed 6000 cases of office hysteroscopy[22]. They also found an increase in success (defined as a satisfactory hysteroscopy), as well as decreased need for anesthesia, while allowing improved ability to perform operative procedures such as polypectomy in the same setting.

DISTENDING MEDIA COMPLICATIONS

While hysteroscopy has a very low rate of significant complications, many that do occur are associated with problems of distending media. It should be no surprise that more reports of such complications are being published as more surgeons become familiar with operative hysteroscopic techniques. The previous pages detail the multiplicity of media available to the hysteroscopic surgeon. In the next pages, we will discuss the dynamics of fluid distention, methods for evaluating intravasation and the differential risks for low- and high-viscosity media. Methods of avoiding distention media complications and treatment of these complications are described.

DYNAMICS OF UTERINE DISTENTION

Evaluation and surgical treatment within the uterine cavity require adequate distention of

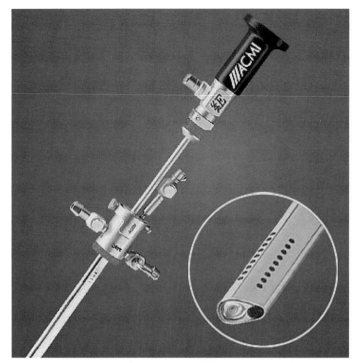

Figure 7 Small hysteroscope with discrete inflow/outflow channels. Courtesy of ACMI Corporation, Southborough, MA, USA

the walls to allow panoramic hysteroscopy to be performed. Methods for achieving distention are discussed in Chapter 2. Adequate uterine distention is usually achieved at 75 mmHg intrauterine pressure, and elevating levels beyond 100 mmHg may increase fluid intravasation risks without beneficial visual improvement. Low-viscosity fluid bags attached to a hysteroscope with large-bore urological tubing will give pressures of 73 mmHg at 1 m and 110 mmHg at 1.5 m above the supine patient[23]. Baker and Adamson used a Cobe CDX pressure transducer to define the intrauterine pressure needed to separate the anterior and posterior uterine walls[24]. They noted a median pressure of 40 mmHg with a range of 25–50 mmHg, consistent with other investigators.

When using continuous-flow systems, such as that with a gynecologic resectoscope, one must balance the need to achieve adequate intrauterine pressure with the requirement for outflow suction. Outflow may be obtained by draining (through gravity) into a calibrated canister or into a perineal drape (Figure 8),

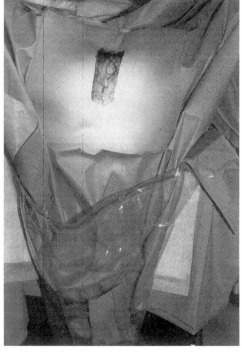

Figure 8 Perineal pouch for collection of fluid run-off

which may then be suctioned into a canister. An alternative would be to attach the outflow directly to a wall suction unit. This allows the surgeon to increase or decrease outflow by manipulation of the outflow valve. The latter method offers the advantage of the media exiting the resectoscope directly into calibrated canisters. It should be noted that even with this setup, a perineal drape and additional suction is placed in an attempt to account for fluid lost from the hysteroscope and around the cervix. The additional factors that affect intrauterine fluid dynamics include loss of fluid transtubally and fluid loss through intravasation (Figure 9). In recent years, we have seen the introduction of several automated devices for more closely tracing fluid inflow and outflow. This has helped in mitigating the inherently difficult task of intraoperatively tracking fluids, given that the commonly used large 3-liter bags of media may not contain precisely 3000 ml. Most new systems use weight-based calibration to assure accuracy of inflow and outflow. Devices such as that seen in Figure 10 are able to demonstrate digitally inflow pressures as well as an ongoing tabulation of fluid deficit. This may more accurately allow the surgeon to set inflow pressures below mean arterial pressure. This type of device may also be helpful to nursing staff, who were previously forced to account for fluids every 10–15 min. In an observational trial, Tomazevic and colleagues evaluated their hysteroscopic experience before and after the introduction of an automated weight-based fluid-deficit system[25]. They noted that in 443 operative hysteroscopic procedures real-time information on intrauterine pressure and fluid deficit aided in improving patient safety.

METHODS FOR EVALUATION OF FLUID LOSS

Besides the extraction of fluid via gravity or suction through the outflow channel and loss from around the instrument, media loss may occur partly through ostial/tubal loss,

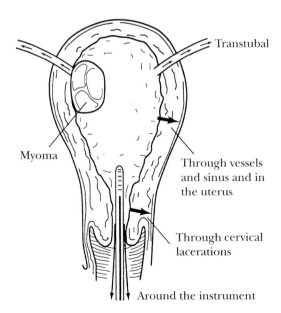

Figure 9 Diagrammatic representation of where media loss occurs

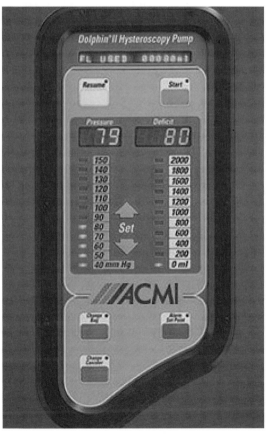

Figure 10 Hysteroscopy pump with ability to demonstrate inflow pressures and to measure fluid deficit. Courtesy of ACMI Corporation, Southborough, MA, USA

and mainly through intravasation. Intrauterine pressures adequate for visualization (75–100 mmHg) will result in little transtubal media passage. Pressures above 100 mmHg are associated with higher levels of transtubal loss. This loss is limited by the closure of the ostium by smooth muscle surrounding the tubal orifice. A similar mechanism is seen during performance of hysterosalpingography, where increased pressure from dye injection causes a contraction of the muscle surrounding the ostium leading to a potential false-positive result of tubal occlusion.

It is not surprising that Baumann and colleagues reported finding glycine in the peritoneal fluid of a patient undergoing transcervical endometrial resection[26]. Although certain rationale exist as to whether tubal occlusion should be performed before or after endometrial ablation, there is no agreement on what effect this has, if any, on the amount of medium intravasation. Magos and colleagues reported a non-statistically significant decrease in fluid loss if tubal occlusion was performed prior to ablation[27], whereas Lomano found no difference in absorption of normal saline in patients undergoing Nd:YAG laser ablation who had previously undergone sterilization[28].

It is likely that transtubal media passage causes increased peritoneal fluid leading to absorption. The clinical significance of this occurrence is mainly that whatever fluid is absorbed by the peritoneum will likely become intravascular and might serve to exacerbate cases of fluid overload. In cases where concurrent laparoscopy is being performed, suction of the fluid may be performed and added to that fluid collected from the hysteroscopic outflow tract.

Most fluid is absorbed via the vascular tree of the uterus. Even at low levels of intrauterine pressure some level of intravasation is difficult to avoid. Although unlikely to be a problem during diagnostic cases, the nature of operative hysteroscopy predisposes to these difficulties. The increased length of time and the dissection of tissue cause endometrial trauma and probably open blood vessels, which under the pressure necessary for adequate visualization allow intravasation. When one considers the amount of vascularity a leiomyoma may have, it is understandable how myoma shaving would create open channels through which media might flow. It does not take a large surface area to have significant fluid loss as demonstrated by the amount of fluid that may be given through a relatively small 20- or 22-gauge intravenous (IV) catheter when the IV bag has a blood pressure cuff surrounding it.

Multiple factors will ultimately impact on the amount of intravasation, but significant variability will still exist between very similar cases. *It is for this reason that fluid monitoring is essential during all operative hysteroscopic cases.* Additional variables that may lead to increased fluid loss include the length of the surgery (which may be less with an experienced surgeon), size of the mass (if a myoma/septum or polyp is present), the size of the endometrial cavity (if endometrial ablation or resection is performed) and the length of the procedure. It is also believed that preoperative treatment with one of the various hormonal agents may improve surgery, in some cases because of the reduction in endometrial or myoma vascularity (see Chapter 5).

Molnar and co-workers retrospectively evaluated 300 patients who underwent endometrial resection to determine the most significant factors predisposing to increased levels of intravasation, in an attempt to devise a scoring system to predict patients at risk from fluid overload[29]. They found that nulliparity, type of preoperative endometrial preparation, increased uterine size, increased cavity length, concurrent hysteroscopic myomectomy and duration of surgery significantly increased the amount of fluid intravasation in patients undergoing endometrial ablation, via resection. In contrast to other reports, tubal patency and the use of an intracervical injection of a vasoconstricting substance had no significant effect on fluid balance.

After evaluation of these multiple factors, their final conclusion was '. . . as it is impossible to predict all cases of fluid overload, it is still imperative that fluid balance is monitored closely in all patients undergoing hysteroscopic surgery'[29].

Garry and colleagues described two different mechanisms by which they believe fluid absorption may occur[30]. Based on studies during Nd:YAG laser ablations, they concluded that when superficial layers of the endometrium are coagulated, fluid absorption is proportional to intrauterine pressure, whereas deep destruction or tissue injury allows larger blood vessels and/or sinus tracts to open, allowing fluid absorption regardless of the level of intrauterine pressure.

Several studies have evaluated fluid loss with controlled pressure systems. In a prospective randomized study, Hasham and co-workers found no fluid absorption when using the Hamou hysteromat (Karl Storz, Endoscopy-America Inc., Culver City, CA, USA) versus 1255 ml per case of absorption in the non-pressure controlled group[31]. (This device is not yet approved for sale in the USA.)

In another interesting study, Vulgaropulos and colleagues evaluated intrauterine pressures and flow rates in an *in vitro* system[32]. They found these parameters were affected by:

(1) Height of the media or pump setting;

(2) Hysteroscope manufacturer;

(3) Amount of cervical dilatation;

(4) Whether the outflow valve was opened or closed.

In an *in vivo* study of 15 patients, they evaluated fluid absorption of 1.5% glycine with 2% ethanol by several methods, including hematocrit, plasma sodium and osmolarity, and blood ethanol levels. Interestingly, they found no significant change in any of these parameters and contrary to other published reports, intrauterine pressure above 200 mmHg did not result in significant fluid absorption. Although previous reports of ethanol use in irrigating fluids have been published in the anesthesiology literature, this was the first application to hysteroscopic surgery[33]. A more recent report evaluated the utility of using 1% ethanol-tagged glycine as a means of evaluating intravasation[34]. The investigators checked serial expired ethanol and venous ethanol levels. Unfortunately,

they concluded that these were insufficient to assess fluid balance and status, and that input/output recording was still necessary.

DISSEMINATION OF ENDOMETRIAL CELLS

For years there has been debate regarding the risk of dissemination of endometrial cancer cells into the peritoneal cavity during dilatation and curettage (D&C) or hysteroscopy. In 1996, Egarter and colleagues reported on a patient with adenocarcinoma who had peritoneal washing immediately prior to hysteroscopy which was negative[35]. A subsequent washing after hysteroscopy was positive. This and other reports led to recent additional investigations to determine actual risk as well as if one type of media would be preferential to another. In an evaluation of 113 consecutive patients with endometrial carcinoma, some of whom had both hysteroscopy and D&C, and some who only had D&C, the authors noted a statistically increased risk of positive peritoneal cytology after fluid hysteroscopy[36]. In a retrospective analysis of CO_2 versus normal saline as media used during hysteroscopy in patients with a subsequent diagnosis of endometrial cancer, Lo and associates concluded that normal saline was associated with an increased rate of positive cytology[37]. Nagele and co-workers performed an interesting prospective randomized cross-over study which evaluated endometrial cell dissemination during hysteroscopy[38]. They performed peritoneal aspirates prior to beginning hysteroscopy, then randomly assigned normal saline or CO_2 as the hysteroscopic media, repeated peritoneal aspirates, then repeated hysteroscopy with the alternate media and again performed peritoneal aspirates. Not surprisingly, aspiration prior to beginning any hysteroscopy had a 7% finding of endometrial cells whereas after hysteroscopy 25% of specimens had endometrial cells. There was no difference between CO_2 or normal saline with each having about a one in four risk of finding endometrial cells.

While these studies suggest that endometrial cells may be disseminated during D&C or hysteroscopy regardless of the media chosen, there remains no substantive clinical data to suggest these results have an impact on subsequent clinical course or outcome.

COMPLICATIONS OF LOW-VISCOSITY MEDIA

The most significant complication of low-viscosity fluids is their ability to cause fluid overload and, in the case of hypotonic fluids, additionally to cause dilution hyponatremia. Decades ago, urologists described a syndrome of dilution hyponatremia later called the post- transurethral resection (TUR) syndrome, because of its association with prostatic resection. This syndrome includes initial bradycardia and hypertension followed by nausea, vomiting, hypertension, seizures, pulmonary edema and cardiac decompensation. Coma and death have now been reported in both the urological and gynecological literature[6].

As previously described, the solutions most commonly used for resectoscopy are hypotonic. An understanding of plasma osmolarity and the impact of sodium levels are critically important. The equation

$$2 \times Na + glucose / 18 + BUN / 28$$

is a close approximation of serum osmolarity. As can be seen from the equation, in the normal physiological state, a significant percentage of the serum osmolarity is accounted for by sodium. During resectoscopic surgery using glycine as a medium, glycine enters the vascular system. It does have an osmolarity (200 mosmol/l), although lower than serum. Because of glycine's short half-life, it is rapidly metabolized, leaving only free water in its place. This helps to explain the clinical scenario of a patient who is stable during the initial postoperative period, becoming symptomatic several hours after the completion of surgery. As the glycine (which has an osmotic effect) is removed from the circulation, the overall osmolarity is decreased (Figure 11). This allows an understanding of why the ideal medium would be isotonic. Isotonicity does not obviate the problem of fluid overload but does decrease the potential of fluid shifts between compartments. This becomes important because of the potential for cerebral edema with hypotonic fluids. The blood–brain barrier allows free movement of water. In situations of plasma hypo-osmolarity and normal brain tissue osmolarity, the flow of water would be into the tissue of higher osmolarity to effect an equilibrium. Unlike other tissues, the brain is almost completely enclosed within the skull. Cerebral edema will cause the brain to press on the cranium, possibly decreasing cerebral blood flow, increasing intracranial pressure, leading to potential tissue hypoxia. Baggish and co-workers reported on two cases of hyponatremia using 3% sorbitol and 1.5% glycine[6]. In one case, the patient's serum sodium was 121 mmol/l, and in the second case it was 102 mmol/l. In both cases, coma, respiratory arrest and death ensued. Postmortem examination revealed cerebral herniation in both cases.

Mannitol has been suggested as a safer fluid because of its higher osmolarity[6]. Although mannitol has no electrolytes and, thus, may also produce hyponatremia, it has a higher endogenous osmotic effect (274 mosmol/l). Evaluation of its metabolism shows it is excreted, essentially unconverted, through the kidneys. This produces an osmotic diuresis, and theoretically, the free water, which would have been left intravascularly, is pulled with the mannitol, allowing a steady-state osmolality and decreasing the potential risks of cerebral edema.

Arieff has suggested that premenopausal women may be at a higher risk from hyponatremia[39]. He believes that the sodium–potassium pump in the brain is altered by the presence or absence of estrogen and cites this as an explanation for the increased morbidity and mortality of hyponatremia in premenopausal women than in men or postmenopausal women. Progesterone has also been suggested as an additional modifier of this system[40]. This

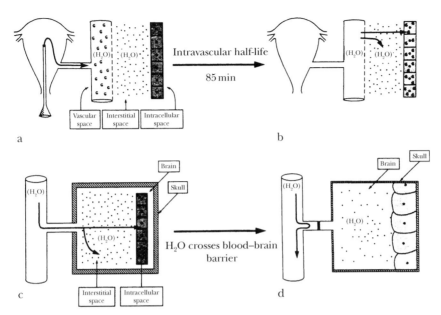

Figure 11 Cerebral edema following absorption of glycine irrigating solution. (a) Intravascular osmolarity is initially maintained by glycine molecules contained in the intravascular space. (b) When glycine moves from the intravascular space into the cell, intravascular osmolarity falls. The concentration of water (H_2O) is greater in the intravascular space than in the interstitial space. As a result, water moves from the vascular space into the interstitial and intracellular space (arrows). (c) Because of the intravascular hypo-osmolar state, water moves across the blood–brain barrier into the interstitial and intracellular space. (d) Cerebral edema develops with compression of the brain against the skull. Water will continue to move into the brain until the hydrostatic pressure of the brain offsets the osmotic force. Reproduced from reference 41 with permission

might have implications as to what pretreatment regimen a patient is placed on.

The relative role of hypo-osmolarity, hyponatremia, or their combination in the level of morbidity remains to be elucidated. Sodium is well known to have many physiological effects, besides being a major constituent of the osmotic pressure. In an animal model, serum osmolarity was held at normal levels while intravascular sodium was markedly decreased[9]. The investigators noted symptoms similar to the TUR syndrome in humans, including lethargy, convulsions and coma.

TREATMENT OF HYPONATREMIA

Early detection and initiation of treatment are important aspects in treating hyponatremia and fluid overload. Table 4 lists the steps in managing cases of acute hyponatremia. If hyponatremia is suspected, surgery should be

immediately stopped. A loop diuretic, such as furosemide (20 mg IV, if there is no renal impairment), should be administered. This initiates rapid diuresis, which aids in decreasing intravascular free water. Although hyponatremia was historically treated by fluid restriction and observation, this is inappropriate for acute surgically induced hyponatremia, which the clinician encounters during or following hysteroscopy. Concomitant with diuretic administration, electrolytes should be sent immediately. Depending on the results, electrolytes should be repeated every few hours until sodium and potassium are normalized. With increasing degrees of volume overload and/or hyponatremia, central monitoring may become important in assessing the complex hemodynamics that may occur. Normal saline may be used for sodium repletion, as hypertonic saline may cause an overshoot of sodium levels with subsequent hypernatremia. Close evaluation of

Table 4 Steps in the treatment of hyponatremia

Stop procedure
Diuretic to reduce hypervolemia
Determine electrolytes status
Central venous monitoring
Normal saline for repletion
Close monitoring of input/output
Steady increases in serum sodium

systemic parameters, including urine output, blood pressure, cardiac status and restriction of input, is necessary.

Serial electrolytes should demonstrate a steady increase and ultimate stabilization of sodium. It is important to note that there is a mortality rate for acute hyponatremia even at levels previously thought to be acceptable. In the report by Baggish and colleagues on media toxicity, one of the deaths occurred in a patient with serum sodium of 121 mmol/l[6].

Treatment should take into account whether the situation is acute (as most surgical cases will be) or chronic (> 48 h). In acute cases, many authors have suggested increases of 1–2 mEq/l per hour for the first 6 h are adequate and may have a significant impact on the level of cerebral edema[41–43]. In cases where hyponatremia is immediately recognized, it is likely that even quicker repletion of sodium is possible.

Cases of chronic hyponatremia appear to have less morbidity and mortality at similar levels. However, it is now well recognized that correcting chronic hyponatremia too rapidly may lead to a clinical entity referred to as central pontine myelinolysis (CPM). A conceptualization of the pathogenesis is presented in Figure 12. As with acute hyponatremia, ineffective repletion of sodium may lead to persistent or worsening symptoms. Chronic hyponatremia, like acute hyponatremia, should be slowly but effectively treated. An increase of 1 mEq/l every 2 h helps to protect against development of CPM. In addition, use of hypertonic saline may predispose the patient to CPM by too quickly correcting serum sodium.

Use of mannitol as a diuretic for acute or chronic hyponatremia remains unclear, since

osmotic diuresis will occur – but at the expense of further exacerbating fluid overload.

COMPLICATIONS OF HIGH-VISCOSITY MEDIA

Because of Hyskon's high molecular weight and extended half-life, fluid problems and treatments associated with intravasation are very different from those associated with low-viscosity fluids. In addition, Hyskon is associated with a number of unique problems. Hyskon is a relatively heterogeneous fluid in which the average molecular weight is 70 kDa; however, it may contain units with both smaller or larger molecular weights. This has metabolic importance, since particles < 50 kDa are renally excreted, whereas larger compounds are metabolized via the reticuloendothelial system. Because of the limited acute metabolism and ability to function as an osmotic particle within the intravascular space, significant increases in intravascular volume may occur, even with limited intravasation. Figure 13 demonstrates the intravascular effect of absorbing 350 ml of Hyskon.

This is the rationale for many authorities recommending that total loss should not exceed 300 ml, and package labelling recommending less than 500 ml total loss.

In contrast to low-viscosity fluids, where intravasation leads to hypo-osmolar plasma, intravasation of Hyskon causes an increase in plasma oncotic pressure, which draws in fluid from the extravascular spaces. In both situations, significant volume overload may occur. The difference lies in the causal mechanism. Multiple reports have demonstrated the ability of Hyskon to induce pulmonary edema through the aforementioned mechanism[44]. What is unclear is at what amount of intravasation do the risks of pulmonary edema become significant? It is likely that age, cardiopulmonary status, renal function and other multiple factors predispose subsets of patients, while most healthy patients would probably tolerate a greater degree of overload. Baggish and co-workers evaluated the relationship between the volume of Hyskon administered and Hyskon

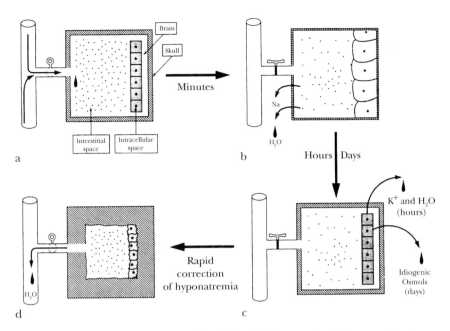

Figure 12 Pathogenesis of central pontine myelinolysis. (a) As a result of intravascular hypo-osmolarity, water moves into the brain. The brain swells and is compressed against the skull. (b) Within minutes, sodium and water are extruded from the extracellular space into the cerebrospinal fluid and, ultimately, into the vasculature. (c) To decrease swelling, the brain cells release potassium and 'idiogenic osmols'. The brain now has decreased the number of osmotically active particles. This response takes up to several days. (d) A rapid increase in plasma osmolarity (as with rapid correction of hyponatremia) leads to movement of water out of the brain and into the vascular space, causing desiccation of the brain. Reproduced from reference 41 with permission

blood levels during hysteroscopy in an attempt to predict a threshold for toxicity[45]. They found a poor correlation between amount of Hyskon used and blood levels at 30 min, and found uptake increased in patients with the greatest myometrial and endometrial damage.

Some authors have suggested a direct effect of dextran on the pulmonary vasculature[46,47]. They believe this toxic effect occurs at the level of the pulmonary capillaries, allowing fluid leakage and subsequent pulmonary edema. While there is evidence for such a cause/effect relationship for several other medications (dextran 40, ritodrine, opiates and salicylates), scientific consensus on this effect for dextran 70 is unclear[48,49].

Treatment for excess intravascular Hyskon, which causes pulmonary edema, is debatable. Use of diuretics, ventilatory support and central venous monitoring are important. Unfortunately, the high-molecular weight of

Hyskon does not allow renal diuresis of the dextran 70 particles. Supportive management until the reticuloendothelial system clears the Hyskon is warranted. Some authors have advocated plasmapheresis for protracted cases with elevated plasma oncotic pressure, such as that produced by excess Hyskon, but little information is available[50]. Such difficult cases are best handled in consultation with nephrologists and intensive-care specialists.

Hyskon has been associated with changes in the coagulation cascade[51]. It has been suggested that such coagulation inhibition may contribute to postoperative bleeding or hemoptysis[52]. While reports of disseminated intravascular coagulation secondary to hysteroscopic use of dextran are rare, reports of changes in clotting factors have been published[53]. Baggish and colleagues found Hyskon decreased fibrinogen with no change in fibrin-split products[45]. A much older report in

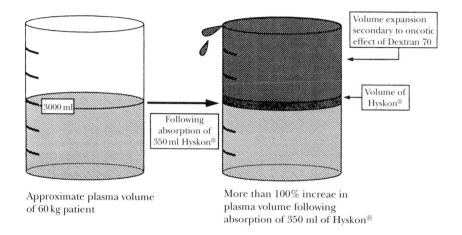

Approximate plasma volume
of 60 kg patient

More than 100% increae in
plasma volume following
absorption of 350 ml of Hyskon®

Figure 13 Plasma volume expansion resulting from the absorption of 350 ml of Hyskon. The volume is increased by 350 ml of Hyskon plus 3000 ml of fluid that is drawn osmotically into the intravascular space. Note that plasma volume is increased by > 100%. Reproduced from reference 41 with permission

the European literature demonstrated that Hyskon caused a reduction in platelet adhesiveness and aggregation[54].

Hyskon has also been associated with anaphylactic or allergic reactions[55]. Even though Hyskon has little immunogenicity, there may be cross-reactivity to the antigen in other dextran-containing substances, such as turnips, beets, or, possibly, bacterial antigens. These idiosyncratic reactions may range from minor allergic manifestations, such as skin changes, to cardiac collapse[23,55]. While often discussed, it is felt that the true incidence of this complication is small[56]. Treatment is similar to that of an allergic reaction.

Because Hyskon is significantly hypertonic, the clinician must carefully monitor the amount of fluid used to decrease the possibility of intravascular absorption. Most authors have recommended total fluid to be used to be between 350 and 500 ml. However, as Figure 13 demonstrated, even a small amount of Hyskon loss leads to significant fluid shifts and volume expansion within the intravascular space. In addition, anaphylactic reactions are unrelated to amount of use, and there seems no effective way to predict who may react to these agents. Interestingly, several patients who exhibited allergic responses were later tested for allergy to

dextran and found to be negative[55,56]. Like low-viscosity fluids, Hyskon may be successfully utilized in a number of clinical scenarios to effectively distend the uterus. Familiarity with the potential problems will allow the astute clinician to avert problems and manage them in an appropriate and timely fashion when they occur.

CLINICAL PEARLS

(1) No perfect medium exists; clinicians must be familiar with a number of media, their risks and benefits.

(2) Carbon dioxide should only be instilled via a dedicated hysteroscopic insulator.

(3) Normal saline and lactated Ringer's are not useful media when using unipolar current, such as with the resectoscope.

(4) Use of sterile water as a medium is inappropriate as it causes hemolysis if intravasation occurs.

(5) Glycine and sorbitol are commonly used distention media when electrosurgery is employed – both are hypotonic and may induce hyponatremia if excess intravasation occurs.

(6) ALWAYS monitor input and output every 10–15 min throughout cases.

(7) NEVER assume that fluid on the floor makes up the deficit.

(8) ALWAYS check electrolytes if overload is suspected.

(9) Hyskon is very hypertonic, and intravasation of small amounts may cause significant intravascular expansion.

(10) Excess intrauterine pressure increases fluid intravasation risk without benefiting distention and visualization.

(11) It is currently difficult to monitor intrauterine pressure, and thus, the least pressure to distend the cavity and facilitate surgery should be used.

(12) Multiple factors may affect the risk of intravasation, including surgeon experience, uterine size, length of the procedure and endometrial preparation.

(13) Chronic hyponatremia should be corrected slowly, but continuously, to decrease the risk of central pontine myelinolysis.

(14) The best method of treatment for hyponatremia is avoidance through close attention to fluid status. Early recognition and prompt treatment with a diuretic are critical.

References

1. Rubin IC. Uterine endoscopy, endometroscopy with the aid of uterine insufflation. *Am J Obstet Gynecol* 1925;10:313

2. Rubin IC. *Uterotubal Insufflation*. St. Louis: CV Mosby, 1947

3. Baggish MS, Daniel JF. Death caused by air embolism associated with neodymium:yttrium aluminum-garnet laser surgery and artificial sapphire tips. *Am J Obstet Gynecol* 1989;161: 877–88

4. Madsen PO, Madsen RE. Clinical and experimental evaluation of different irrigating fluids for transurethral surgery. *Invest Urol* 1965;3: 122–9

5. Dequesne J. Hysteroscopic treatment of uterine bleeding with the Nd–YAG laser. *Lasers Med Sci* 1987;2:73–6

6. Baggish MS, Brill AI, Rosensweig B, *et al.* Fatal acute glycine and sorbitol toxicity during operative hysteroscopy. *J Gynecol Surg* 1993;9: 137–43

7. Weiner J, Gregory L. Absorption of irrigating fluid during transcervical resection of endometrium. *Br Med J* 1990;300:748–9

8. Roesch RP, Stoelting RK, Lingeman JE, *et al.* Ammonia toxicity resulting from glycine absorption during transurethral resection of the prostate. *Anesthesiology* 1983;58:577–9

9. Berstein GT, Loughlin KR, Gittes RE. The physiologic basis for the TURP syndrome. *J Surg Res* 1989;46:135–41

10. Mizutam AR, Parker J, Katz J, Schmidt J. Visual disturbances, serum glycine levels, and transurethral resection of the prostate. *J Urol* 1990; 144:697–9

11. Duffy S, Sharp F, Reid P. Irrigation solutions and blood: the electrical events during electrosurgery. *Gynecol Endocrinol* 1992;1:11–14

12. Edstrom K, Fernstrom I. The diagnostic possibilities of a modified hysteroscopic technique. *Acta Obstet Gynecol Scand* 1970;49:327–30

13. Amin HK, Neuwirth RS. Operative hysteroscopy utilizing dextran as a distending medium. *Clin Obstet Gynecol* 1983;26:277–84

14. Loffer ED. Preliminary experience with the VersaPoint bipolar resectoscope using a vaporizing electrode in a saline distending medium. *J Am Assoc Gynecol Laparosc* 2000;7:498–502

15. Vilos GA. Intrauterine surgery using a new coaxial bipolar electrode in normal saline solution (Versapoint): a pilot study. *Fertil Steril* 1999;72:740–3

16. Kung RC, Vilos GA, Thomas B, *et al.* A new bipolar system for performing operative hysteroscopy in normal saline. *J Am Assoc Gynecol Laparosc* 1999;6:331–6

17. Marwah V, Bhandari SK. Diagnostic and interventional microhysteroscopy with use of the coaxial bipolar electrode system. *Fertil Steril* 2003;79:413–17

18. Bettocchi S, Ceci O, DiVenere R, *et al.* Advanced operative office hysteroscopy without anaesthesia: analysis of 501 cases treated with a 5 Fr. bipolar electrode. *Hum Reprod* 2002;17: 2435–8

19. Munro MG, Weisberg M, Rubinstein E. Gas and air embolization during hysteroscopic electrosurgical vaporization: comparison of gas generation using bipolar and monopolar electrodes in an experimental model. *J Am Assoc Gynecol Laparosc* 2001;8:488–94

20. Pellicano M, Guida M, Zullo F, *et al.* Carbon dioxide versus normal saline as a uterine distension medium for diagnostic vaginoscopic hysteroscopy in infertile patients: a prospective, randomized, multicenter study. *Fertil Steril* 2003;79:418–21

21. Nagele F, Bournas N, O'Connor H, *et al.* Comparison of carbon dioxide and normal saline for uterine distension in outpatient hysteroscopy. *Fertil Steril* 1996;65:305–9

22. Perez-Medina T, Bajo JM, Martinez-Cortes L, *et al.* Six thousand office diagnostic-operative hysteroscopies. *Int J Gynecol Obstet* 2000;71:33–8

23. Loffer FD. Complications from uterine distention during hysteroscopy. In Corfman KS, Diamond MP, DeCherney A, eds. *Complications in Laparoscopy and Hysteroscopy*. Boston: Blackwell Scientific Publications, 1993:177–86

24. Baker VL, Adamson GD. Minimum intrauterine pressure required for uterine distention. *J Am Assoc Gynecol Laparosc* 1998;5:51–3

25. Tomazevic T, Savnik L, Dintinjana M, *et al.* Safe and effective fluid management by automated gravitation during hysteroscopy. *J Soc Laparosc Surg* 1998;2:51–5

26. Baumann R, Magos AC, Kayo JOS, Turnbull AC. Absorption of glycine irrigating fluid during transcervical resection of the endometrium. *Br Med J* 1990;300:304–5

27. Magos AL, Baumann R, Turnbull AC. Safety of transcervical endometrial resection. *Lancet* 1990; 355:44

28. Lomano JM. Photocoagulation of the endometrium with the Nd-YAG laser for the treatment of menorrhagia. *J Reprod Med* 1986;31: 148–50

29. Molnar BG, Broadbent JAM, Magos AL. Fluid overload risk score for endometrial resection. *Gynecol Endocrinol* 1992;1:133–8

30. Garry R, Mooney P, Hasham F, Kokri M. A uterine distention system to prevent fluid absorption during Nd-YAG laser endometrial ablation. *Gynecol Endocrinol* 1992;1:23–7

31. Hasham F, Garry R, Kokri MS, Mooney P. Fluid absorption during laser ablation of the endometrium in the treatment of menorrhagia. *Br J Anaesth* 1992;68:151–4

32. Vulgaropulos SP, Haley LC, Hulka JF. Intrauterine pressure and fluid absorption during continuous flow hysteroscopy. *Am J Obstet Gynecol* 1992;167:386–91

33. Hahn RG. Ethanol monitoring of irrigating fluid absorption in transurethral prostatic surgery. *Anesthesiology* 1988;68:867–73

34. Molnar BG, Magos AL, Kay J. Monitoring fluid absorption using 1% ethanol-tagged glycine during operative hysteroscopy. *J Am Assoc Gynecol Laparosc* 1997;4:357–62

35. Egarter C, Krestan C, Kurz C. Abdominal dissemination of malignant cells with hysteroscopy. *Gynecol Oncol* 1996;63:143–4

36. Obermair A, Geramou M, Gucer F, *et al.* Does hysteroscopy facilitate tumor cell dissemination? Incidence of peritoneal cytology from patients with early stage endometrial carcinoma following dilation and curettage (D&C) versus hysteroscopy and D&C. *Cancer* 2000;88:139–43

37. Lo KW, Cheung TH, Yim SF, *et al.* Hysteroscopic dissemination of endometrial carcinoma using carbon dioxide and normal saline: a retrospective study. *Gynecol Oncol* 2002;84:394–8

38. Nagele F, Wieser F, Deery A, *et al.* Endometrial cell dissemination at diagnostic hysteroscopy: a prospective randomized crossover comparison of normal saline and carbon dioxide uterine distension. *Hum Reprod* 1999;14:2739–42

39. Arieff AI. Hyponatremia, convulsions, respiratory arrest, and permanent brain damage after elective surgery in healthy women. *N Engl J Med* 1986;314:1529–35

40. Berl T. Treating hyponatremia: what is the controversy about? *Ann Intern Med* 1990;113:417–19

41. Witz CA, Silverberg KM, Burns WN, *et al.* Complications associated with the absorption of hysteroscopic fluid media. *Fertil Steril* 1993; 60:745–56

42. Sterns RH. The management of symptomatic hyponatremia. *Semin Nephrol* 1990;10:503–14

43. Sterns RH. The treatment of hyponatremia: first, do no harm. *Am J Med* 1990;88:557–60

44. Schinagl EF. Hyskon (32% dextran 70) hysteroscopic surgery and pulmonary edema. *Anesth Anal* 1990;70:223–4

45. Baggish MS, Davaulur C, Rodriguez F, Comporesi E. Vascular uptake of Hyskon (dextran 70) during operative and diagnostic hysteroscopy. *J Gynecol Surg* 1992;8:211–17

46. Zbella EA, Moise J, Carson SA. Noncardiogenic pulmonary edema secondary to intrauterine instillation of 32% dextran 70. *Fertil Steril* 1985;43:479–80

47. Leake J, Murphy AA, Zacur H. Noncardiogenic pulmonary edema: a complication of operative hysteroscopy. *Fertil Steril* 1987;48:497–9

48. Kaplan AI, Sabin S. Dextran 40: another cause of drug-induced noncardiogenic pulmonary edema. *Chest* 1975;68:376–7
49. Benedetti TJ. Maternal complications of parenteral β-sympathomimetic therapy for premature labor. *Am J Obstet Gynecol* 1983;145: 1–6
50. Moran M, Kapsner C. Acute renal failure associated with elevated plasma oncotic pressure. *N Engl J Med* 1987;317:150–3
51. Ljungstrom KG. Safety of 32% dextran for hysteroscopy. *Am J Obstet Gynecol* 1990;163: 2029–30
52. Siegler AM, Valle RF, Lindemann HJ, Mencaglia L. In *Therapeutic Hysteroscopy Indications and Techniques*. St. Louis: CV Mosby, 1990:51

53. Jedekin R, Kessler I, Olsfanger D. Disseminated intravascular coagulopathy and adult respiratory distress syndrome: life-threatening complications of hysteroscopy. *Am J Obstet Gynecol* 1990; 162:44–5
54. Cronberg S, Robertson B, Nilsson IM, Nilehn JE. Suppressive effect of dextran on platelet adhesiveness. *Thromb Diath Haemorrh* 1966;16: 384–92
55. Trimbos-Kemper TCM, Veering BT. Anaphylactic shock from intracavitary 32% dextran 70 during hysteroscopy. *Fertil Steril* 1989;51:1053–4
56. Ahmed N, Falcone T, Tulandi T, Houle G. Anaphylactic reaction because of intrauterine 32% dextran 70 instillation. *Fertil Steril* 1991; 55:1014–16

7

Uterine septa

R. F. Valle

A septate uterus distorts the symmetry of the uterine cavity and may interfere with normal reproduction. When surgical treatment is required, it can be provided transcervically via the hysteroscope utilizing a variety of methods. These include mechanical hysteroscopic scissors, thermal energies via the resectoscope and laser energy via fiberoptic lasers.

EMBRYOLOGY AND ANATOMY

The Fallopian tubes and the uterus are of Müllerian origin; in early embryological development, the paramesonephric ducts fuse caudally and distally to form the upper vagina and uterus, while the remaining upper segments result in the Fallopian tubes. This process begins at 4–6 weeks of embryological life and usually is completed at 12–14 weeks of gestational age. In the absence of Müllerian inhibiting factor (MIF) produced by the testes, the paramesonephric or Müllerian ducts will progress to normal development. The uterine septum usually completes its reabsorption by 19–20 weeks of embryological life. Failure to reabsorb will result in a septate uterus with partial or complete septation[1].

The anatomy resulting from arrest at fusion, canalization, or reabsorption will depend on the degree and stage at which the arrest occurs. Because there is no failure of fusion with the septate uterus, the uterine body is uniform externally, differentiating this anomaly from the bicornuate uterus, in which there is lack of fusion and an external division remains.

The septation of the uterine body encompasses various lengths and widths of the septum. While some septa are thin, others are broad and produce thinner and smaller uterine cavities. Some only partially divide the uterine cavity and others extend the entire length of the uterine corpus and, occasionally, the entire length of the uterine cervix. In 20–25% of these patients, concomitant septation of the vagina occurs; occasionally, bicornuate uteri have an additional septation of the uterus[2] (Figure 1).

INDICATIONS FOR TREATMENT

The majority of women with uterine septa reproduce successfully; only 20–25% suffer pregnancy wastage – usually late first-trimester or early second-trimester miscarriages initiated by minilabors and bleeding.

The relationship between the septate uterus and infertility remains controversial; the consensus is that this type of uterine anomaly does not cause infertility. Nonetheless, as the therapeutic approach to this anomaly has evolved, patients with primary infertility requiring assisted reproductive technologies or difficult treatments for infertility have been considered candidates for treatment of the uterine septation.

Since the presence of a uterine septum may not be the basis of a reproductive problem, preoperative evaluation is important. Hysterosalpingography is the most accurate and effective method of diagnosing a septate uterus, particularly division of the uterine cavity.

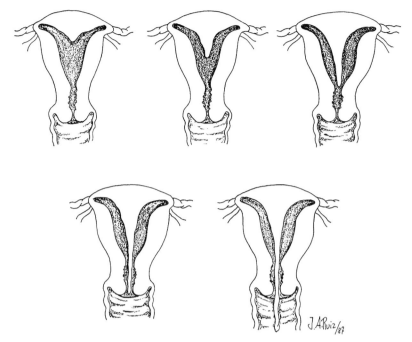

Figure 1 Diagrammatic representation of uterine septa ranging from partial to complete

Nonetheless, it is important to evaluate other factors that may cause pregnancy wastage before deciding on surgical treatment of the uterine septum. Karyotyping should be performed in both husband and wife, and a normal maturation of the endometrium should be evaluated with a late luteal phase endometrial biopsy and midluteal phase serum progesterone. Endocrine conditions, such as hypothyroidism, should be evaluated with a thyroid stimulating hormone (TSH) assay.

Autoimmune and alloimmune conditions must be ruled out with a lupus anticoagulant factor study and partial thromboplastin time (PTT), as well as anticardiolipin antibodies (ACA) and antinuclear antibodies (ANA). Chronic endometritis is best ruled out with endometrial biopsy.

Finally, because of the close embryological relationship of Müllerian structures with the mesonephric ducts, when these anomalies occur, renal anomalies should be ruled out. Although these urinary tract anomalies are not as marked and frequent with the septate uterus,

duplication of calyceal systems, renal ptosis and other such anomalies have been described. Therefore, it is valuable to evaluate these patients by a screening intravenous pyelogram (IVP)[3,4].

METHODS OF TREATMENT

In the past, invasive surgical treatments requiring laparotomy and hysterotomy were performed only in habitual aborters – women experiencing more than three spontaneous miscarriages in the early or mid-second trimester of pregnancy. With new, less-invasive approaches, such as hysteroscopic treatment, the indications have been liberalized to focus attention on each individual patient and her unique reproductive failure[5].

Until the introduction of the hysteroscopic approach, surgical treatment of the symptomatic uterine septum was by abdominal metroplasty of the Jones or Tompkins type.

The Jones abdominal metroplasty involves the transfundal excision of the septum by removing a cuneiform portion of the fundal myometrium with subsequent surgical repair[6]. This technique has resulted in over 80% viable pregnancies and has been used as the standard for success of procedures to correct the symptomatic septate uterus. Disadvantages with this procedure are the need for laparotomy, hysterotomy and the possibility of postoperative adhesions, particularly at the tubal ovarian regions, sometimes resulting in secondary infertility. Once the patient has a hysterotomy, the waiting period before attempting pregnancy is prolonged (3–6 months). Should a pregnancy occur and be carried to term, a Cesarean section is mandatory.

The Tompkins procedure involves bisection of the uterus in the anteroposterior plane and transverse division of the uterine septum without excision of myometrial tissue[7]. This technique bleeds less than the Jones procedure and results in a more uniform uterine cavity that is not reduced in size. For this reason, most practitioners prefer the Tompkins approach to treat the septate uterus. Nonetheless, hysterotomy carries the disadvantage of the need for a 3- to 6-month waiting period until pregnancy is permitted. A Cesarean section is required when the pregnancy is carried to term to prevent possible uterine dehiscence.

HYSTEROSCOPIC METROPLASTY

Hysteroscopic treatment provides a less-invasive approach to divide the uterine septum. In a hysteroscopic approach, as with the Tompkins type of abdominal metroplasty, the septum is divided under direct vision, the avascular consistency of this embryological remnant inhibiting significant bleeding. Resection of the septum is not necessary as the septal remnants are pulled into the uterine musculature. The hysteroscopic approach permits this condition to be treated as an ambulatory procedure with minimal discomfort to the patient as well as minimal morbidity[8–12]. Because the uterine wall is not invaded, a Cesarean section is required only for obstetric indications. The healing process with re-epithelialization of the uterine

cavity takes only 4–5 weeks, so patients are allowed to conceive sooner than with abdominal metroplasty. Hospitalization is not required, so expenses are markedly reduced.

There are three different approaches to the hysteroscopic metroplasty (Figure 2): mechanical division with hysteroscopic scissors, resectoscopic division with electrosurgery, and fiberoptic laser division of the uterine septum.

Hysteroscopic metroplasty with scissors

Hysteroscopic metroplasty with scissors is the most commonly used method. An operative hysteroscope with a 7.0 Fr operative channel is required. A continuous-flow system to measure fluids infused and recovered is ideal to monitor non-recovered fluid and prevent excessive intravasation. Hysteroscopic scissors can be flexible, semirigid or rigid. Flexible scissors are difficult to manipulate. Semirigid scissors are most commonly used as they permit a targeted division of the tissue, they can be selectively directed to the area in need of dissection, and they can be retrieved at will when a better panoramic view is required. The semirigid scissors can be directed easily without much force or manipulation through the operating channel of the hysteroscope, facilitating hysteroscopic surgery, but they must be sharpened and tightened frequently. Scissors of the hook type are most helpful to divide the uterine septum, particularly when reaching the broad fundal area where small superficial cuts must be made on the remaining septum to sculpture this fundal area and avoid deep penetration (Figures 3–5).

Rigid scissors, often called optical scissors and fixed to the end of the hysteroscope, can also be used to divide fibrotic and broad septa. When using the fixed instrument, it is important to have a perfect panoramic view while performing the division. The scissors should be introduced with utmost care to avoid uterine damage as their sharp tips can easily perforate the uterus if force is exerted against the uterine wall.

With the use of mechanical tools in operative hysteroscopy, the best medium to distend the uterine cavity is one that contains electrolytes,

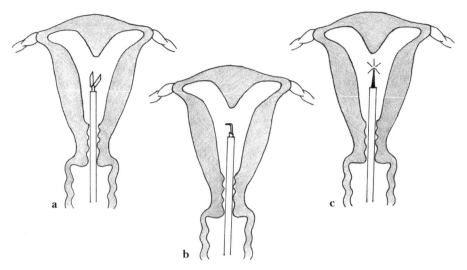

Figure 2   Hysteroscopic metroplasty: (a) scissors; (b) resectoscope; (c) fiberoptic laser

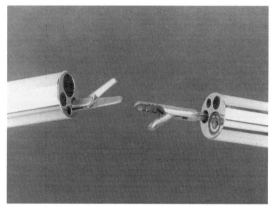

Figure 3   Weck-Baggish hysteroscope with double operating channels (scissors on left, grasping forceps on right)

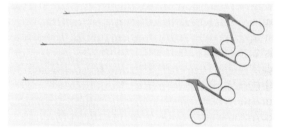

Figure 4   Semirigid hysteroscopic intruments

particularly sodium (Na), permitting more volume to be intravasated during a procedure without the development of hyponatremia. Normal saline, 5% dextrose in half normal saline (D_5 0.45% NaCl) or Ringer's lactate, a balanced solution, can be safely used with good visualization properties.

The technique of uterine septal division with hysteroscopic scissors involves dividing the septum exactly at the midline, where tissue is more fibrotic and avascular. The novice approaching this operation tends to drift to the posterior uterine wall in an anteverted uterus or the anterior wall in a retroverted uterus. When this occurs, vessels from myometrial tissue may reach the septum, causing unnecessary bleeding. The division is performed systematically from side to side, cutting small portions of the septum with each bite. Once the uterotubal cones are visualized, the cuts become more shallow and the small vessels crossing the septum from the myometrium should be closely observed to avoid penetrating myometrial tissue. With the laparoscope in place and the light dimmed, an assistant observes the translucency of the hysteroscopic light through the uterine wall, warning the hysteroscopist of any increase in translucency as the division progresses in this fundal area. Once the septal division is completed, and before the

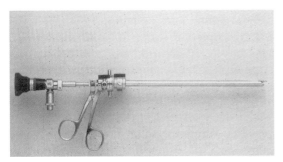

Figure 5 Operating hysteroscope (Olympus) with rigid fixed scissors in place

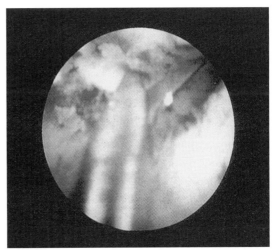

Figure 6 Hysteroscopic division of partial uterine septum

instruments are removed, the uterine fundal area is observed hysteroscopically while decreasing the intrauterine pressure. This is done to observe significant bleeding. In the presence of arterial bleeding, selective coagulation is performed (Figure 6).

There are several advantages to dividing the uterine septum with scissors (Table 1). This simple technique can be performed quickly and is applicable to practically all septa. The scissors can easily be guided into the recessed areas of the septum. Because no electricity is used, the medium to distend the uterine cavity may contain electrolytes. This gives a safety margin for utilization of fluids since more volume may be used as compared with fluids devoid of electrolytes. Finally, no additional expense of energy is required.

There are a few disadvantages to using this technique. Small scissors can become easily dulled and loose and may not cut precisely, so they should be exchanged periodically and repaired. Also, if division of the septum is not maintained in the midline, bleeding may occur. Sharp scissors may cause perforation if not controlled in the uterine fundal and cornual regions. Finally, not all hysteroscopes have perfect continuous flow; therefore, a washing effect cannot be provided unless a double-channel hysteroscope is available.

Resectoscopic division of the uterine septum

Resectoscopic division of the uterine septum provides hemostasis if a true midline incision is

Table 1 Hysteroscopic division of uterine septa with scissors

Advantages
Simple
Quick
Applicable to all septa
Media with electrolytes can be used
No energy sources required

Disadvantages
Scissors get dull
Bleeding if not in midline
Possible perforation
No washing effect unless double-channel
   hysteroscope used

not maintained but may involve more lateral tissue destruction. A gynecological resectoscope, 8–9 mm outer diameter, with a narrow and thin electrode (cutting loop, preferably pointed forward, knife electrode, or wire electrode), can be used to divide the septum by contact electrosurgery. Knives and electrodes have been modified for this purpose and are available from the various manufacturing companies. Whether they are thinner or thicker depends upon the thickness of the tissue to be divided. The resectoscope allows a perfect continuous-flow system that permits exact measurement of the volume of fluid infused and recovered, and provides continuous washing of the uterine cavity and a clear view, removing bubbles and debris during the procedure (Figures 7–10).

Because electricity is used with the resectoscope, only fluids devoid of electrolytes can be utilized (see Chapter 6). A specific amount of non-recovered fluid must be maintained during the procedure because excessive fluid intravasation can occur, causing fluid overload that is worsened by the lack of electrolytes and results in hyponatremia.

The uterine septum is divided, beginning at its apex or nadir, by short and brief contacts of the loop or knife with the septum. This is the only time the resectoscope is used cutting forward rather than with the shaving motion toward the operator commonly used in polyp, myoma or endometrial resection. Extra care should be used in determining the exact depth of penetration and direction of the electrode. Laparoscopic or sonographic monitoring is mandatory. It is important to observe the symmetry of both uterotubal cones and, with laparoscopy, the transillumination the resectoscope's light produces through the uterine wall. The resectoscopic electrode will coagulate any vessel encountered, so on reaching the fundal area, it is of utmost importance to avoid resection into the myometrial tissue. The contact of the electrode should become even more superficial and the resectoscopic transillumination more clearly observed by the assistant (Figures 11–13).

While performing the division of the uterine septum utilizing electrosurgery, it is important to observe periodically, from a distance, the uterine cavity symmetry at the level of the internal os. During the division of the septum, this symmetry may not be evident while working close to the tissue.

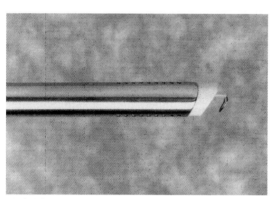

Figure 7 Distal end of resectoscope (Storz) with resecting loop in place

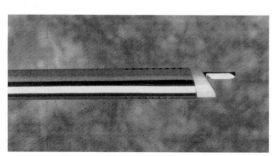

Figure 8 Distal end of resectoscope (Storz) with knife electrode

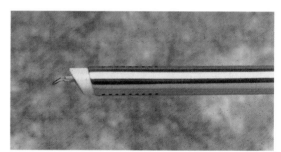

Figure 9 Distal end of resectoscope (Storz) with forward-cutting loop

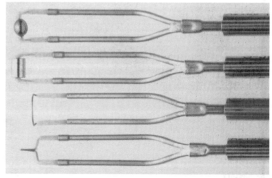

Figure 10 Electrodes for use with resectoscope. Top to bottom: rollerball, rollerbar, resecting loop, cutting knife (Olympus)

With resectoscopic division of the uterine septum, bleeding is decreased; owing to the coagulating effect of the electrical energy, the cuts are easy and the uterine cavity is washed by the continuous flow of distending fluid through the resectoscope[13,14]. Visualization is excellent and manipulation is easy.

Disadvantages are that monopolar electrical current is necessary and peripheral coagulation of adjacent normal endometrium, a reservoir for future re-epithelialization of the area, may occur. Furthermore, at the juxtaposed myometrium, the landmarks are lost because the coagulating power of the electrical energy may not allow for observation of the small arterial bleeders usually observed with mechanical division.

The fluids used for these procedures cannot contain electrolytes in order to permit electrosurgery. Therefore, care must be taken to avoid hyponatremia if excessive intravasation occurs. Occasionally, a broad septum may make manipulation of the resectoscope difficult and these septa may be difficult to divide with the resectoscope (Table 2).

Hysteroscopic metroplasty with fiberoptic lasers

Hysteroscopic metroplasty with fiberoptic lasers is similar in many ways to resectoscopic methods. The septum can be divided with fiber-

optic lasers, particularly the Nd:YAG with an extruded or sculptured fiber of the sharp type to permit cutting. The Argon or KTP-532 can also

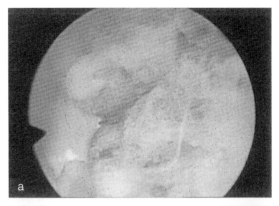
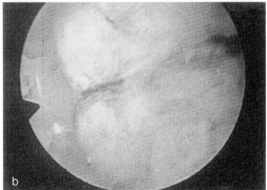

Figure 12 Resectoscopic division of uterine septum with electric knife: (a) initial division; (b) deeper cutting. See also Color Plates II and III, respectively

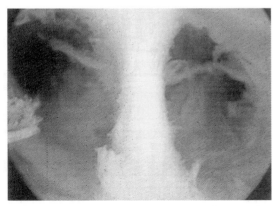

Figure 11 Hysteroscopic view of complete uterine septum. See also Color Plate I

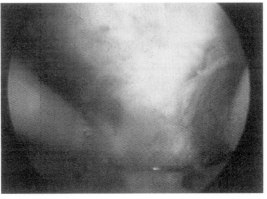

Figure 13 Resectoscopic division of uterine septum with 180° loop. See also Color Plate IV

be used in this manner, although the lower power produced by these lasers makes cutting more tedious. Extruded fibers are usually used in the uterus. Coaxial fibers with sapphire tips need to be cooled continuously, either by fluids or gases. Fluid coolant may be used, but gases should never be used in the uterus to cool the sapphire tips because of the high flow required of about 1 l/min (Figures 14 and 15). Because lasers are not conductive, electrolyte-containing fluids should be used to distend the uterine cavity. Normal saline, 5% dextrose in normal saline and Ringer's lactate are most useful to distend the uterine cavity and obtain clear visualization. It is important to have some outflow with these hysteroscopic techniques to remove the debris and bubbles produced with the activated laser; therefore, a continuous-flow hysteroscope or one with inflow and outflow channels is most advantageous.

Division of the uterine septum should begin at the nadir of the septum in the midline, dividing the septum from side to side. Care must be taken to move the fiber continuously to prevent boring into one hole. Because division of the septum with fiberoptic lasers may be somewhat tedious, the division should be systematic from side to side. The same precautions should be used as with division of the septum with electrocoagulation. Avoid invading the juxtaposed fundal myometrium as the

coagulating power of the laser will also seal small arterial vessels at the fundal uterine wall.

There are advantages to the hysteroscopic division with fiberoptic lasers. Bleeding is avoided because of the coagulating power of the laser. This energy source cuts well and is easy to manipulate, perhaps even more easily manipulated than the resectoscope. Since there is a lack of conductivity, fluids with electrolytes can be used.

However, there are disadvantages. The laser is an expensive energy source and needs special protective glasses. Back-scattering of these fiberoptic lasers can damage the retina. The possibility of lateral scattering makes lasers potentially damaging to normal endometrium

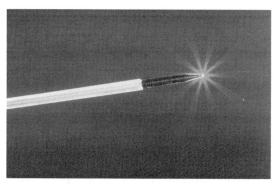

Figure 14 Quartz-sculpted conical fiber for contact precise cutting and coagulating (tip size, 300 μm) (Laser Sonics)

Table 2 Hysteroscopic division of uterine septa with resectoscope

Advantages
No bleeding
Cuts easily
Washing of uterine cavity
Excellent visibility
Easy manipulation

Disadvantages
Electrosurgery required (monopolar)
Possible lateral coagulation
Landmarks of myometrium lost
Fluids without electrolytes must be used
Difficult to divide septa with small uterine cavities

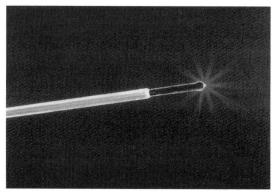

Figure 15 Quartz-sculpted ball-shaped tip fiber for enhanced coagulation (tip size, 1200 μm) (Laser Sonics)

peripheral to septum. Damage of this peripheral endometrium may slow epithelialization of the newly denuded area[15]. Finally, lasers require special maintenance and assistants, including a laser safety officer for operating the unit and appropriate eye protection for the assisting personnel.

Because the procedure may be tedious, excessive amounts of fluids may be required[16]. Should the hysteroscope lack continuous-flow system or a double channel, to collect the returning fluid after cleansing the cavity from bubbles and debris, excessive fluid may be intravasated. In the absence of a perfect monitoring system for the inflow and outflow, the intravasated fluid may not be adequately measured, thereby endangering the patient with pulmonary edema secondary to fluid overload, despite the use of fluids with electrolytes. Therefore, it is important to monitor the fluid infused and maintain the intrauterine pressure so as not to exceed the mean arterial pressure of about 100 mmHg[17] (Table 3).

INTRAOPERATIVE AND POSTOPERATIVE MANAGEMENT

Prophylactic antibiotics are commonly used to prevent infection in the uterine cavity, and specifically in the Fallopian tubes, when intrauterine manipulation is required. Intravenous cephalosporins can be used intraoperatively and continued for 3–4 days postoperatively in an oral form. Kefzol® 1 mg intravenously piggyback is used 30 min prior to surgery, followed by Keflex® 500 mg orally four times a day for 3 or 4 days following the procedure. While the use of high doses of conjugated estrogens, such as Premarin®, is controversial, this medication may allow better and faster re-epithelialization of the denuded area left by division of the septum. High doses, such as Premarin 2.5 mg orally twice daily for 30 days, can be used and terminal progesterone added in the form of Provera® 10 mg each day in the last 10 days of this artificial cycle. Once the patient completes withdrawal bleeding from hormonal therapy, a hysterosalpingogram can be performed to assess the symmetry of the uterine cavity.

Table 3 Hysteroscopic division of uterine septa with fiberoptic lasers

Advantages
No bleeding
Cut well
Easy manipulation
Fluids with electrolytes can be used

Disadvantages
Expensive
Special protective glasses needed
Possible lateral scattering
Require special maintenance and assistance (laser safety officer)

The woman may attempt pregnancy when a satisfactory result is obtained. Because of the axis by which the uterine cavity is observed, hysterosalpingography becomes an excellent method to assess the surgical results. Hysteroscopy, which looks for symmetry from the cervical axis, may provide an alternative appraisal of the uterine fundus. Either method can be utilized as long as the practitioner is aware of the drawbacks. It is not unusual to see a small central fundal residual septal projection on hysterosalpingography following hysteroscopic division of the uterine septum. Nonetheless, when a small residual septum < 1 cm in length is observed, no additional therapy is performed, as this residual septum has no clinical significance.

RESULTS

Reproductive outcome following hysteroscopic treatment of the symptomatic septate uterus has not only equalled but has surpassed the results obtained with traditional abdominal metroplasties, with over 85% viable pregnancies[12]. Furthermore, the patient is spared a laparotomy and hysterotomy, eliminating the potential for pelvic adhesions as well as the associated pain, disability and expense. Patients treated hysteroscopically need wait only one spontaneous menses before attempting conception and do not require a mandatory Cesarean section[18–21].

While more experience with hysteroscopic division of the uterine septum utilizing hysteroscopic scissors has been accumulated, the results obtained utilizing fiberoptic lasers, such as Argon, KTP-532 and the Nd:YAG, seem to equal the reproductive outcome obtained with hysteroscopic scissors[22-24]. The original studies reporting on division of the uterine septum utilizing the resectoscope with a cutting loop eliminated 30% of the patients because of inability to divide all septa, particularly broad ones[13]. This restricted treatment may have been associated with the type of electrode used, particularly the 90° resecting loop. The new electrodes are thinner and better designed to reach these areas, and the feasibility rate seems to equal that obtained with hysteroscopic scissors and fiberoptic lasers. Although the choice of instrument depends in part on the familiarity and experience of the operator with various modalities, historically, the use of hysteroscopic scissors for division of the uterine septum has been favored by the majority of physicians performing this type of operation[25,26] (Tables 4 and 5)

Vaporizing electrodes that can be activated in saline solutions are being used as well to divide uterine septa. However, similar concerns arise as with the use of electrosurgery with thick electrodes. Scattering may damage peripheral endometrium; therefore, when used, only those of a sharp conical tip should be selected.

CONCURRENT PROCEDURES

The laparoscope is an excellent adjunct in monitoring the surgical treatment of the symptomatic septate uterus. It allows visualization of the external uterine pathology (ruling out a bicornuate uterus), and myometrial thickness (by transillumination), as well as revealing tubal–peritoneal pathology and monitoring the division of the uterine septum in order to decrease the risk of uterine perforation.

Table 4 Comparison of methods of hysteroscopic division of uterine septa

Feature	Scissors	Resectoscope	Fiberoptic lasers
Simplicity	++	+	+
Speed	+++	++	+
Hemostasis	+	+++	+++
Applicable to all septa	++	+	++
Evaluation of juxta-posed myometrium	+++	+	+
Expense	+	++	+++
Possible uterine perforation	+	++	++
Required skill	+++	+++	+++
Fluid overload	+	++	++

Sonography has also been used for this purpose, but maintaining the transducer on the same plane with the hysteroscope is cumbersome. Maintaining appropriate uterine planes where the uterine wall, septum and dissecting instrument can be seen simultaneously is difficult, particularly when the uterus moves as the hysteroscopist proceeds with the division of the septum. Nonetheless, intraoperative sonography will increase the safety of performing these procedures, should laparoscopy be contraindicated. No additional benefit to visualize the pelvic structures can be added by sonography, except in observing enlargement of the ovaries and evaluation of possible ovarian cysts.

Pathology associated with the septate uterus requires the same treatment as that for lesions alone. Nonetheless, it is advantageous to treat other lesions, such as polyps or myomas, before the uterine septum is divided. This is performed to allow more perfect visualization of the symmetry of both uterine cavities. Occasionally, the septum has to be excised first to permit better visualization of the lesions in a unified uterine cavity.

Table 5 Hysteroscopic metroplasty. Data in parentheses are expressed as percentage of total number of pregnancies achieved. Modified from reference[25]

Study	No. of patients	Medium	Technique	IUD	Estrogen/ progesterone	Anti-biotics	Pregnancy Term	Premature	Abortion	In progress
Edstrom, 1974	2	dextran 70, 32%	rigid biopsy forceps	+	—	—	—	19 weeks	—	—
Chervenak and Neuwirth, 1981	2	dextran 70, 32%	scissors adjacent to hysteroscope	+	+	+	1	—	—	—
Rosenberg et al., 1981	1	dextran 70, 32%	flexible scissors	NA	NA	NA	NA	—	—	—
Daly et al., 1983	25	dextran 70, 32%	—	—	+	—	7	—	1	2
Perino et al., 1985	11	CO_2	flexible, semirigid scissors	+	—	—	NA	—	—	—
DeCherney et al., 1986	72	dextran 70, 32%	resectoscope	—	—	—	58	—	4	4
Corson and Batzer, 1986	18	dextran 70, 32% CO_2	resectoscope and rigid scissors	—	—	—	10	1	2	2
Fayez, 1986	19	dextran 70, 32%	rigid scissors	Foley catheter	—	+	14	—	—	—
March and Israel, 1987	91	dextran 70, 32%	flexible scissors	+	+	—	44	4	7	7
Valle, 1987	59	5% dextrose in water dextran 70, 32%	flexible, semirigid, rigid scissors	—	+	+	44	2	5	—
Choe and Baggish, 1992	19	dextran 70, 32%	Nd:YAG with bare or sculptured fibers	Foley catheter ($n = 3$)	+	+	10	1	1	3
Fedele et al., 1993	102	dextran 40, 10% in normal saline	semi-rigid scissors ($n = 80$) argon laser ($n = 10$) resectoscope ($n = 12$)	21	39	+	45	10	11	NA
Valle, 1996	124	5% dextrose in 0.5 normal saline glycine 1.5%	semi-rigid scissors ($n = 98$) resctoscope ($n = 20$) Nd:YAG laser ($n = 6$)	—	+	+	84	7	12	—
Total	545						317 (78.5)	26 (6.4)	43 (10.6)	18 (4.5)

IUD, intrauterine device; NA, not applicable

References

1. Moore KL. *The Urogenital System*, 4th edn. Philadelphia: WB Saunders, 1988: 246–85
2. Rock JA, Zacur HA. The clinical management of repeated early pregnancy wastage. *Fertil Steril* 1983;39:123–40
3. Carp HJA, Toder V, Mashiach S, *et al.* Recurrent miscarriage: a review of current concepts, immune mechanisms, and results of treatment. *Obstet Gynecol Surv* 1990;45:657–69
4. Buttram VC, Gibbons WE. Mullerian anomalies: a proposed classification (an analysis of 144 cases). *Fertil Steril* 1979;32:40–6
5. Valle RE. Clinical management of uterine factors in infertile patients. In Speroff L, ed. *Seminars in*

Reproductive Endocrinology. New York: Georg Thieme Verlag, 1985;3:149–67

6. Jones AW, Jones GES. Double uterus as an etiologic factor in repeated abortions: indications for surgical repair. *Am J Obstet Gynecol* 1953;65:325–39

7. Tompkins P. Comments on the bicornuate uterus and twinning. *Surg Clin N Am* 1962; 42:1049–62

8. Daly DC, Walters CA, Soto-Albors CE, *et al.* Hysteroscopic metroplasty: surgical technique and obstetric outcome. *Fertil Steril* 1983;39:623–8

9. Valle RF, Sciarra JJ. Hysteroscopic treatment of the septate uterus. *Obstet Gynecol* 1986;676:253–7

10. Perino A, Mencaglia L, Hamou J, *et al.* Hysteroscopy for metroplasty of uterine septa: report of 24 cases. *Fertil Steril* 1987;48:321–3

11. Daly DC, Tohan N, Walters C, *et al.* Hysteroscopic resection of the uterine septum in the presence of a septate cervix. *Fertil Steril* 1983;39:560–3

12. March CM, Israel R. Hysteroscopic management of recurrent abortion caused by septate uterus. *Am J Obstet Gynecol* 1987;156:834–42

13. DeCherney AH, Russell JB, Graebe RA, *et al.* Resectoscopic management of Müllerian fusion defects. *Fertil Steril* 1986;45:726–8

14. Rock JA, Murphy AA, Cooper WH. Resectoscopic techniques for the lysis of a class V: complete uterine septum. *Fertil Steril* 1987;48:495–6

15. Candiani GB, Vercellini P, Fedele L, *et al.* Repair of the uterine cavity after hysteroscopic septal incision. *Fertil Steril* 1990;54:991–4

16. Candiani GB, Vercellini P, Fedele L, *et al.* Argon laser versus microscissors for hysteroscopic incision of uterine septa. *Am J Obstet Gynecol* 1991;164:87–90

17. Garry R, Hasham F, Kokri MS, *et al.* The effect of pressure on fluid absorption during endometrial ablation. *J Gynecol Surg* 1992;8:1–10

18. Daly DC, Maier D, Soto-Albors C. Hysteroscopic metroplasty: six years experience. *Obstet Gynecol* 1989;73:201–5

19. Siegler AM, Valle RF, Lindemann HJ, *et al. Therapeutic Hysteroscopy. Indications and Techniques.* St Louis: CV Mosby, 1990:62–81

20. Hassiakos DK, Zourlas PA. Transcervical division of the uterine septa. *Obstet Gynecol Surv* 1990;45: 165–73

21. Fayez JA. Comparison between abdominal and hysteroscopic metroplasty. *Obstet Gynecol* 1986; 68:399–403

22. Daniell JF, Osher S, Miller W. Hysteroscopic resection of uterine septi with visible light laser energy. *Colposc Gynecol Laser Surg* 1987;3: 217–20

23. Choe JK, Baggish MS. Hysteroscopic treatment of septate uterus with neodymium-YAG laser. *Fertil Steril* 1992;57:81–4

24. Fedele L, Arcaini L, Parazzini F, *et al.* Reproductive prognosis after hysteroscopic metroplasty in 102 women: lifetable analysis. *Fertil Steril* 1993;59:768–72

25. Siegier AM, Valle RF. Therapeutic hysteroscopic procedures. *Fertil Steril* 1988;50:685–701

26. Valle RF. Hysteroscopic treatment of partial and complete uterine septum. *Int J Fertil* 1996;41: 310–15

8

Intrauterine adhesions

R. F. Valle

Intrauterine adhesions may interfere with both normal reproduction and menstrual patterns. When surgical treatment is undertaken, results are much improved if the corrective surgery is performed under direct visualization using a hysteroscope.

ETIOLOGY

Intrauterine adhesions are scars that result from trauma to a recently pregnant uterus. In over 90% of cases, they are caused by curettage[1-3]. Usually, the trauma has occurred because of excessive bleeding requiring curettage 1–4 weeks after delivery of a term or preterm pregnancy or after an induced abortion. During this vulnerable phase of the endometrium, any trauma may denude or remove the basalis endometrium, causing the uterine walls to adhere to each other and form a permanent bridge, distorting the symmetry of the uterine cavity. In rare circumstances, conditions such as abdominal metroplasties or myomectomies may cause intrauterine adhesions, but these adhesions are usually due to misplaced sutures rather than the true coaptation of denuded areas of myometrium that occurs following postpartum or postabortal curettage[3].

The type and consistency of these adhesions vary: some are focal, some extensive, some mild and some thickened and dense, with extensive fibromuscular or connective tissue components. The extent and type of uterine cavity occlusion correlate well with the extent of trauma during the vulnerable phase of the endometrium following a recent pregnancy. Some adhesions are focal, others completely occlude the uterine cavity. Consistency usually follows the longevity and duration of these adhesions, the older ones being thickened and dense and formed by connective tissue[4-7].

Reproductive outcome seems to correlate well with the type of adhesions and the extent of uterine cavity occlusion. Therefore, it is useful to have a way of classifying these adhesions as filmy and composed endometrial tissue, fibromuscular, or those composed of connective tissue. The degree of uterine cavity occlusion is also important. Attempts to classify intrauterine adhesions by hysterosalpingo-graphy give a good appraisal of the extent of uterine cavity occlusion, but it is impossible to determine by hysterosalpingography the type of adhesions that are present. When using hysteroscopy alone, it is difficult to assess the extent of uterine cavity occlusion by visualization because the axis to the hysteroscopist is from the cervix to the fundus and not perpendicular to the uterine body as it is in hysterography, outlining the uterine cavity from a different axis. For this reason, the combination of hysterosalpingography and hysteroscopy has been used most commonly to assess not only the extent of uterine cavity occlusion, but also the type of adhesions found by hysteroscopy at the time of treatment. Valle and Sciarra[3] utilized a three-stage classification of the extent and severity of intrauterine adhesions (mild, moderate and severe) based on the degree of involvement shown on hysterosalpingography and the extent and type of adhesions found on hysteroscopy. Three stages of intrauterine adhesions are defined: mild adhesions are filmy adhesions composed of basalis endometrial tissue producing partial or complete uterine cavity occlusion; moderate adhesions are fibromuscular adhesions, characteristically thick, still covered with endometrium that may bleed upon division, which partially or totally occlude the uterine cavity; and severe adhesions are composed of connective tissue only, lacking any endometrial lining, and not likely to bleed upon division, they may partially or totally occlude the uterine cavity[3].

Recently, the American Fertility Society (now the American Society of Reproductive Medicine) has proposed a classification of intrauterine adhesions based on the findings at hysterosalpingography and hysteroscopy, and their correlation with menstrual patterns[8]. Using a uniform classification for intrauterine adhesions greatly enhances our ability to evaluate, report and compare results of different treatments of intrauterine adhesions, particularly when utilizing these modalities by the hysteroscopic approach.

INDICATIONS FOR TREATMENT

Intrauterine adhesions frequently result in menstrual abnormalities, such as hypomenorrhea or even amenorrhea, depending upon the extent of uterine cavity occlusion. Patients with long-standing intrauterine adhesions may also develop dysmenorrhea. Over 75% of women with moderate or severe adhesions will have either amenorrhea or hypomenorrhea. Patients with significant uterine cavity occlusion secondary to intrauterine adhesions experience menstrual abnormalities, particularly amenorrhea (37%) and hypomenorrhea (31%). Patients with minimal or focal intrauterine adhesions may not demonstrate obvious menstrual abnormalities and may continue to have normal menses[9].

Patients may also exhibit problems in reproduction, particularly pregnancy wastage, should the adhesions not totally occlude the uterine cavity. When total amenorrhea and total uterine cavity occlusion exist, the patient will generally be infertile. Other problems associated with intrauterine adhesions are premature labor, fetal demise and ectopic pregnancy. When pregnancy is carried to term, placental insertion abnormalities, such as placenta accreta, percreta or increta, may occur. Schenker and Margalioth[9] evaluated 292 patients who did not receive treatment for intrauterine adhesions. Of these, 133 women (45.5%) conceived 165 times, and of these, only 50 (30%) achieved a term pregnancy; 38 (23%) had preterm labor, and 66 aborted spontaneously (40%). In 21 patients (13%), placenta accreta occurred and in 12 patients (7.3%) other complications, such as ectopic pregnancy and abnormal placental presentations, were diagnosed.

The most important clue to the diagnosis of intrauterine adhesions is a history of trauma to the endometrial cavity, particularly following delivery or abortion. Secondary to that is a history of amenorrhea or hypomenorrhea. Because intrauterine adhesions are not related to hormonal events, an intact hypothalamic–pituitary–ovarian axis should result in a biphasic basal body temperature curve demonstrating ovulation; failure to withdraw from a progesterone challenge test in a patient who is amenorrheic will strengthen the diagnosis. Uterine sounding has been used to ascertain obstruction of the internal cervical os, but this test should be abandoned because of an increased danger of uterine perforation as well as inaccuracy of diagnosis. The most useful screening test for intrauterine adhesions is hysterosalpingography. It provides evaluation of the internal cervical os and uterine cavity, delineation of the adhesions, and information about the condition of the rest of the uterine cavity if adhesions do not completely occlude this area. About 1.5% of hysterosalpingograms performed for infertility evaluation demonstrate intrauterine adhesions[10]. When hysterosalpingograms are performed for repeated abortions, about 5% demonstrate intrauterine adhesions[9]. A history compatible with intrauterine adhesions will increase the yield of hysterosalpingography for intrauterine adhesions in about 39% of patients[11]. These adhesions are star-like, stellate irregular-shaped, filling defects, with ragged contours and variable locations in the uterine cavity. They are most commonly found in the central corporeal cavity and less frequently at the uterotubal cones and lower uterine segment.

Despite the usefulness of hysterosalpingography as a screening method for patients suspected of having intrauterine adhesions, the final diagnosis is determined only by direct visualization with hysteroscopy because about 30% of abnormal hysterosalpingograms may be excluded and corrected by hysteroscopy[12]. The diagnosis can be confirmed by visualization, and the appropriate treatment can be provided once the adhesions are observed endoscopically.

Hysterosalpingography is useful in determining the extent of uterine cavity occlusion, but it cannot provide an appraisal of the consistency and type of intrauterine adhesions. For this reason, hysteroscopy becomes a useful adjunct to hysterosalpingography by confirming the extent and type of intrauterine adhesions.

Other techniques, such as ultrasonography and magnetic resonance imaging (MRI), have been used to make this diagnosis, but their accuracy is not well determined, and not enough experience exists with these techniques to supplant the hysterosalpingogram and hysteroscopy[13,14]. Furthermore, the cost of MRI may be prohibitive.

METHODS OF TREATMENT

Treatment of intrauterine adhesions is surgical, consisting of removing the adhesions by division. In the past, blind methods of division were used with curettes, probes or dilators, or hysterotomy-assisted division of these adhesions under direct vision, but these techniques have failed to produce acceptable results and have been largely abandoned. Introduction of modern hysteroscopy has permitted transcervical division of adhesions under visual guidance; hysteroscopic methods have used mechanical means, such as hysteroscopic scissors, the resectoscope and fiberoptic lasers.

Treatment of intrauterine adhesions with hysteroscopic scissors is the most common method employed. Because intrauterine adhesions, in general, are avascular and divided (not removed), the treatment has been similar to that for division of a uterine septum. The adhesions are divided centrally, allowing the uterine cavity to expand upon division of the adhesions. This is performed utilizing flexible, semirigid and, occasionally, rigid or optical scissors. The most commonly used method is the semirigid hysteroscopic scissors because of the increased facility manipulating the scissors, selectively dividing the adhesions when they retract upon cutting. Occasionally, thick connective tissue adhesions are present that form very thick stumps and benefit not only from division but also from removal. To achieve this effect, sharp punch-biopsy forceps become most useful when lateral thick adhesions are present, and the technique involves not only division of the adhesions but also removal. It is important to use sharp biopsy forceps to selectively sculpture the uterine cavity to achieve a uniform symmetry. This technique is also useful at the uterotubal cones, particularly at the junction of the tubal openings and the uterus (Figures 1–4).

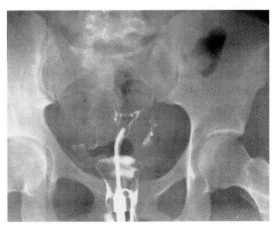

Figure 1 Hysterosalpingogram shows extensive uterine cavity occlusion by adhesions

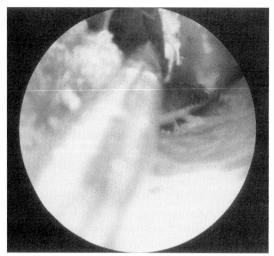

Figure 2 Hysteroscopic division of extensive intra-uterine adhesions using semirigid scissors

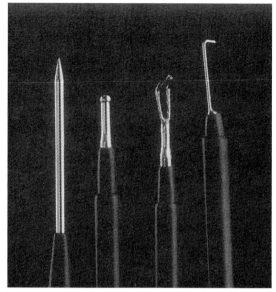

Figure 4 Electrodes for use through hysteroscopic operating channel (6.0 Fr, 2 mm). Left to right: point tip, ball tip, loop tip, hook tip. Courtesy of Cook Ob/Gyn, Spencer, IN, USA

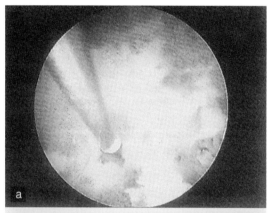

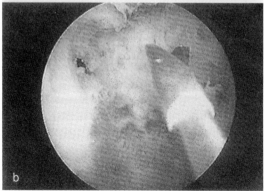

Figure 3 Hysteroscopic division of extensive fundal intrauterine adhesions: (a) initial division of adhesions; (b) right uterotubal cone is visible. See also Color Plates V and VI

While the semirigid and flexible scissors are most useful for the division of adhesions by hysteroscopy, the rigid optical scissors are less helpful in this endeavor. Because of the thick, sturdy configuration of these adhesions, when the uterine wall is thin and sclerotic, there is greater chance of uterine perforation, particularly because a panoramic view is impaired. Targeted dissection, which is easily obtained with the flexible and semirigid scissors, is hampered and difficult with optical scissors.

Fluids with electrolytes should be used when dividing these adhesions mechanically with scissors, because of the increased chance of intravasation and because the adhesions are cut close to the myometrial tissue, and the extensive area of denudation may predispose to fluid intravasation. Normal saline, 5% dextrose in half normal saline and Ringer's lactate are most appropriate. Care must be taken to measure the amount of fluid used and the amount recovered when using the hysteroscope, particularly if the instrument has inflow and outflow, permitting an estimate of the amount of fluid that has not been recovered. In the absence of a continuous-flow system, care must be taken to measure the total inflow of fluids and ascertain that the intrauterine pressure does not exceed the mean arterial pressure of about 100 mmHg. These procedures must be expedited to avoid excessive intravasation of fluid.

Depending upon the extent of uterine cavity occlusion, division is performed under visual control by cutting the adhesions in the middle to avoid uterine damage at the level of the uterine wall. When there is total uterine cavity occlusion, selective dissection of adhesions begins at the internal cervical os until a neocavity is created and then the dissection progresses until the uterotubal cones are free. When extensive adhesions are present, the hysteroscopist should be alert to perforation. Concomitant laparoscopy should be considered in all cases. Upon completion of the procedure, indigo carmine is injected transcervically to test for tubal patency[3,15].

The advantages of using hysteroscopic scissors for the division of intrauterine adhesions are those of mechanical methods. Mechanical tools provide excellent landmarks when dividing adhesions, particularly when approaching the juxtaposed myometrium. Bleeding may be observed at the myometrium, and this warns the hysteroscopist to stop the dissection to avoid perforation. No scattering of energies is produced to damage the small areas of healthy endometrium, which are the reservoir for future re-epithelialization. This is an important consideration because no extensive healthy endometrium can be found when extensive intrauterine adhesions are present. The disadvantages are that it may sometimes be difficult to manipulate semirigid instrumentation, particularly to the lateral walls of the uterine cavity. Scissors may not provide the sharpness or mechanism to cut the adhesions, as the scissors do not close well distally and need to be readjusted and sharpened frequently.

Treatment of intrauterine adhesions utilizing the resectoscope is an alternative to mechanical tools. The resectoscope can be used to divide intrauterine adhesions either with a resecting loop, a loop bent forward, or with specifically designed electrodes that can be directly applied to the adhesions dividing them easily. These are in the form of knives or wires that must be specifically and selectively directed to the adhesions, particularly those in the lateral portion of the uterus or at the uterotubal cones. When utilizing the resectoscope, fluids without electrolytes must be used, e.g. 5% dextrose in water, 1.5% glycine, 3.5% sorbitol and 5% mannitol, which provide excellent visualization and are useful distending media. When dividing these adhesions, the resectoscopic loop may not be the appropriate electrode to use because it is designed to resect rather than to selectively divide the adhesions centrally. When the resectoscopic loop has been used for this purpose, several complications have occurred, particularly due to future sacculations of the uterus, dehiscences and perforations. Ascertaining where the adhesions finish and where normal myometrium begins is difficult, and resections may be so deep that a portion of the myometrium may be shaved during division of the adhesions. Electrodes, such as the knife or wire types that can selectively be directed to the adhesions and divide them systematically, have been specifically designed for this purpose. Nonetheless, concern remains about scattering energy and damaging the peripheral healthy endometrium. With the use of specific electrodes, this effect may be somewhat decreased. It is important to monitor the operation with concomitant laparoscopy or sonography because the landmarks of junction between adhesions and myometrium may be lost, and the coagulating effect this energy may produce in the myometrium may obscure view of small vessels that, when bleeding, warn the hysteroscopist to stop further dissection.

Use of the resectoscope has several advantages. Bleeding is decreased during dissection because of the electrical coagulating effect. The resectoscopic continuous-flow system allows estimation of the deficit of fluid, thus decreasing the chances of fluid overload.

There are also disadvantages. Monopolar energy must be used. Only fluids devoid of electrolytes can be used. Additionally, electrosurgical damage of peripheral endometrium and loss of landmarks while coagulating close to the myometrium, resulting in inadvertent invasion of this area, may occur. Finally, electrical damage to surrounding organs with or without perforation is a risk[16].

Fiberoptic lasers, such as the Nd:YAG, Argon and KTP-532, can also be used to divide intrauterine adhesions. However, their application has been somewhat limited. The Nd:YAG laser with sculptured or extruded fibers can be a useful tool to divide intrauterine adhesions selectively, particularly those that are lateral and fundal[15]. Care must be taken to use these fibers by contact and selectively to be aware of the overall symmetry of the uterine cavity because the coagulating power of the laser may cause a similar effect to electrosurgery; that is, coagulation and cutting, and landmarks of the juxtaposed myometrium may be lost while dividing adhesions. Small arteries that cross the myometrium may not bleed, so dissection may proceed further than necessary. The hysteroscopic manipulation of the fiberoptic lasers is very easy and is facilitated with the use of foroblique telescopes. The Argon and KTP-532 utilize the sharpest fibers to cut rather than to coagulate[17].

Because lasers are not conductive, fluids with electrolytes should be used. Normal saline, 5% dextrose in half normal saline or Ringer's lactate provide excellent visualization and contain sodium if excessive fluids are absorbed. The utilization of these electrolyte-containing fluids will not prevent pulmonary edema but will decrease the risk of hyponatremia; therefore, more fluid may be used than when using fluids without electrolytes. Ideally, a hysteroscope with a continuous-flow system should be used – or one with true inflow and outflow – to monitor the injected fluid and have a perfect account of the deficit or non-recovered fluid[18].

Use of the laser is attractive and has the benefit of easy manipulation, but requires more time than use of mechanical tools, such as hysteroscopic scissors. It is important, therefore, when utilizing this type of energy to expedite the procedure as much as possible, so as to avoid excessive fluid being intravasated.

Recently, vaporizing electrodes have been introduced in an attempt to use them with electrolytic solution distending the uterus. Similar concerns as with electrosurgery apply, particularly without evaluation of the penetration and scattering that these electrodes produce when applied to tissues.

The treatment of severe intrauterine adhesions remains a challenge and other methods have been suggested to simplify the treatment, such as concomitant fluoroscopy or sonography, transfundal uterine injection of dyes, coaxial injection of radiopaque material, vital dyes to distinguish fibrous adhesions from residual endometrium, endometrial electrosurgical scoring, blind lateral sounding of the uterine cavity, and hysterotomy for transfundal dissection of adhesions. However, all of the above have been used in a limited fashion and have not proved their efficacy consistently[19].

INTRA- AND POSTOPERATIVE MANAGEMENT

The principal goal of therapy is to remove adhesions surgically. Because most of these patients have a sclerotic or destroyed endometrium, they need other adjunctive therapy to promote re-epithelialization and a mechanical separation of the uterine walls to prevent reformation of adhesions. These adjuncts are intrauterine splints, prophylactic antibiotics and estrogens, to promote re-epithelialization.

Prophylactic antibiotics are used routinely in these patients because of the traumatized endometrium and the extensive manipulation these patients usually require. The antibiotics used are in the form of cephalosporins, Kefzol® 1 mg intravenously piggyback 30 min before the procedure, to be followed with Keflex® 500 mg orally four times a week for 1 week, should an intrauterine splint be placed. Additionally, in those patients with extensive intrauterine adhesions, an indwelling number 8 pediatric Foley catheter is inserted and 3–3.5 ml of a solution instilled. It is left in place for 1 week to prevent reformation of adhesions. Adjunctive hormonal therapy consists of conjugated estrogens in the form of Premarin® 2.5 mg twice daily for 30 or 40 days, depending on the extent of uterine cavity occlusion and the type of adhesions found. The more extensive and older are the adhesions, the more prolonged the required hormonal treatment. In the last 10 days of this artificial cycle, medroxyprogesterone acetate (Provera®) 10 mg a day are given orally for 10 days, to induce withdrawal bleeding. Upon completion of the hormonal treatment, and once withdrawal bleeding has ceased, a hysterosalpingogram is performed to assess the results of the operation and decide upon further therapy or initiation of attempts to conceive. Those patients with filmy, focal adhesions may not require hysterosalpingography but may require an office hysteroscopy to assess uterine cavity symmetry[3,19].

RESULTS

The results of hysteroscopic treatment of intrauterine adhesions have correlated well with the extent of uterine cavity occlusion and the type of adhesions present. Normal menstruation is restored in over 90% of patients[3,19]. The reproductive outcome correlates well with the type of adhesions and the extent of uterine cavity occlusion. Of 187 patients treated hysteroscopically by Valle and Sciarra[3], removal of mild, filmy adhesions in 43 cases gave the best results, with 35 (81%) term pregnancies; in 97 moderate cases of fibromuscular adhesions, 64 (66%) term pregnancies occurred, and in 47 severe cases of connective tissue adhesions, 15 (32%) term pregnancies occurred. Overall

Table 1 Results of hysteroscopic lysis of intrauterine adhesions. Modified from reference 20

| | | | | | Normal menses | | Reproductive outcome | | | |
| | | | | | | | Pregnant | | Term | |
Study	No. of patients	IUD	Estrogen/ progesterone	Antibiotics	n	%	n	%	n	%
Edstrom, 1974	9	+	—	—	2		1		1	
March et al., 1981	38	+	+	+	38	100	38	100	34	89.5
Neuwirth et al., 1982	27	+	+	+	20	74	14	51.8	13	48.1
Sanfilippo et al., 1982	26	+	+	—	26	100	26	100	13	50
Siegler and Kontopoulos, 1981	25	Foley catheter	+	—	13	52	11	44	6	24
Hamou et al., 1983	69	+	+	—	59	85.5	20	29	15	21.7
Sugimoto et al., 1984	258	+	+	—	180	69.7	107	41.4	64	24.8
Wamsteker, 1984	36	+	+	+	34	94.4	17	47.2	12	33.3
Friedman et al., 1986	30	—	+	—	27	90	24	80	23	76.6
Valle and Sciarra, 1987	187	+ Foley catheter	+	+	167	89.3	143	76.4	114	60.9
Zuanchong and Yulian, 1986	70	+	+	+	64	91.4	30	42.9	17	24.2
Lancet and Kessler, 1988	98	Hyskon	flexible scissors electrosurgery		98	100	86	87.8	77	78.6
Pabuuccu et al., 1999	40	glycerine	Murphy probe scissors		33	82.5	27	67.5	23	57.5
Feng et al., 1999	365	5% dextrose	biopsy forceps/ scissors		294	80.5	156*	83.8	145	78.0
Total	1278				1060	87.5	718	72.3	603	87.2

*Of 186 desiring pregnancy, 156 conceived; IUD, intrauterine device

restoration of menses occurred in 90% of patients, and the overall term pregnancy rate was 79.7%. These results demonstrate a much better reproductive outcome than was previously obtained with blind methods of therapy[20-24] (Table 1).

Results following treatment of intrauterine adhesions utilizing the resectoscope have been similar; nonetheless, the reported postoperative complications may be serious and should be kept in mind when utilizing this type of instrument[16]. A few series report lysis of adhesions with fiberoptic lasers, but when the lasers are used appropriately, results should not vary significantly from those reported with electrosurgery.

SUMMARY

Hysteroscopic surgery has been greatly facilitated and enhanced by the use of the gynecological resectoscope. No single technique, used exclusively, can accomplish all tasks. Used in combination with other available techniques for hysteroscopic surgery, however, the gyneco-logical resectoscope enhances our ability to treat different conditions that would previously have required major surgery. The treatment of the symptomatic septate uterus, as well as the treatment of intrauterine adhesions, can be accomplished by three different techniques: scissors, resectoscope and fiberoptic lasers. All have advantages and disadvantages and must be used with knowledge of each particular technology and its limitations. Each technique should be tailored not only to the anatomy, embryology and etiology of each process, but also to the experience and knowledge of the operator. The operator should select the appropriate method and technique for each patient. The goals of therapy should be a successful pregnancy for those patients with impaired reproduction, keeping in mind the safety of the patient, with the least morbidity possible, the absence of complications, the overall effectiveness, and diminution of unnecessary cost. Versatility plays a significant role in the selection of therapeutic alternatives; the surgeon has intelligently to select the best method for each individual patient.

References

1. Asherman JG. Amenorrhea traumatica (atretica). *J Obset Gynaecol Br Emp* 1948;55: 23–30
2. Asherman JG. Traumatic intrauterine adhesions. *J Obstet Gynaecol Br Emp* 1950;57:892–6
3. Valle RF, Sciarra JJ. Intrauterine adhesions: hysteroscopic diagnosis, classification, treatment, and reproductive outcome. *Am J Obstet Gynecol* 1988;158:1459–70
4. Foix A, Bruno RO, Davidson T, *et al.* The pathology of postcurettage intrauterine adhesions. *Am J Obstet Gynecol* 1966;96:1027–33
5. Siegler AM, Kontopoulos VG. Lysis of intrauterine adhesions under hysteroscopic control: a report of 25 operations. *J Reprod Med* 1981; 26:372–4
6. March CM, Israel R, March AD. Hysteroscopic management of intrauterine adhesions. *Am J Obstet Gynecol* 1978;130:653
7. Siegler AM, Valle RF. Therapeutic hysteroscopic procedures. *Fertil Steril* 1988;50:685–701
8. The American Fertility Society. Classifications of adnexal adhesions, distal tubal occlusion, tubal occlusion secondary to tubal ligation, tubal pregnancies, Mullerian anomalies, and intrauterine adhesions. *Fertil Steril* 1988;49:944–55
9. Schenker JG, Margalioth EJ. Intrauterine adhesions: an updated appraisal. *Fertil Steril* 1982;37:593–610
10. Dmowski WP, Greenblatt RB. Asherman's syndrome and risk of placenta accreta. *Obstet Gynecol* 1969;34:288–99

11. Klein SM, Garcia CR. Asherman's syndrome: a critique and current review. *Fertil Steril* 1973; 24:722–35

12. Valle RF, Sciarra JJ. Current status of hysteroscopy in gynecologic practice. *Fertil Steril* 1979;32:619–32

13. Confino E, Friberg J, Giglia RV, *et al.* Sonographic imaging of intrauterine adhesions. *Obstet Gynecol* 1985;66:596–8

14. Vartiainen J, Kajanoja P, Ylostalo PR. Ultrasonography in extended placental retention and intrauterine adhesions: a case report. *Eur J Obstet Gynecol Reprod Biol* 1989;30:89–93

15. Neuwirth RS, Hussein AR, Schiffman BM, *et al.* Hysteroscopic resection of intrauterine scars using a new technique. *Obstet Gynecol* 1982;60: 111–13

16. Friedman A, Defazio J, DeCherney AH. Severe obstetric complications following hysteroscopic lysis of adhesions. *Obstet Gynecol* 1986;67:864–7

17. Newton JR, Mackenzie WE, Emens MJ, *et al.* Division of uterine adhesions (Asherman's syndrome) with the Nd-YAG laser. *Br J Obstet Gynaecol* 1989;96:102–4

18. Valle RF. Intrauterine adhesions (Asherman's syndrome). In Blanc B, Marty R, eds. *Office and Operative Hysteroscopy.* New York: Springer-Verlag, 2002:229–42

19. March CM, Israel R. Gestational outcome following hysteroscopic lysis of adhesions. *Fertil Steril* 1981;36:455

20. Seigler AM, Valle RF, Lindeman HJ, *et al.*, eds. *Therapeutic Hysteroscopy. Indications and Techniques.* St Louis: CV Mosby, 1990:103

21. Intrauterine adhesions. In Siegler AM, Valle RF, Lindemann HJ, *et al.* eds. *Therapeutic Hysteroscopy. Indications and Techniques.* St Louis: CV Mosby, 1990:82–105

22. Lancet M, Kessler I. A review of Asherman's Syndrome, and results of modern treatment. *Int J Fertil* 1988;33:14–24

23. Pabuccu R, Atay V, Orhon E, *et al.* Hysteroscopic treatment of intrauterine adhesions is safe and effective in the restoration of normal menstruation and fertility. *Fertil Steril* 1997;68: 1141–3

24. Feng ZC, Yang B, Shoo J, *et al.* Diagnostic and therapeutic hysteroscopy for traumatic intrauterine adhesions after induced abortions: a clinical analysis of 365 cases. *Gynaecol Endosc* 1999;8:95–8

9

Removing intrauterine lesions: myomectomy and polypectomy

F. D. Loffer

Prior to hysteroscopy, many intrauterine polyps and myomas went undiagnosed until the patient came to hysterectomy. Blind procedures, such as endometrial biopsies and dilatation and curettage, do not detect the majority of intrauterine growths[1,2]. Imaging procedures are more helpful. Unfortunately, the false-positive rate may be high, and lesions identified at a hysterogram are proven hysteroscopically or by hysterectomy in only 43–69% of cases[3–5]. Diagnostic techniques, such as ultrasound, are better tools than hysterograms for determining the nature of an intrauterine lesion[6–9]. The expense of magnetic resonance imaging (MRI) precludes its use for this purpose. Finally, none of the imaging techniques provide tissue for pathological diagnosis.

Hysteroscopy is an excellent method for not only identifying intrauterine lesions but also for removing them. The first suggestion of a transcervical approach using a resection loop was in 1957[10]. Although the instrument was not clearly described, specific reference was made that it was not a urological resectoscope. The first reported gynecological use of a resection loop was in 1978, when a urological resectoscope was used[11]. Subsequent to that time, other reports have been published[12–32].

ANATOMY

It is necessary to understand the anatomy of the intrauterine lesions that will be found and treated in order to select what cases are appropriate for hysteroscopic management and in what manner the resectoscope will be used. Intrauterine growths are defined as being either pedunculated or sessile. This distinction is based on their attachment to the uterine wall. A pedunculated structure is attached by a stalk or pedicle, while a sessile structure is attached by a broad base.

A polypoid structure may be a leiomyoma, adenomyoma, or an endometrial polyp. The differentiation between pedunculated and sessile leiomyoma is a matter of the size of the stalk. Leiomyomas are intimately related to myometrium and are demarcated by a false or pseudocapsule. This capsule is less well demonstrated in those leiomyomas that are pedunculated. Pedunculated adenomyomas of the uterus are a mixture of normal endometrium and uterine musculature, which contain endometrial glands without any surrounding endometrial stroma. Like leiomyomas, they also may be sessile. They frequently occur in young patients and may be the basis of infertility. Endometrial polyps originate from the middle or basal third of the endometrium and may or may not be covered by functioning endometrium.

Sessile leiomyomas and adenomyomas lie partially embedded in the myometrium. The amount embedded can be estimated by the angle the leiomyoma makes with the endometrium at its attachment to the uterine wall.

A simple grading scale has been proposed[33]. Those leiomyomas that lie primarily or completely within the uterine wall are intramural and not approachable by hysteroscopic techniques. Subserosal leiomyomas, which lie beyond the uterine cavity on the abdominal side of the uterus, are also not suitable for hysteroscopic management.

Although very uncommon, both endometrial polyps and leiomyomas may show malignant changes. This author found two cases of uterine sarcoma in his first 200 patients. Both patients presented as postmenopausal bleeding. The risk of malignancy in leiomyomas would appear to range between 1% and 1.4%[34]. There are no specific characteristics to identify malignancy prior to tissue being sent for pathological review. However, the onset of bleeding from submucosal fibroids in postmenopausal patients should raise concern.

Sessile and pedunculated lesions can arise from anywhere in the uterine cavity. On occasion, pedunculated lesions in the lower uterine segment may prolapse through the cervix and be visible on vaginal examination.

Hysteroscopists often discuss the maximum size of a myoma that can be successfully resected. It is this author's opinion that the size of the submucous myoma is relatively self-limiting. If it is primarily intramural, it can grow to any size since it will enlarge the uterus and further distort the uterine cavity. Intramural myomas are not managed by hysteroscopy. However, when the myoma is primarily intrauterine, it can grow until it reaches a size at which time it would most likely prolapse through the cervical canal (Figure 1). Although myomas larger than 5–6 cm may be identified by ultrasound to be projecting into the cavity, they are probably primarily intramural and, therefore, may not be good candidates for hysteroscopic resection.

INDICATIONS FOR HYSTEROSCOPIC SURGERY

Patients with intrauterine lesions will generally present with either abnormal bleeding, pregnancy wastage/infertility, or both. Occa-

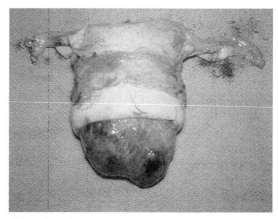

Figure 1 The size of submucous myomas is probably self-limiting. This fibroid measuring approximately 6 cm could no longer be contained in the uterine cavity. See also Color Plate VII

sionally, a pelvic ultrasound performed for pelvic pain or to evaluate the adnexa or the size of uterine leiomyoma may identify an as yet asymptomatic intrauterine lesion.

The usual history given by premenopausal patients who present with abnormal bleeding is progressively heavier periods associated with increasing pre- and postmenstrual spotting and length of flow. Some of the heaviest menstrual bleeding patients experience is related to submucous leiomyomas. Postmenopausal patients may present with postmenopausal bleeding or excessively heavy withdrawal bleeding from hormonal replacement therapy.

The initial evaluation of premenopausal patients presenting with significant menorrhagia or menometrorrhagia is usually not surgical. If the bleeding is of recent onset and not severe, short observation may be indicated to see if it is a transient problem. When the bleeding is related to anovulation, endocrine causes should be ruled out. If no underlying correctable problem is identified, cyclic progesterone or oral contraceptives can be given to regulate and decrease the menstrual flow. A diagnostic hysteroscopy is indicated when the menorrhagia or menometrorrhagia fails conservative treatment, is persistent, severe, or occurs in a postmenopausal patient. This hysteroscopic evaluation can usually be performed in an office setting.

Some patients who want hysteroscopic surgical management of their bleeding problems and in whom infertility is not a concern may choose not to have an office hysteroscopy. They can first be evaluated by hysteroscopy in an outpatient facility prior to the expected definitive surgery. This alternative is feasible since the cause of the bleeding is usually from a submucous leiomyoma or a normal-appearing endometrial cavity, and the menorrhagia can usually be managed at the time of the initial diagnosis. If a lesion is present, it can be removed. If no lesion is present, endometrial ablation can be performed. It is important that patients who choose this route understand that there may be findings that preclude any hysteroscopic management. This risk can be minimized by a preoperative endometrial biopsy, which will determine ovulation and rule out premalignant changes. Sounding of the uterus can determine size of the cavity and, if large, suggests a submucous or intramural myoma. An ultrasound will also provide further information.

In patients whose only complaint is infertility or pregnancy wastage, screening hysteroscopy has little value[4]. Initial evaluation should generally be by hysterosalpingography. If a filling defect is found, it can then be evaluated and managed hysteroscopically. Most patients with pregnancy wastage or infertility secondary to an intrauterine lesion will have associated menorrhagia, and clinical suspicion will be raised that an intrauterine lesion may exist.

SURGICAL METHODS

Intrauterine lesions have been removed by a variety of methods. Enucleation of lesions with scissors has been described[35]. The Nd:YAG laser has been successfully used with sapphire tips (Surgical Laser Technology Corporation, Malvern, PA) (Loffer F.D., unpublished observations) and bare Nd:YAG fibers[36–38]. The energy from the Nd:YAG laser can be used to transect the base of polypoid lesions, transect sessile lesions into small pieces, or necrose larger lesions. Polyp snares may also be used in pedunculated lesions[39]. Hysteroscopic

evaluation of the uterine cavity to identify the location of the lesions followed by wide dilatation with laminaria will also allow ring forceps to be placed in the uterine cavity and the lesion to be evulsed from the uterine cavity[40].

However, it is the unipolar or bipolar resectoscopes that are most ideally designed to remove intrauterine lesions. Although the resectoscope requires more dilatation than scissors, snares or the Nd:YAG laser, it is generally more versatile. It requires less cervical dilatation and is, therefore, probably less potentially damaging to the cervix than the evulsion technique. It is suitable for all operable lesions and, when appropriate waveform and power settings are used, will limit the area of surrounding tissue destruction (see Chapter 2). The continuous-flow resectoscope should always allow adequate visualization, even when patients are bleeding heavily. Hemostasis from the transected area is easily obtained, and chips can be sent to pathology for histological review. Because of these features, most hysteroscopists are now using the resectoscope for the removal of uterine leiomyomas and endometrial polyps.

TECHNIQUES OF USING THE RESECTOSCOPE

Patient preparation prior to surgery does not need to be extensive. A few authors use laminaria to soften and dilate the cervix prior to the procedure[24,26]. Prophylactic antibiotics are often used by some authors[12,13,16,18,22,26,30,31], but, many others do not use them and have not reported increased infections[21,23–25,28]. However, antibiotic prophylaxis would appear to be advantageous in patients with a past history of pelvic inflammatory disease[41]. When a very large fibroid is to be resected, an attempt to reduce its size can be made with the use of leuprolide acetate (TAP Pharmaceutical, Inc., Lake Forest, IL, USA) (see Chapter 5).

The most commonly used resectoscopes are monipolar instruments, in which case the uterine cavity is distended with a low-viscosity non-electrolyte-containing fluid, such as sorbitol, glycine or mannitol. A 5% mannitol solution is almost iso-osmolar and acts as a diuretic. These two qualities are not shared by glycine or sorbitol, thus 5% mannitol has significant advantages when non-electrolyte solutions for unipolar equipment are used. A diluted dextran 70 solution or dextrose and water can also be used. Undiluted dextran 70 and CO_2 are not suited for use with the continuous-flow resectoscope. Water should not be used as intravasation will cause intravascular hemolysis.

A bipolar resectoscope is available which has the safety of bipolar energy and must be used with normal saline as a distending medium. This significantly decreases the risks associated with non-electrolyte distending media[42].

Traditional resectoscopic equipment has been described in detail elsewhere (see Chapter 2). The usual telescope used has a foroblique lens with an angle of view ranging between 12° and 30°. A zero degree endoscope can also be used[18]. It is this author's preference to use a 30° telescope. Although this makes observation of the fully extended electrode more difficult, it does make it easier to look behind polyps and myomas, and to see where they lie in the uterine cavity.

Traditional unipolar resectoscopic technique

The usual electrode used is a 90° loop. The electrode is advanced beyond the end of the telescope by moving the thumb ring forward. When fully extended, it may start to leave the field of view. When pressure on the thumb ring is relaxed, the built-in tension of the instrument will cause the loop to traverse back towards the end of the telescope and to be withdrawn into the insulated end of the resectoscope. In order to resect the largest amount of tissue possible at any given time, the loop electrode will have to be placed behind the material to be cut. It is often troubling to the novice hysteroscopist that the loop is then hidden by the tissue to be resected. It must be remembered that the loop is electrically activated only when being brought towards the end of the telescope. Therefore, only the tissue lying

between the outstretched loop and the end of the telescope will be transected (Figure 2). Very occasionally, in order to undercut a piece of tissue, the electronically activated loop may be advanced for a short distance under direct vision.

If there is any question as to where the loop lies relative to other structures, such as the tubal ostia, it is possible, using a 30° telescope, to advance the loop only slightly beyond the end of the telescope and to place it under direct vision. Then the loop is advanced at the same speed that the resectoscope is withdrawn. This results in the loop staying in its original position even though it is fully extended from the end of

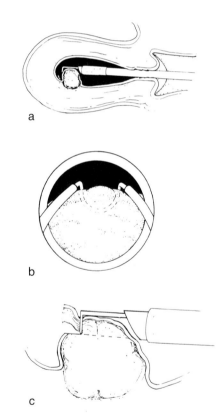

Figure 2 Placement of the loop electrode to maximize the size of the chip. (a) In order for the largest possible chip to be obtained, it is necessary to place the loop behind the lesion to be transected. (b) Although the loop is out of sight, the depth is limited by the supporting arms of the electrode. (c) The only tissue that will be cut is that which lies between the end of the resectoscope and the electrode

the resectoscope. This maneuver allows a full cut to be obtained (Figure 3).

In the above descriptions, while cutting chips only the electrode is moved. The resectoscope does not move relative to the uterine cavity. At times, when a lesion is particularly large, it is advantageous to start the resection as described above, and when the loop is approximately halfway towards the end of the telescope, the whole resectoscope can be withdrawn a short distance before the electrode is allowed to close into the end of the instruments (Figure 4).

As tissue is cut, it will frequently pull up against the end of the telescope and momentarily obstruct view. When this occurs, visualization can be achieved by advancing the electrode without any electrical current being applied. Another troublesome problem is that tissue will frequently stick to the electrode. When this

occurs, it may fall free when the loop is repositioned for the next resection. If it does not, it will separate as soon as the next resection is begun.

Generally, power settings of 100–110 W of a continuous (cut) current provide a good cutting effect. Since the electrode is literally cutting through tissue on a bed of sparks, the operator should feel little resistance as the loop comes back towards the resectoscope (see Chapter 12). In order to facilitate this arcing, the foot pedal of the generator should be keyed just prior to the electrode making contact with the tissue to be resected. If the operator feels that the electrode is dragging as it passes through the tissue, either the power setting is too low or the electrode is being drawn too quickly through the tissue. A blend waveform is not necessary since bleeding from the transected surfaces is seldom a problem. Occasionally, however, a smaller arterial bleeder will be visualized as a small geyser of blood. The loop can be placed against this and a short burst of 40 W of a modulated (coagulating) current will be sufficient to stop the bleeding.

Bubbles and other small debris can be a problem, especially when working on the anterior surface of the uterine cavity. It is the continuous flow design of the gynecological resectoscope that allows the cavity to be quickly cleaned by a rapid turnover of the distending medium.

It is this author's preference to use gravity to distend the uterus with low-viscosity media. Mechanical pumps may be used, but they do not provide additional safety. Fluid monitoring devices, however, are extremely important. Manual tracking of fluids is frought with many potential errors. In this set-up the bag of distending medium is raised approximately 1 m above the level of the patient. A wide-bore Y-shaped urological tubing must be used. This generates a pressure of approximately 50–75 mmHg with an adequate flow rate and allows for changing of new bags without disruption of flow of distending medium. The outflow part of the resectoscope is connected to wall suction. This not only allows measurement of the amount of fluids removed from the uterus

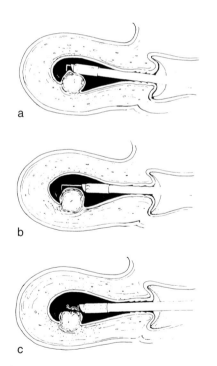

Figure 3 Placing the electrode under direct vision. (a) The electrode is placed under direct vision; (b) the resectoscope is withdrawn at the same speed that the electrode is advanced. This results in the loop being fully extended without altering the placement of the electrode. (c) Resection can now be performed

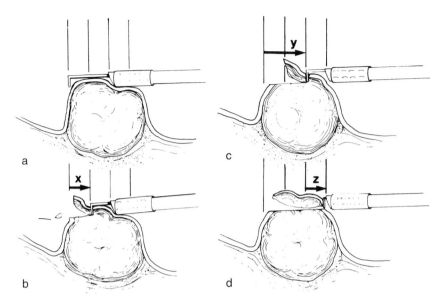

Figure 4 Increasing the length of chips removed by movement of both the electrode and the resectoscope. (a) The loop is placed fully extended (see Figure 2a and b); (b) the loop is partially closed resecting a portion (x) of the chip; (c) the resectoscope is then withdrawn without further closing of the loop thus enlarging the length of the chip to y; (d) finally, the loop is closed into the resectoscope completing the formation of a long chip by resecting to z

but also facilitates cleansing of the cavity. The outflow is generally kept partially closed to reduce the amount of fluid used. When necessary to clear the cavity of bloody bubbles or debris rapidly, it can temporarily be opened fully.

When sessile lesions are at the top of the uterine fundus, it may be difficult to shave them down with a 90° electrode; 180° electrodes are available. No thumb action is required with a 180° electrode except to advance the tip beyond the end of the telescope to provide adequate visualization. Movement of the scope from one side to the other will then allow the electrode to shave the fundal fibroid to the level of the uterine cavity.

When a polypoid structure is being removed, it is possible to transect the base by dropping the 90° electrode into the stalk. It may be necessary to do this in more than one side of the stalk. Frequently, part of the stalk remains after the body of the polypoid structure is removed. It can then be shaved off at the level of the uterine wall after the polyp has been taken out of view. Care must be taken that the

pedunculated lesion is either soft and pliable enough or small enough to be removed through the cervix. A large pedunculated leiomyoma might be easily transected and then be very difficult to remove from the uterine cavity. Larger pedunculated lesions should be shaved into smaller portions. Lesions have been left in the uterine cavity; however, this does not allow histological evaluation, is troublesome to the patient, and is less than optimal in infertility patients.

Unless they are small, sessile leiomyomas are generally not resected unless at least 40–50% is projecting into the uterine cavity. When < 40–50% of the leiomyoma is projecting into the cavity, it becomes difficult to determine how large the remaining portion is that needs to be resected. Fibroids are not always round, and the depth of the intramural portion may be rather extensive (Figure 5). Concomitant laparoscopy is generally not used since it is neither necessary nor wise actually to resect below the level of the endometrial cavity. Perforation should not occur if this principle is not violated.

In those leiomyomas where a significant portion is intramural, a technique initially described by this author can be used to facilitate complete removal (Figure 6). In order to avoid the risk of perforation of the uterus, the leiomyoma is shaved only to the level of the

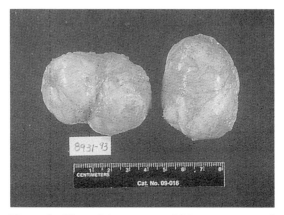

Figure 5 These leiomyomas, which were removed intact through an abdominal incision, show that the shape of leiomyomas is not always round. More may lie intramural than is apparent on hysteroscopic view. A grading scale as proposed[36] would probably have correctly identified the degree of intramural extension for the leiomyoma on the right. However, the constricted area as seen on the specimen on the left could have given the impression that the intramural portion was smaller than that projecting into the uterine cavity. See also Color Plate VIII

uterine cavity. When the uterus is allowed to contract for the removal of the chips, the leiomyoma will be literally squeezed by the contracting uterine musculature out of its intramural location. This author has not found it necessary to use medication to facilitate the uterus contracting. Using this technique, all of the intramural portion can usually be removed. Occasionally with very large growths, a repeat procedure may be necessary.

This process of removing large sessile myomas is facilitated if the edges, as they enter the intramural portion, are initially resected, thus 'pedunculizing' the myoma. After the extent of the intramural portion has been identified, and in large part removed, that portion of the leiomyoma projecting into the cavity can then be shaved into smaller pieces[43].

As the intramural portion is extruded into the uterine cavity, its white, firm and smooth capsule is readily visible and appears differently from the surrounding myometrium. The latter generally appears as criss-crossing bands of myometrium with large, open channels.

When the leiomyoma is relatively large, numerous chips are created and, eventually, the resectoscope will have to be removed and the chips retrieved before the case can continue. Removal of these chips is a nuisance. Usually, a large one can be trapped against the

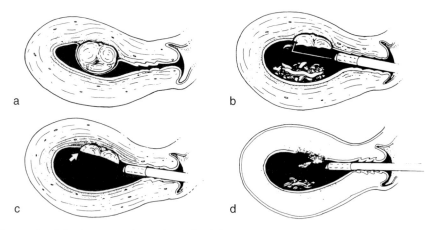

a   b

c   d

Figure 6 Removal of the intramural portion of a leiomyoma. (a) The sessile myoma before resection; (b) resection is carried down to the level of the uterine cavity; (c) each time the uterus is allowed to empty, the intramural portion is pushed further into the uterine cavity; (d) finally, the base is level with the uterine cavity and can be completely removed. Adapted from reference 20. © Copyright 1990, with permission from American College of Obstetricians and Gynecologists

end of the telescope by the loop electrode as the instrumentation is removed from the uterus. Polyp forceps and small curettes are then used to remove the remaining free chips. However, even when the uterine cavity appears to have been completely explored by these blind methods, there often are numerous chips remaining.

New biopolar resectoscope technique

The equipment and techniques are similar to the unipolar resectoscope technique. The significant benefits of this instrumentation as compared to traditional unipolar resectoscopic equipment are its bipolar safety and the fact that physiological normal saline can and must be used as the distending medium. There is a traditional loop electrode which is used in the same fashion. The greatest difference, however, is a block-shaped vaporizing electrode. This author has found this to extend his ability to remove larger sessile fibroids at a single surgery[42]. In a sessile myoma this technique is accomplished by vaporizing a large section down the middle. This effectively cuts it into two halves. Then the attached base is vaporized and a large piece is removed for histological evaluation. The other half can be vaporized or similarly removed. The procedure can be finished more quickly because there are no large number of chips to remove.

Concomitant endometrial ablation

In those patients in whom fertility is not an issue, consideration should be given also to performing an endometrial ablation along with removal of the leiomyoma. This author has found this has greatly improved long-term results. Possible reasons for this observation are that other factors, such as adenomyosis, may be contributing to the heavy menstrual flow and a cavity made smaller by endometrial ablation may be less prone to develop new submucosal myoma. When endometrial ablation is performed, this author prefers to use a rolling technique before the actual resection

of the uterine lesion. The reasons for this are that the endometrial surface is much more easily visualized, and missed areas of ablation are less likely to occur. In addition, there are not yet any vascular spaces open, and intravasation of the distending medium is much less of a problem.

RISKS

Fluid intravasation is the single greatest risk during the resection of intrauterine lesions (see Chapters 6 and 20). Some intravasation will occur with all hysteroscopic cases[42]. It is increased when vascular channels are open, such as during resection procedures. Cases of long duration will allow more fluid to intravasate than shorter ones. Excessive distending pressure will drive fluid faster into these channels. Removal of intrauterine lesions is often of long duration, in which cases numerous vascular channels are open. This predisposes these procedures to a high risk of intravasation.

The hysteroscopist has little control over the size of the lesion and the number of vascular channels that are opened. Since there is some control over the length of the procedure, the surgeon should make every effort to progress through the surgery as rapidly as is safely possible. The one factor that the surgeon has complete control over is the amount of pressure used to distend the uterus. Pressure of 60–70 mmHg is quite adequate for appropriate uterine distention. Higher pressures are not necessary. They do not provide better visualization or cleaning of the uterine cavity! They do significantly increase the risks of intravasation. Since some intravasation is inevitable, strict intake and output of the low-viscosity fluids used should always be maintained. Preferably a fluid monitor will be used and fluid management guidelines followed[45].

It has been this author's experience that the deficit between the fluid used and retrieved is infrequently a problem when 60–75 mmHg pressure is used. However, when the deficit approaches 1000 ml, it most likely will rapidly exceed that amount. Routine electrolytes and diuretics are not necessary. However, when the deficit is approximately 1500 ml, 20 mg of intravenous furosemide is given and serum electrolytes drawn. A slightly greater deficit can be accepted if mannitol is used, since it is almost iso-osmolar and has diuretic action. Preparation should be made for the case to be brought to a conclusion, even if the lesion has not been completely resected. Using these criteria, this author has not had significant problems. When the bipolar resectoscope is used over 2000 ml of normal saline can be allowed provided that a diuretic is used and the amount of fluid intravasated is never allowed to exceed measured outflow and urinary outflow by 2000 ml.

Cervical lacerations occur from either the tenaculum or the dilatation of the cervix to accommodate these large-diameter instruments. Single-tooth tenacula easily tear the cervix. It is this author's preference to use a Jacob tenaculum, which secures the cervix better than a single-tooth tenaculum. Some authors use laminaria the night before the surgery to dilate the cervix, thus not only avoiding tearing the tenaculum off the cervix during dilatation but also reducing the risk of lacerating the upper cervix and lower uterine segment. Small lacerations of the cervix and lower uterine segment are commonly seen and may account for some of the intravasation experienced. However, many cervices are soft and require little dilatation. This is especially so if the patient has been bleeding heavily and passing clots.

Perforation of the uterus should be an infrequent problem, since transection of the lesion is never carried out below the level of the uterine cavity. Perforation may occur during dilatation and entrance of the resectoscope, or if the operator becomes disoriented. Obturators are available with all sheaths and are often helpful in introducing instruments. The resectoscope and telescope can then be introduced afterwards. The visual obturator (Circon ACMI, Southborough, MA, USA) is especially helpful in that it allows obturation under direct visualization.

Electrical injuries are always a potential risk[46]. However, they seldom occur since a continuous (cutting) waveform will have minimal spread to adjacent tissue, and injury should occur only with a perforation. Electrical injuries at the ground plate can be avoided if a REM-type system is used. Damage beyond the uterine cavity can rarely occur if the loop is not placed below the level of the uterus or advanced blindly. Therefore, most authors do not believe laparoscopic guidance need be routinely used.

Postoperative bleeding is generally not a problem. Most patients have an initial brisk and heavy flow of blood immediately following the procedure. Some of this volume is from the distending medium and makes the blood loss appear greater than it actually is. Generally, the uterus quickly contracts and the bleeding slows and stops just as it does in a postpartum uterus. This process can be facilitated by injecting into the cervix a diluted Pitressin® solution (0.3 units in 10 ml of normal saline). Foley catheters and balloons are available to tamponade the uterus, but in this author's experience, they are seldom necessary.

Postoperative adhesions in the patient desiring fertility can occur. This is probably an increased problem if two fibroids have been removed and the raw surfaces are in that position. Estrogens can be used to facilitate covering the surface if this risk appears to be high.

POSTOPERATIVE MANAGEMENT

Postoperatively, these patients will experience minimal discomfort. The need for considerable pain relief should alert the surgeon to the possibility that an intra-abdominal injury may have occurred. Pre- and postoperative non-steroidal anti-inflammatory drugs are helpful. These and several oxycodone tablets are sufficient to control uterine cramping. Recovery appears to be related more to the amount of distending medium intravasated and the length of the anesthesia than to any other factor. Patients are told that they can expect a bloody, watery discharge that should not be heavy. It should become progressively less over the period of time until the next menses.

RESULTS

Results of this procedure can be assessed by considering the peer review literature. There were 17 series found that gave results for the resection of leiomyomas. Indications for the surgery and whether concomitant endometrial ablation was used are listed in Table 1. The majority of cases were performed for problems of abnormal bleeding. Only a few patients were done solely because of infertility/pregnancy wastage. The exact number who had both abnormal bleeding and fertility problems was often difficult to determine.

Results of resectoscopic removal of intra-uterine lesions are listed in Table 2. Pregnancy rates for patients ranged from 33.3 to 66.6% and the control of bleeding occurred in from 73.4 to 100% of patients. It is difficult to obtain exact figures, since some reports do not differentiate between results achieved by only the resection of lesions and those in which only ablation procedures were performed. In addition, some authors do not state if patients were trying to become pregnant before hysteroscopic removal of the lesion or only afterwards. Finally, the figures concerning results in some reports are not consistent throughout the articles. Nevertheless, very good results appear to consistently achieved.

Other reports in the literature suggest a pregnancy rate of 47–52.8% after removal of a submucosal myoma and of 78.3% after removal of an endometrial polyp[47–49]. Failure to control bleeding may be immediate and result from incomplete resection or concomitant problems, such as adenomyosis, or they may be long term, resulting from the same problems that occur early as well as the growth of new fibroids. Infertility patients may fail to achieve a pregnancy because of coexisting problems in addition to intrauterine lesion.

Complications experienced by those surgeons with considerable experience have been few, indicating that this can be a safe procedure (Table 3). The risk of excessive fluid intravasation always exists; the literature

Table 1 Indications for removal of intrauterine lesions with or without associated endometrial ablation

| Study | Indications | | | | No. with ablation |
	No. of cases	AUB	Infertility	Both	
Derman et al., 1991[29]	108*	79	15	0	NS
Haning et al., 1980[12]	1	1	0	0	0
DeCherney and Polan, 1983[13]	14	14	0	0	0
Lim et al., 1986 and 1988[16,17]	31	31	0	0	11
Hallez, 1995[18]	284	253	31	NS	0
Corson and Brooks, 1991[21]	92	80	12	NS	0
Serden and Brooks, 1991[22]	120	120	NS	NS	30
Indman, 1993[23]	51	51	NS	NS	38
Wortman and Daggett, 1991[24]	26	26	NS	NS	22
Townsend et al., 1993[25]	95	95	0	0	50
Itzkowic, 1993[26]	37†	36	0	1	9
Hamou, 1993[27]	103	69	34	0	36
Pace, 1993[28]	126	108	18	0	0
Wamstecker et al., 1993[30]	51	39	0	12	0
Istre et al., 1993[31]	21	21	0	0	21
Emanuel et al., 1999[32]	285	285	0	0	0
Loffer	200	175	5	15	75

*14 cases lost to follow-up; †1 case lost to follow-up; AUB, abnormal uterine bleeding; NS, not stated

Table 2 Successful results (%) obtained using the resectoscope for removal of intrauterine lesions. Data in parentheses are numbers of patients

Study	Infertility/pregnancy wastage		Abnormal bleeding	
Derman et al., 1991[29]	NS		73.4	(58/79)
Haning et al., 1980[12]	NS		100	(1/1)
DeCherney and Polan, 1983[13]	NS		100	(14/14)
Lim et al., 1986 and 1988[16,17]	0		96.7	(30/31)
Hallez, 1995[18]	56.3	(18/32)	67.6	(68/73)
Corson and Brooks, 1991[21]	66.6	(8/12)	81.3	(65/80)
Serden and Brooks, 1991[22]	NS		91.6	(98/107)
Indman, 1993[23]	NS		94.1	(48/51)
Wortman and Daggett, 1991[24]	0		95.5	(21/22)
Townsend et al., 1993[25]	0		97.9	(93/95)
Itzkowic, 1993[26]	NS		91.9	(34/37)
Hamou, 1993[27]	55.9	(19/34)	92.7	(64/69)
Pace, 1993[28]	NS		98.0	(99/101)
Wamstecker et al., 1993[30]	33.3	(4/12)[†]	94.1	(48/51)
Istre et al., 1993[31]	NS		81.0	(17/21)*
Emanuel et al., 1999[32]	NS		90.3	—
Loffer	46.6	(7/15)	88	(175/200)
Total	46.4	(39/84)	89.4	(829/927)

*At 106 months; [†]estimated, exact figures not given; NS, not stated

Table 3 Complications occurring with resectoscopic removal of intrauterine lesions

Study	No. of cases	Complication					
		Excess fluid absorption	Uterus perforation	Electrical injury	Bleeding	Infection	Resulting laposcopy
Derman et al., 1991[29]	108	0	0	0	4	0	2
Haning et al., 1980[12]	1	0	0	0	0	0	0
DeCherney and Polan, 1983[13]	14	0	0	0	0	0	0
Lim et al., 1986 and 1988[16,17]	31	0	0	0	0	0	0
Hallez, 1995[18]	284	NS	1	0	0	0	1
Corson and Brooks, 1991[21]	92	0	3	0	1	1	0
Serden and Brooks, 1991[22]	120	1	1	0	4	2	0
Indman, 1993[23]	51	2	0	0	1	0	0
Wortman and Daggett, 1991[24]	26	0	0	0	2	0	0
Townsend et al., 1993[25]	95	0	0	0	0	0	0
Itzkowic, 1993[26]	37	1	0	0	8	1	1
Hamou, 1993[27]	103	NS	NS	NS	NS	NS	NS
Pace, 1993[28]	126	0	0	0	1	0	0
Wamstecker et al., 1993[30]	51	0	1	0	0	0	0
Loffer	200	4	3	0	2	1	0

NS, not stated

contains many reports[43], and many others are never reported. Strict intake and output of distending media must be maintained. Occasional perforation of the uterus during dilatation, insertion of the scope, or retrieval of chips may occur. Perforation with an activated electrode should be very uncommon. The risk of serious bleeding requiring some management, such as with an intrauterine balloon, occurred in only 2.2% of cases. Transfusions were generally not necessary.

In reviewing case series reports, it is clear that those patients presenting with infertility or pregnancy wastage are frequently helped, although there are often coexisting factors. Menorrhagia is controlled in the majority of patients, but since the uterus remains, a failure rate can be expected and patients should be aware of this.

After reviewing the long-term results of his own series, this author has concluded that concomitant ablation in those patients not desiring fertility may significantly improve the results obtained in controlling bleeding. The benefits may result from constricting the cavity, thus decreasing the chance of further submucous fibroid growth. It may also improve results in those patients who have adenomyosis. This author has further concluded that those patients in whom pain is a significant component of their problem are probably not well served by undergoing resection with or without ablation since only the discomfort of the passage of blood clots can be guaranteed to be controlled.

CLINICAL PEARLS

(1) Most submuous myomas and clinically significant endometrial polyps are not identified by blind procedures, such as a dilatation and curettage, or endometrial biopsy.

(2) Patients with significant dysmenorrhea should understand that their pain may not be helped by removal of the polyp or fibroid.

(3) Although the risk of malignancy is low, tissue removed should always undergo pathological evaluation.

(4) Resection of myoma should not be carried below the level of the uterine cavity.

(5) The intramural portion can frequently be completely removed by allowing the uterus to contract and, thus, project the remaining part of the myoma into the cavity.

(6) Resectoscopic removal of submucous myomas may be accomplished by significant fluid intravasation.

References

1. Gimpleson RJ, Rappold HO. A comparative study between panoramic hysteroscopy with directed biopsies and dilatation and curettage. *Am J Obstet Gynecol* 1988;158:489–92
2. Loffer FD. Hysteroscopy with selective endometrial sampling compared with D&C for abnormal uterine bleeding: the value of a negative hysteroscopic view. *Obstet Gynecol* 1989;73:16–20
3. Kessler I, Lancet M. Hysterography and hysteroscopy: a comparison. *Fertil Steril* 1984;46:709–10
4. Snowden EU, Jarrett JC II, Dagwood MY. Comparison of diagnostic accuracy of laparoscopy, hysteroscopy and hysterosalpingography in evaluation of female infertility. *Fertil Steril* 1984;41:708–13
5. Valle RF, Sciarra JJ. Current status of hysteroscopy in gynecologic practice. *Fertil Steril* 1979;32:619–32
6. Fedele L, Bianchi S, Dorta M, *et al.* Transvaginal ultrasonography versus hysteroscopy in the diagnosis of uterine submucous myomas. *Obstet Gynecol* 1991;77:745–8
7. Goldstein SR, Nachtigall M, Snyder JR, *et al.* Endometrial assessment by vaginal ultrasonography before endometrial sampling in patients with postmenopausal bleeding. *Am J Obstet Gynecol* 1990;163:119–23

8. Randolph JR, Ying YK, Maier DB, *et al.* Comparison of real-time ultrasonography, hysterosalpingography, and laparoscopy/hysteroscopy in the evaluation of uterine abnormalities and tubal patency. *Fertil Steril* 1986;46:828–32

9. Widrich T, Bradley L, Mitchinson AR, *et al.* Comparision of saline infusion sonography with hysteroscopy for the evaluation of the endometrium. *Am J Obstet Gynecol* 1996;174:1327–34

10. Norment WB, Sikes, Berry FX, *et al.* Hysteroscopy. In Turcle R, ed. *Surgical Clinics of North America.* Chicago: WB Saunders, 1957:1377–86

11. Neuwirth RS. A new technique for an additional experience with hysteroscopic resection of submucous fibroids. *Am J Obstet Gynecol* 1978;131: 91–4

12. Haning RV, Harkins PG, Uehling DT. Preservation of fertility by transcervical resection of a benign mesodermal uterine tumor with the resectoscope and glycine distending media. *Fertil Steril* 1980;33:209–10

13. DeCherney AH, Polan ML. Hysteroscopic management of intrauterine lesions and intractable uterine bleeding. *Obstet Gynecol* 1983; 61:392–7

14. Neuwirth RS. Hysteroscopic management of symptomatic submucous fibroids. *Am J Obstet Gynecol* 1983;62:509–11

15. Loffer FD. Hysteroscopic management of menorrhagia. *Acta Eur Fertil* 1986;17:463–5

16. Lin BL, Miyamoto N, Aoki R, *et al.* Transcervical resection of submucous myoma. *Acta Obstet Gynecol Jpn* 1986;38:1647–52

17. Lin BL, Miyamoto N, Tomomater M, *et al.* The development of a new hysteroscopic resectoscope and its clinical applications on transcervical resection (TCR) and endometrial ablation (EA). *Jpn J Obstet Gynecol Endosc* 1988;4:56–61

18. Hallez JP. Single stage total hysteroscopic myomectomies: indications, techniques and results. *Fertil Steril* 1995;63:703–8

19. Brooks PG, Loffer FD, Serden SP. Resectoscopic removal of symptomatic intrauterine lesions. *J Reprod Med* 1989;34:435–7

20. Loffer FD. Removal of large symptomatic intrauterine growths by the hysteroscopic resectoscope. *Obstet Gynecol* 1990;76:836–40

21. Corson SL, Brooks PG. Resectoscopic myomectomy. *Fertil Steril* 1991;55:1041–4

22. Serden SP, Brooks PG. Treatment of abnormal uterine bleeding with the gynecologic resectoscope. *J Reprod Med* 1991;36:676–9

23. Indman PD. Hysteroscopic treatment of menorrhagia associated with uterine leiomyomas. *Obstet Gynecol* 1993;81:716–20

24. Wortman M, Daggett A. Hysteroscopic management of intractable uterine bleeding. A review of 103 cases. *J Reprod Med* 1991;38:505–10

25. Townsend DE, Fields G, McCausland A, *et al.* Diagnostic and operative hysteroscopy in the management of persistent postmenopausal bleeding. *Obstet Gynecol* 1993;82:419–21

26. Itzkowic D. Submucous fibroids: clinical profile and hysteroscopic management. *Aust NZ J Obstet Gynecol* 1993;33:63–7

27. Hamou J. Electroresection of fibroids. In Sutton CJG, Diamond M, eds. *Endoscopic Surgery for Gynecologists.* London: WB Saunders, 1993: 327–30

28. Pace S. Transcervical resection of benign endocavitary lesions. *Gynecol Endosc* 1993;2:165–9

29. Derman SG, Rehnstrom J, Neuwirth RS. The long-term effectiveness of hysteroscopic treatment of menorrhagia and leiomyomas. *Obstet Gynecol* 1991;77:591–4

30. Wamstecker K, Emanual MH, deKruix JH. Transcervical hysteroscopic resection of submucous fibroids for abnormal uterine bleeding: results regarding the degree of intramural extension. *Obstet Gynecol* 1993;32:736–40

31. Istre O, Skajaa K, Holm-Nielsen P, *et al.* The second-look appearance of the uterine cavity after resection of the endometrium. *Gynecol Endosc* 1993;2:159–63

32. Emanuel MH, Wamstecker K, Hart AAM, *et al.* Long term results of hysteroscopic myomectomy for abnormal uterine bleeding. *Obstet Gynecol* 1999;93:743–8

33. Wamstecker K, deBlok S. Diagnostic hysteroscopy: technique and documentation. In Sutton CJH, Diamond M, eds. *Endoscopy Surgery for Gynecologists.* London: WB Saunders, 1993: 263–76

34. Emanuel MH, Wamsteker K, Eastham WN, *et al.* Leiomyosarcoma or cellular leiomyoma diagnosed after hysteroscopical transcervical resection of a presumed leiomyoma. *Gynecol Endosc* 1992;1:161–4

35. Valle RF. Hysteroscopic removal of submucous leiomyomas. *J Gynecol Surg* 1990;6:89–96

36. Dequesne J, DeGrandi P. Focal treatment of uterine bleeding and infertility with Nd:YAG laser and flexible hysteroscopy. *Gynecol Surg* 1989;5:177–82

37. Baggish MS, Sze EHM, Morgan G. Hysteroscopic treatment of symptomatic submucous myomata uteri with the Nd:YAG laser. *J Gynecol Surg* 1989; 5:27–36

38. Donnez J, Gillerst S, Bourgonjon D, *et al.* Neodymium:YAG laser hysteroscopy in large submucous fibroids. *Fertil Steril* 1990;54: 999–1003

39. McLucas B. Diathermy polyp snare: a new modality for treatment of myomas and polyps. *Gynecol Endosc* 1992;1:107–10

40. Goldrath MH. Vaginal removal of the pedunculated submucous myoma: the use of laminaria. *Obstet Gynecol* 1987;70:670–2

41. McCausland VM, Fields GA, McCausland AM, *et al.* Tubo-ovarian abscesses after operative hysteroscopy. *J Reprod Med* 1993;38:198–200

42. Loffer FD. Preliminary experiences with VersaPoint bipolar resectoscope using a vaporizing electrode in a saline distending media. *J Am Assoc Gynecol Laparosc* 2000;7:498–502

43. Lim B-L, Iwata Y, Liu KH. Removing a large submucosal fibroid hysteroscopically with the two-resectocope method. *J Am Assoc Gynecol Laparosc* 1994;1:259–63

44. Loffer FD. Complications from uterine distention. In Corfman RS, Diamond MP, DeCherney AL, eds. *Complications of Laparoscopy and Hysteroscopy.* Boston: Blackwell Scientific Publications, 1993:177–86

45. Loffer FD, Bradley LD, Brill AI, *et al.* Hysteroscopic fluid monitoring guidelines. *J Am Assoc Gynecol Laparosc* 2000;7:167–8

46. Sullivan B, Kenney P, Seibel M. Hysteroscopic resection of fibroid with thermal injury to sigmoid. *Obstet Gynecol* 1992;80:546–7

47. Giatras K, Berkeley AS, Noyes N, *et al.* Fertility after hysteroscopic resection of submucous fibroids. *J Am Assoc Gynecol Laparosc* 1999;6:155–8

48. Goldenberg M, Sivan E, Sharabia Z, *et al.* Outcome of hysteroscopic resection of submucous myomas on infertility. *Fertil Steril* 1995;64:714–16

49. Varasiteh NN, Neuwirth RS, Levin B, *et al.* Pregnancy rate after hysteroscopic polypectomy and myomectomy in infertile women. *Obstet Gynecol* 1999;94:168–71

10

Tubal catheterization and falloposcopy

E. Confino

INTRODUCTION

For many years physicians have evaluated Fallopian tubes during laparotomy and using hysterosalpingography. More recently, this approach has shifted to endoscopic evaluation. Endoscopic imaging of the Fallopian tubes is an invasive method whereby distention of the abdominal wall allows proper visualization of the Fallopian tubes, uterus and ovaries. Physicians have consistently sought alternative, less-invasive methods of visualization of the uterine cavity and Fallopian tubes.

X-ray imaging of the uterus and Fallopian tubes requires the transcervical injection of contrast material. Early attempts to identify appropriate contrast materials required the use of iodinated media[1,2]. Hysterography is a fast and simple procedure which renders a projected image of the uterine cavity and Fallopian tubes. This procedure to evaluate the Fallopian tubes and the uterus remains widely practiced. Water-soluble and oil-based media are used with excellent radiological imaging of the reproductive tract and minimal complications due to contrast material intolerance. Different imaging techniques have been explored over the past decade, using alternative radiological methods, such as radioactive materials[3] and, more recently, high-resolution ultrasound with sonographic contrast materials[4]. Although the amount of radiation absorbed by the ovaries and Fallopian tubes is low and clinically negligible[5], the medical profession has continued its quest to eliminate radiation. Recent improvements in magnetic resonance imaging (MRI) technology are promising, but expensive. MRI equipment may delay or impede the conversion of this technology into a routine and cost-effective screening test[6].

Questions remain regarding the clinical relevance of endoscopic evaluation of the Fallopian tubes. The diagnostic algorithm involving invasive endoscopic procedures, such as laparoscopy, performed to evaluate the uterus and Fallopian tubes is less frequently applied[7].

Improvements in fiberoptic technology resulted in the development of falloposcopes and microendoscopes. These improved methods of endoscopic assessment did not change the medical assessment of the best means to evaluate the uterus and Fallopian tubes[8,9]. Variations on non-invasive imaging technology, including microlaparoscopy and hydrolaparoscopy, are also evolving[10].

Contrast ultrasound imaging of the uterine cavity has been widely accepted, displacing office hysteroscopy[11]. However, ultrasound-guided recanalization of the Fallopian tubes remains experimental and, to date, is not widely accepted[12].

This chapter focuses on endoscopic transcervical tubal catheterization performed to evaluate and treat the Fallopian tubes.

ENDOSCOPIC TRANSCERVICAL ACCESS TO THE FALLOPIAN TUBE

Pioneering transcervical catheterization of Fallopian tubes recanalized proximally occluded Fallopian tubes using wire guides under X-ray imaging[13]. Shortly after this early report of transcervical wire recanalization, transcervical balloon tuboplasty (Figure 1) was reported for the first time, following hysteroscopic recanalization of a proximally occluded Fallopian tube[14]. The early case report was followed by a pilot study which involved a series of hysteroscopic catheterizations and balloon tuboplasty cases with a first successful pregnancy[15]. Radiological wire recanalization of tubes was reported with similar results[16].

Hysteroscopic recanalization of the Fallopian tube requires visualization of the tubal ostia using a hysteroscope with an operating channel[17]. The ostium of the Fallopian tube is cannulated with a flexible catheter introduced through the operative channel of the hysteroscope (Figure 2). This catheter is wedged into the internal os and chromotubation is performed. A laparoscopic team observes the fimbriated end of the Fallopian tube to document patency following the injection of dye. Frequently, hydrotubation during proximal tubal cannulation results in patent Fallopian tubes observed during laparoscopy[18]. Separated adhesions and hydrostatic pressure dislodge endotubal plugs. An alternative pathology treated by proximal tubal cannulation is a spasm of the Fallopian tubes[19]. These two pathological conditions may be recanalized because of the hydrostatic pressure created at the tip of the catheter or falloposcope, introduced during hysteroscopy into the interstitial portion of the Fallopian tube, that successfully dislodges microplugs of proteinaceous debris[20].

The follow-up study of the transcervical balloon tuboplasty multicenter clinical trial revealed that long-term tubal patency following transcervical balloon tuboplasty occurred in three-quarters of the patients, with a lasting effect on tubal patency[21]. Tubal cannulation became the treatment of choice in patients with bilateral proximal tubal occlusion, thus replacing microsurgical tubal cornual anastomosis.

ANATOMICAL CONSIDERATIONS DURING HYSTEROSCOPIC TRANSCERVICAL TUBAL CATHETERIZATION

The performance of concomitant laparoscopy during hysteroscopic tubal cannulation allows evaluation of the anatomy of the distal Fallopian tube[15]. Laparoscopy identifies hydrosalpinges with severe peritubal and periovarian damage.

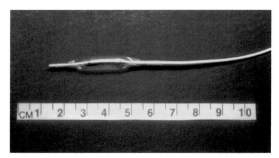

Figure 1 A transcervical balloon tuboplasty catheter equipped with a 3-mm balloon (Cook/Gyn, Bloomington, IN, USA). This catheter allowed introduction of the balloon into the cornual area and lateral stretching of the walls to achieve tubal recanalization. The size of the balloon was reduced subsequently to allow interstitial balloon tuboplasty of tubal occlusions and strictures

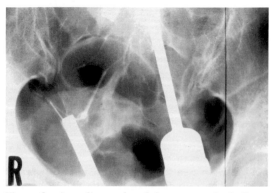

Figure 2 A radiograph of hysteroscopic balloon tuboplasty demonstrating the balloon catheter protruding from the tip of the hysteroscope in the lower field

Patients with a previous diagnosis of proximal occlusion later diagnosed with distal damage to the Fallopian tubes are re-routed to *in vitro* fertilization (IVF), frequently with a recommendation to perform salpingectomy to enhance their IVF pregnancy rates[22]. The additional advantage of concomitant laparoscopy during tubal cannulation is the ability of the laparoscopic team to stretch the Fallopian tube and ease the access of the wire guide or balloon catheter throughout the length of the Fallopian tube. Prior radiological knowledge of the level of tubal obstruction often improves the performance of this combined procedure (Figure 3). Table 1 describes the steps of endoscopic tubal catheterization.

Anatomical variations of the proximal Fallopian tube involve sharp angles of the interstitial portion of the Fallopian tube. An acute angle of the proximal Fallopian tube exceeding 90° makes tubal cannulation difficult, and risks tubal perforation with the wire guide. These perforations are usually of little clinical importance[23]. Once the interstitial proximal portions of the Fallopian tubes are catheterized and recanalized, there is no need to cannulate and advance the wire guide into the distal portion of the Fallopian tube[24]. The presence of surgically manageable peritubal adhesions causing proximal tubal occlusion can be detected during a combined laparoscopic–hysteroscopic approach. An external stricture of the Fallopian tube can be relieved using laparoscopic adhesiolysis. Selective injection of dye into that Fallopian tube performed by the hysteroscopic team will verify the success of adhesiolysis in recanalizing proximally occluded Fallopian tubes.

The narrow, fibrotic Fallopian tube represents an anatomical variant of proximal tubal occlusion. Indirect evidence derived from pressure studies of these Fallopian tubes suggests that narrow Fallopian tubes may benefit either from ballooning or dilatation, in cases with segmental stricture or rapid conversion to IVF[25,26]. Pressure profiles of narrow Fallopian tubes suggest that these tubes differ in physiology from normal Fallopian tubes. Follow-up of women with normal tubal perfusion pressures shows significantly higher pregnancy rates than occur in women with elevated tubal perfusion pressures[26].

In 5–10% of patients, tubal perforation will occur during tubal cannulation[9]. Tubal perforation usually occurs in the proximal portion of the Fallopian tube. Since the

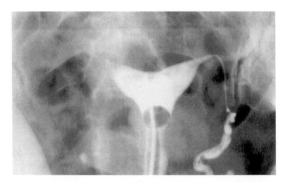

Figure 3 A radiograph depicting transcervical balloon tuboplasty performed under radiological guidance. An area of tubal stricture was catheterized in the isthmoampullary region. This patient demonstrates that in the absence of peritubal stricture, the radiological transcervical catheterization may offer some advantages in selected patients with interstitial stenosis or occlusion

Table 1 The steps involving hysteroscopic tubal cannulation in patients with proximal occlusion

Access hysteroscopically the endometrial cavity under saline distention

Identify the ostium of the Fallopian tubes

Introduce and wedge a curved catheter into the internal os

Inject water-soluble dye through the catheter into the Fallopian tube and observe the laparoscopic appearance of the proximal and distal Fallopian tube

Identify the presence of expelled mucus plugs from the fimbriae

If peritubal pathology is present and deemed relevant to tubal function, perform laparoscopic adhesiolysis and reinject dye through the proximal tube

If proximal occlusion is not relieved during selective injection of dye, advance a wire guide or a small balloon catheter into the proximal occlusion. Upon withdrawal of the wire guide or balloon catheter, selective injection of dye will verify successful recanalization of the Fallopian tube

diameter of wire guides is less than 1 mm, tubal perforation is unlikely to cause any significant bleeding or damage to adjacent organs. The laparoscopic team should identify the area of perforation to detect potential injury or bleeding[15].

Postprocedural infection is a potential complication. Postprocedural salpingitis is observed in fewer than 1% of procedures. Since this complication is rare, there is no need for antibiotic prophylaxis in patients prescreened for sexually transmitted diseases[23].

TRANSCERVICAL FALLOPOSCOPY

Endoscopic imaging of the Fallopian tube can be performed during laparoscopic evaluation of infertile patients[27,28]. Evaluation of salpingoscopy findings compared with fine anatomical architecture of the Fallopian tube reinforced the value of salpingoscopy[29]. The performance of salpingoscopy requires fimbrial cannulation of the Fallopian tube using saline distention with a small-diameter endoscope. Since only 10–20% of patients suffer from proximal tubal disease, the combination of laparoscopy and salpingoscopy allows a thorough evaluation of the Fallopian tube prior to corrective surgery[30]. If previous knowledge of tubal patency exists or chromotubation during laparoscopy reveals unilateral tubal patency, complete evaluation of the Fallopian tube requires integration of hysterosalpingogram and hysteroscopy[31].

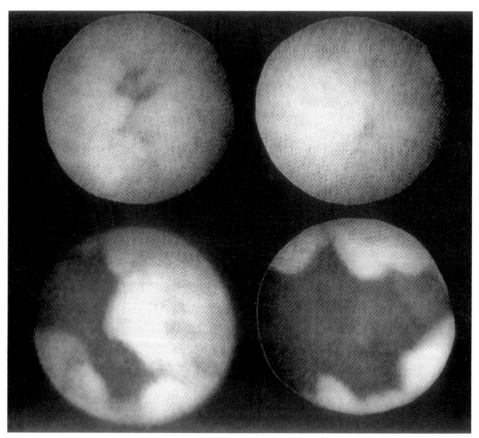

Figure 4 Falloposcopy images of the proximal Fallopian tube demonstrating a progression from the isthmic portion of the Fallopian tube in the upper portion of the figure to the endotubal folds typical of the proximal ampullary portion of the lower portion of the figure

Improvements in fiberoptic technology in the late 1980s reduced the endoscopic diameter to less than 1 mm, permitting transcervical tubal cannulation without concomitant laparoscopy[32] (Figure 4). The technique of transcervical falloposcopy requires introduction of a guide wire throughout the Fallopian tube and passage and advancement of the falloposcope over the guide wire[33]. An alternative method uses a linear eversion technology to unfold the catheter into the Fallopian tubes[34]. Clinical evaluation of falloposcopy revealed that additional endotubal pathology could be identified and classified in many patients[35]. This additional microendoscopic information could not be obtained based solely on the results of hysterosalpingogram or salpingoscopy. The advancement of the falloposcope into the tube was also potentially therapeutic. An early case of falloposcopic diagnosis and possible treatment of tubal pregnancy was reported[36]. The diagnosis of hydrosalpinx could be made during falloposcopy without the need to perform concomitant laparoscopy. Those patients with falloposcopically diagnosed hydrosalpinx could be re-routed to IVF, eliminating laparoscopic evaluation of the Fallopian tubes.

Although falloposcopy is non-invasive and well tolerated[37], the technique was never widely accepted because of the special expertise required; difficulty in imaging the Fallopian tube occurred because of 'white outs' caused by the proximity of the tubal walls. Many fertility clinics were reluctant to invest in the relatively expensive equipment. The limited therapeutic benefit of falloposcopy, combined with its complexity, required that this technique be simplified and made 'user friendly'. Falloposcopy and salpingoscopy continue to be under-utilized in the clinical evaluation of the Fallopian tubes, but this may change over time.

THE FUTURE OF TUBAL ENDOSCOPY

Endoscopic evaluation and treatment of the Fallopian tube are not used to their greatest potential in today's infertility practices. Improved pregnancy rates following *in vitro* fertilization make *in vivo* reproduction less attractive. Changing treatment algorithms which resulted in early re-routing of patients into IVF, regardless of the status of the Fallopian tubes, transformed this area from vibrant work in progress to a dormant alternative procedure. Practitioners infrequently use Fallopian tubes for assisted reproduction due to the superiority of uterine transfer of embryos, compared to tubal placement of gametes and embryos[38,39]. Notwithstanding the decreased interest in Fallopian tubes, the evaluation and use of the Fallopian tubes will remain a paramount factor in the practice and treatment of infertility.

References

1. Rubin IC. X-ray diagnosis in gynecology with the aid of intrauterine collargol injection. *Surg Gynecol Obstet* 1915;20:435
2. Sicard JA, Forestier J. Methode d'exploration radiologique par l'huile iodee (Lipiodol). *Bull Mem Soc Radiol Med* 1923;11:148
3. Antuaco TL, Boyd CM, London SN, *et al.* Technetium 99-m hysterosalpingography in infertility: an accurate alternative to contrast hysterosalpingograpy. *Radiographics* 1989;9:115
4. Dijkman AB, Mol BW, van der Veen F, *et al.* Can hysterosalpingocontrast-sonography replace hysterosalpingography in the assessment of tubal infertility? *Eur J Radiol* 2000;35:44–8
5. Hedgpeth PL, Thurmond AS, Fry R, *et al.* Radiographic fallopian tube recanalization: absorbed ovarian radiation dose. *Radiology* 1991; 180:121–2
6. Pelleritos JS, McCarthy SM, Doyle MB, *et al.* Diagnosis of uterine anomalies: relative accuracy of magnetic resonance imaging, endovaginal sonography and hysterosalpingography. *Radiology* 1992;183:795–800

7. Ayida G, Chamberlin P, Barlow D, *et al.* Is routine diagnostic laparoscopy for infertility still justified? *Hum Reprod* 1997;12:1436–9

8. Lundberg S, Rasmussen C, Berg AA, *et al.* Falloposcopy in conjunction with laparoscopy: possibilities and limitations. *Hum Reprod* 1998; 13:1490–2

9. Rizquez C, Confino E. Transcervical tubal cannulation, past, present, and future. *Fertil Steril* 1993;60:211–26

10. Brosens I, Campo R, Gordts S. Office hydro-laparoscopy for the diagnosis of endometriosis and tubal infertility. *Obstet Gynecol* 1999;11:371–7

11. Sankpal RS, Confino E, Matzel A, *et al.* Investigation of the uterine cavity and fallopian tubes using three-dimensional saline sono-hysterosalpingography. *Int J Gynecol Obstet* 2001; 73:125–9

12. Stern JJ, Peters AJ, Coulam CB. Transcervical tuboplasty under ultrasonographic guidance: a pilot study. *Fertil Steril* 1991;56:359–61

13. Platia MP, Krudy AG. Transcervical fluoroscopic recanalization of proximally occluded oviduct. *Fertil Steril* 1985;44:704–6

14. Confino E, Friberg J, Gleicher N. Transcervical balloon tuboplasty. *Fertil Steril* 1986;46:963–6

15. Confino E, Friberg J, Gleicher N. Preliminary experience with transcervical balloon tuboplasty (TBT). *Am J Obstet Gynecol* 1988;159:370–5

16. Thurmond AS, Novy MJ, Uchida BT, *et al.* Fallopian tube obstruction: selection salping-ography and recanalization. *Radiology* 1987;163: 511–14

17. Daniell JF, Miller W. Hysteroscopic correction of cornual occlusion with resultant term pregnancy. *Fertil Steril* 1987;48:490–4

18. Sulak PJ, Letterie GS, Hayslip CC, *et al.* Hysteroscopic cannulation and lavage in the treatment of proximal tubal occlusion. *Fertil Steril* 1987;48:493–5

19. Thurmond A, Novy M, Rosch J. Terbutaline in diagnosis of interstitial fallopian tube obstruc-tion. *Invest Radiol* 1986;23:209–10

20. Kerin JF, Surrey ES, Williams DB, *et al.* Fallopo-scopic observations of endotubal isthmic plugs as a cause of reversible obstruction and their histological characterization. *J Laparoendosoc Surg* 1991;1:103–10

21. Gleicher N, Confino E, Coulam C, *et al.* The multicentre transcervical balloon tubo-plasty study: conclusions and comparison to alternative technologies. *Hum Reprod* 1993;8: 1264–71

22. Surrey ES, Schoolcraft WB. Laparoscopic management of hydrosalpinges before in-vitro fertilization-embryo transfer: salpingectomy versus proximal tubal occlusion. *Fertil Steril* 2001;75:612–17

23. Confino E, Tur-Kaspa I, DeCherney A, *et al.* Transcervical balloon tuboplasty: a multicenter study. *J Am Med Assoc* 1990;264:2079–82

24. Wiedemann R, Montag M, Sterzik K. Proximal tubal occlusion. A modern approach to the diag-nosis and treatment of proximal tubal occlusion. *Hum Reprod* 1996;11:1823–5

25. Jessup MJ, Grainger DA, Kluzak TR, *et al.* Diagnosing proximal tubal obstruction: evaluation of peak intrauterine pressures using four common cannula techniques in extirpated uteri. *Obstet Gynecol* 1993;81:732–5

26. Karande V, Pratt DE, Rabin DS, *et al.* The limited value of hysterosalpingography in assessing tubal status and fertility potential. *Fertil Steril* 1995; 6:1167–71

27. Cornier E, Reintuch MJ, Doucarra L. La fibro-tuboscopic ampullaire. *J Gynecol Obstet Biol Reprod* 1984;13:49

28. Brosen I, Boeckx W, Delattin P, *et al.* Salpingo-scopy: a new pre-operative diagnostic tool in tubal infertility. *Br J Obstet Gynaecol* 1987;94: 768–73

29. Herschlag A, Seifer DB, Carcanigiu ML, *et al.* Salpingoscopy: light microscopic and electron microscopic correlations. *Obstet Gynecol* 1991; 77:399–405

30. Henry-Suchet J, Loffredo V, Tesuier PJ. Endoscopy of the tube (= tuboscopy); its prognostic value of tuboplasty. *Acta Eur Fertil* 1985;16:139

31. Fayez JA, Mutie G, Schneider PJ. Clinical articles: the diagnostic value of hysterosalpingography and hysteroscopy in infertility investigation. *Am J Obstet Gynecol* 1987;156:558–60

32. Kerin J, Daykhovsky L, Grundfest W, *et al.* Falloposcopy: a microendoscopic transvaginal technique for diagnosing and treating endo-tubal disease incorporating guide wire cannulation and direct balloon tuboplasty. *J Reprod Med* 1990;35:606–12

33. Kerin J, Daykhovsky L, Segalwitz J, *et al.* Falloposcopy: a microendoscopic technique for visual exploration of the human fallopian tube from the uterotubal ostium to the fimbria using a transvaginal approach. *Fertil Steril* 1990;54: 390–400

34. Bauer O, Diedrich K, Bacich S, *et al.* Trans-cervical access and intra-luminal imaging of the fallopian tube in the non-anaesthetized patient; preliminary results using a new tech-nique for fallopian access. *Hum Reprod* 1992;7(Suppl 1):7–11

35. Kerin JF, Williams DB, San Roman GA, *et al.* Falloposcopic classification and treatment of fallopian tube lumen disease. *Fertil Steril* 1992; 57:731–41

36. Risquez J, Pennehoaut G, Foulot H, *et al.* Transcervical tubal cannulation and fallopo-

scopy for the management of tubal pregnancy. *Hum Reprod* 1992;7:274–5

37. Scudamore I, Dunphy B, Cooke I. Outpatient falloposcopy: intra-luminal imaging of the fallopian tube by trans-uterine fibre-optic endoscopy as an outpatient procedure. *Br J Obstet Gynaecol* 1992;99:829–35

38. Jansen RPS, Anderson JG, Radomic I, *et al.* Pregnancies after ultrasound guided fallopian tube insemination with cryostored donor semen. *Fertil Steril* 1988;49:920–2

39. Bauer O, Van der Ven H, Diedrich K, *et al.* Preliminary results on transvaginal tubal embryo stage embryo transfer (TV-TEST) without ultrasound guidance. *Hum Reprod* 1990;5:553–6

11

Hysteroscopic sterilization

J. A. Abbott and T. G. Vancaillie

INTRODUCTION

Female sterilization is the most common form of contraception worldwide. It is estimated that there are more than 100 million women who rely on permanent sterilization as a form of contraception[1]. There are a plethora of methods described for tubal sterilization, and transcervical techniques have been described since the middle of the 19th century, when chemical cautery was used to stenose the tube and induce sterility[2].

Initial reports of electrosurgical sterilization in the 1920s were associated with high morbidity, although the procedure was performed with hysteroscopic guidance[3]. There followed a quiescent period for hysteroscopic sterilization until the 1970s, when renewed interest in both blind and hysteroscopic techniques emerged as possible treatments to induce permanent sterilization. Whilst the morbidity from these procedures was not as high, success rates were low, and this approach to sterilization lost favor.

The 'third wave' of hysteroscopic sterilization arrived at the beginning of the 21st century, and technological advances have paved the way for new techniques that are easier to perform and may have greater efficacy than previous hysteroscopic sterilization techniques.

This chapter will review hysteroscopic sterilization through its evolution, to the present day, when the third wave has brought renewed hope that it will provide the advantages of permanent contraception, without the attendant risks associated with the transabdominal approach.

HISTORICAL PERSPECTIVE

Hysteroscopy has been described since 1869, when a woman was investigated for resistant vaginal bleeding[4]. The first reported use of the hysteroscope for sterilization was described in 1927, when animals were sterilized in this manner. The use of high-molecular weight fluid as a distention medium was not described until 1970[5]; CO_2 was introduced into widespread use 4 years later[6], although this method was initially reported in 1925[7].

The approaches to tubal sterilization are summarized below:

(1) Access may be:

    (a) Blind;

    (b) Radiological;

    (c) Visual (hysteroscopic).

(2) The methods for tubal occlusion are:

    (a) Chemical (caustic substances);

    (b) Mechanical (tubal blocking devices);

    (c) Thermal (electrosurgical and laser).

All combinations of access and occlusion methods have been attempted to try to effect high rates of closure, with low complication rates.

There follows a description of these methods for tubal occlusion followed by a review of the next generation of hysteroscopic sterilization techniques – the 'third wave'. The third wave of hysteroscopic sterilization techniques brings a new dimension, absent in previous attempts. Soft tissue implants are used to stimulate a tissue in growth response by the host, which eventually leads to occlusion of the tubal lumen.

CHEMICAL

Sclerosing chemicals have been described for many years as a possible means of occluding the Fallopian tubes. The main issue with sclerosing chemicals is that they may not be retained within the tube for a sufficient length of time to cause tubal occlusion. In addition, it is imperative that there should not be any loss of these substances into the peritoneal cavity, where their action would have deleterious effects. Some chemicals with powerful actions also have toxic side-effects and therefore may not be suitable for tubal occlusion.

The first description of chemical occlusion was by Zipper and colleagues[8], who described blind instillation of quinacrine into the uterine cavity to occlude the tubes. The most significant issue with this approach was the need for repeated applications of the substance to ensure that tubal occlusion occurred. Quinones and co-workers refined this technique by using hysteroscopic guidance and tubal catheterization to deliver a localized dose of quinacrine to the tube[9]. Despite these changes, there was a universally poor tubal occlusion rate, even with repeated applications of quinacrine and the technique has been abandoned.

Other chemical methods include the blind instillation of a phenol and atabrine paste into the uterine cavity[10]. The high success rates reported by the authors have not been confirmed in any other studies of this technique, which is not used outside South East Asia. Tetracycline has been demonstrated to produce poor results in the single reported human study[11].

Methyl cyanoacrylate (MCA) is a tissue adhesive that has been studied as a possible chemical sclerosant to induce tubal occlusion. The compound is injected into the tubes, where it polymerizes on contact with water and binds the tube closed. As it is degraded and removed from the tube it releases several products including formaldehyde, which permanently fuses the tube. The MCA method of occlusion was developed in conjunction with a delivery device, the Femcept® (BioNexus Inc., Raleigh, NC, USA), that was designed to instil a measured amount of MCA to the tube. Initial reports from Richart and co-workers demonstrated an 89% tubal occlusion rate after two instillations of MCA via the Femcept[12].

MECHANICAL

Numerous techniques for mechanical occlusion by permanent or semipermanent devices have been described. These devices may be either pre-formed or formed in place and have had variable success.

Pre-formed

Of the pre-formed devices, only a few have reached clinical investigation in humans. The first is the ceramic plug, which has been investigated only in women immediately prior to hysterectomy[13]. This rigid plug is found to require considerable skill to place, and technical difficulties are commonly a cause for failure of device placement. Uterine perforation has been reported and the device is not currently being investigated further.

Brundin's hydrogelic tubal plug[14], or P-block device, has a nylon skeleton with nylon anchors to prevent tubal migration immediately after placement. The gel contains MCA to aid tubal occlusion. Initial reports on this device are poor, with bilateral tubal occlusion reported in only 43% of women in whom it was fitted. Further work on this device (now in its ninth version) has resulted in an increased diameter of the plug which has led to an increase in success. For this version, 191 women were treated with significantly higher success rates, although plug migration and pregnancies have both been reported[14].

Hamou and colleagues described an intra-tubal device[15] that consists of a nylon thread with loops at both ends to prevent migration, and also allows for device retrieval with the intention of producing a reversible contra-ceptive effect. The device does not occlude the tube *per se* and whilst it has a high rate of successful placement, pregnancies have been reported[16].

Hosseinian and associates described a poly-ethylene plug delivered to the tubal ostia via a specialized cannula. The plug is placed into the tube, with migration being prevented by four anchoring metal spines that penetrate into the surrounding myometrium[17]. Tubal occlusion has been reported in 90% of tubes, although pregnancy occurred in six of 44 women. Plug removal is possible and tubal patency following removal is reported to be 90%.

Sugimoto described a pre-formed silicone plug, which is delivered to the tube under hysteroscopic guidance[18]. Initial reports of high success rates for this device have not had long-term follow-up.

A recent report describes the use of a hysteroscopically placed screw to achieve tubal occlusion[19]. The procedure has been through a number of technical changes to its current level, although clinical studies have not yet been reported.

Figure 1 illustrates a number of these differ-ent occlusive devices.

Formed in place

The use of silicone to occlude the tubes mechanically was first described in 1966[20]. This technique involves the instillation of liquid silicone under hysteroscopic guidance into the tube, with a rubber obturator placed at the uterine ostium after injection. The obturator

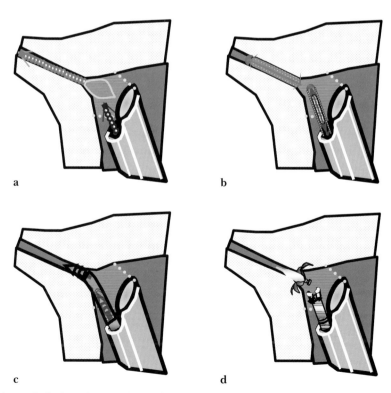

Figure 1 Pre-formed devices for mechanical occlusion. a, Intratubal device; b, hydrogelic tubal plug; c, silicon plug; d, polyethylene plug

binds to the silicone and a flexible plug, larger at both ends than in the middle, is formed[21]. A loop embedded into the obturator makes removal of the plug possible, although the patency of the tube following the removal of the preformed plug is not guaranteed[22]. Pregnancies have been reported following removal of the plugs[23].

The procedure requires specialized equipment to mix and dispense the liquid silicone and to pump it into the tubal lumen under hysteroscopic control. The procedure can be completed in the office under paracervical block[22,23]. The advantages of this system are that it does not require electrosurgical instruments and obviates any thermal injury to adjacent pelvic structures. Additionally, the silicone conforms to the shape of the tube rather than being a rigid or pre-formed plug that may not suit all tubal lumens. Despite this fact, there have been recorded cases of extravasation of the silicone into the paratubal or myometrial tissues[21–23]. The disadvantages of the system include the need for a follow-up X-ray at 3 months to ensure correct tubal positioning, the possibility of plug fracture and migration into the uterus or the peritoneal cavity, and a repeat procedure rate of approximately 15–20%, mostly due to tubal spasm[21–23].

In studies of this technique, 1146 women have had the procedure performed with 27 pregnancies occurring (0.02%) during 15 085 woman months. Short-term complications include uterine cramping, perforation of the uterus, silicone extravasation and pelvic pain[21–23].

THERMAL OCCLUSION

Using thermal energy to occlude the proximal tube for sterilization purposes has been described since 1916[24]. Hyams described a method for blind cautery of the tubal ostia in 1934[25], although the failure rate was approximately 40%[26]. It was not until the 1970s, however, that thermal coagulation by electro-diathermy was utilized and extensively studied by Quinones and associates[9]. In 1972, studies using the technique reported a reduction in

apparent morbidity and an increase in the tubal occlusion rate demonstrated by post-procedure hysterosalpingography[27]. Bilateral tubal occlusion has been reported in approximately 83% of patients undergoing the procedure[9], although pregnancy following the procedure has been reported, including ectopic and cornual pregnancies.

Following these initial reports, which sparked renewed interest in the technique of hysteroscopic sterilization, a review of 773 cases of hysteroscopic electrocoagulation of the tubes for sterilization, reported that there is a significant failure rate[28]. Ten centers were involved, and of 524 tested cases post-sterilization, failure was reported in 35.5% (186/524). This included patent tubes demonstrated by hysterosalpingography in 175 cases, and 11 pregnancies[28]. Of the 249 cases that were not tested, 59 pregnancies were reported including intrauterine, ectopic, miscarriage and cornual pregnancy. The total pregnancy rate in these cases was 23.7%.

Possibly more significant than the pregnancies from this series was the 3.2% morbidity rate associated with the procedure, including uterine perforations (1%), bowel damage and peritonitis (0.4%), acute peritonitis alone without bowel injury (0.5%) and a 1% ectopic pregnancy rate. There was one reported death from bowel perforation and peritonitis.

It would seem from this analysis that the experience of the surgeon is an important factor in increasing tubal occlusion rates and decreasing morbidity. March and Israel reported a high failure rate early in the development of the procedure, with both tubal patency as demonstrated by cornual sinuses in many patients, and a number of pregnancies in their small series of 27 patients[29].

The Nd:YAG laser has been investigated as a possible instrument to occlude the tubes and induce sterilization. Failure of sterilization was noted in 76% of an initial study by Brumsted and associates[30]. Donnez and co-workers described a 100% success rate of tubal occlusion demonstrated by Nd:YAG laser at 3-months post-procedure on hysterosalpingography. In the description of the technique, the endometrium surrounding the tubal cornua is ablated by the laser fiber as well as the intramural portion of the tube. The exact mechanism by which tubal occlusion occurs is not apparent[31]. Despite this, the recommendation from the authors is that the technique should be reserved for women over the age of 40, because of its irreversibility.

Thermal energy used alone to destroy part of the tubes hysteroscopically has not proved as successful as its laparoscopic counterpart and has been almost abandoned as a method for sterilization in clinical practice.

THE 'THIRD WAVE' OF HYSTEROSCOPIC STERILIZATION

Essure™

The Essure pbc (permanent birth control) device (Conceptus Inc., San Carlos, CA, USA) is a hybrid metallic and fiber coil that is placed into the tube under hysteroscopic control. The device has an inner coil made from stainless steel and an outer coil made from nickel titanium alloy. Running along and through the inner coil are polyethylene terephthalate (PET) fibers. Figure 2 illustrates the Essure device and deliver catheter.

The device is maintained in a 'low profile' position, where the outer coil is tightly opposed to the inner coil, which is maintained by a release wire and the hydrophilic delivery catheter. The device is delivered to the tube under hysteroscopic control and placed into the tubal lumen aided by a single-handed control mechanism. Once the guide wire is released, the outer coil rapidly unwinds and expands into the tubal lumen to anchor the device in place. The PET fibers then elicit a benign tissue ingrowth, with fibrous tissue causing complete tubal occlusion within 3 months[32].

The device can be placed under local anesthetic (paracervical block) with intravenous sedation as required. There have been a number of studies reporting the outcomes from phase II and pivotal trials, which are summarized here[33–35]. Of 871 women involved in the studies, 745 (85%) have had the procedure attempted with a placement rate of 627/745 (84%). Of the 603/627 (96%) women

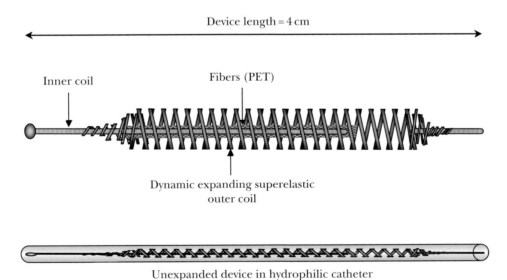

Figure 2 The Essure™ permanent birth control device

with correctly placed devices, bilateral tubal occlusion was demonstrated at 3 months by hysterosalpingography, with 99.5% achieving bilateral tubal occlusion at 12 months. There were no reported pregnancies in the 193 women relying on the device for contraception for more than 1 year, and no pregnancies reported in women with the device for less than 1 year.

The procedure was well tolerated in more than 90% of women; with total procedure time approximately 35 min and total hysteroscopy time approximately 18 min. In these studies, 92% of patients had the procedure performed under local anesthesia, with or without intravenous sedation. Satisfaction with the procedure was high, and long-term comfort with the device was 99% at 18 months.

Adverse events during these studies included device breakage, uterine perforation with subsequent incorrect placement noted, and distal placement of the device. These events may or may not have prevented reliance on the device for contraception.

The advantages of this system include the immediate anchoring effect generated by the unwinding of the outer coil. The elasticity of this anchoring mechanism allows the device to conform to different-shaped tubes. The narrowest portion of the tubal lumen in the intramural area has the narrowest expansion of the coils, with restriction of movement either into the uterus or into the peritoneal cavity. The ingrowth of tissue into the device causes complete obliteration of the tubal lumen and permanently anchors the device in position.

Disadvantages of this system include the absolute irreversibility of the procedure. Once placed, the device is very difficult to remove and a misplaced distal device may not provide contraception, and may not be retrievable. It is probable that placement of the device is not feasible in every woman, although improving design appears to be addressing some of the early issues. Tubal occlusion by spasm or partial obliteration from prior endometritis or pelvic inflammatory disease may prevent placement of the device at the first attempt. Further assessment then needs to be undertaken by hysterosalpingography to assess the tubal status. A second procedure may become necessary for device placement. Tubal perforation during the procedure can occur, and non-recognition of this may prevent sterilization. Hysteroscopic skills for correct placement of the device are essential, and guidance and supervision are recommended for initial training with the technique.

Adiana

The Adiana sterilization method (Adiana, Redwood City, CA, USA) is a combination of controlled thermal damage of the endosalpinx and insertion of a biocompatible matrix within the tubal lumen. The thermal injury to the endosalpinx is aimed at removing the epithelium. Healing brings fibroblasts in direct contact with the matrix, which soon becomes colonized. Tissue ingrowth achieves occlusion of the lumen and at the same time anchors the matrix in place. The procedure is performed under hysteroscopic control and lasts about 10 min. Patients require local anesthesia with occasional intravenously administered sedation. Figure 3 illustrates the Adiana device and delivery catheter.

The method has been tested in animals as well as in patients scheduled to undergo hysterectomy. Histology results show incorporation of the matrix within a 12-week span after the procedure.

An investigational device exemption study commenced in November 2002, the results of which are still pending. Interim reports, however, reveal an access rate over 94% and absence of notable complications or side-effects.

CONCLUSION

Hysteroscopic sterilization has been through a number of phases of development since its

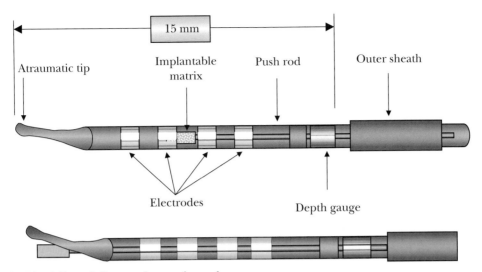

Figure 3 The Adiana delivery catheter: electrode array

inception, and with increasing improvements in technology and experience, there has been a resurgence in this technique as an alternative to transabdominal sterilization (Table 1). The initial treatments that relied on single factor tubal occlusion, have given way to the third wave of combined occlusive procedures. Two phenomena have contributed to the apparent success of the third wave methods. First, and foremost, is the departure from the obsession of developing a reversible method of contraception. This can be directly attributed to the current predictably high success rate of *in vitro* fertilization. The other factor is the introduction of know-how acquired in the field of soft tissue implants.

The fundamentals of hysteroscopic sterilization include efficacy of the procedure in preventing pregnancy, safety for the woman, ability to perform under local anesthesia,

cost-efficacy and availability. What will determine the role of hysteroscopic sterilization into the future is the ability of these new procedures to meet these demands. The initial results are encouraging and further, ongoing research is essential to evaluate fully these devices. Once efficacy and acceptability have been established, then cost-effectiveness of outpatient transcervical sterilization versus laparoscopic sterilization in a standard setting must be investigated to determine the possible benefit to health-care providers in both the developed and developing worlds.

It is probable that this approach to sterilization may only be possible in about 90–95% of an unselected population, and will never fully replace the transabdominal approach to sterilization. However, its development offers choice and an alternative to the risks of traditional approaches of permanent sterilization.

Table 1 Approaches to female sterilization

Approach to tube	Technique	Authors	Advantages	Disadvantages
Chemical				
Blind/ hysteroscopic	quinacrine	Zipper et al.[8] Quinones et al.[9]	simple, non-surgical, inexpensive	repeated applications necessary, tubal occlusion variable and low
Blind	phenol/ atarbine paste	Kang et al.[10]	simple, non-surgical, inexpensive	high success rates reported in single centers not repeated elsewhere
Blind	tetracycline	Zaneveld and Goldsmith[11]	not currently used	very low success rate
Blind (Femcept)	methyl cyanoacrylate	Richart et al.[12]	simple, non-surgical, inexpensive, tubal occlusion rate 89%	repeated applications necessary to achieve effect
Mechanical				
Hysteroscopic	pre-formed ceramic plug	Craft[13]	not currently used	difficulty inserting, perforation of uterus
Hysteroscopic	P-block hydrophilic plug	Brundin[14]	reportedly high success rates, possible reversibility	plug migration, tubal perforation
Hysteroscopic	nylon intratubal device	Hamou et al.[15]	reversible, reported high success rates	migration/expulsion of device
Hysteroscopic	polyethylene plug	Hosseinian et al.[17]	reversible, myometrial anchor, reported high success rates	local inflammatory response at anchor sites, migration
Hysteroscopic	silicone	Sugimoto[18]	ease of insertion	no long-term follow-up
Hysteroscopic	polytetrafluoro-ethylene screw	Hart and Magos[19]	unknown	unknown
Hysteroscopic	ovabloc	Cooper[23] Houck et al.[36] Loffer[22]	non-surgical, high success, silicone conforms to shape of tube	tubal spasm may require repeat applications, fracture of plug with migration may occur
Thermal				
Hysteroscopic	electrosurgical	Neuwirth et al.[27] Quinones et al.[9] Darabi et al.[28]	ease of access, moderate success rates	significant complications including death reported
Hysteroscopic	Nd:YAG laser	Brumsted et al.[30] Donnez et al.[31]	reports of 100% success at sterilization contrasted with significant failure	non-repeated high success rates, expense of equipment
Third wave				
Hysteroscopic	Essure™ pbc	Kerin et al.[34] Cooper[35] Valle et al.[33]	reported high success rates, well tolerated under local anesthesia, no pregnancies to date	disposable device, irreversibility
Hysteroscopic	Adiana	Vancaillie (personal communication)	unknown	unknown

References

1. World Health Organization. *Female sterilization. A guide to provision of services.* New York: World Health Organization, 1992
2. Friorep R. Zur Vorbengung der Nothwendigkeit des Kaiserschnitts und der perforation. *Notizen aus dem Gebiete der Natur und Heilkunde,* 1849; 11:9–10
3. Schroeder C. Uber den Avsbau und die Leistungen der Hysteroskopie. *Arch Gynecol Obstet* 1934;156:407
4. Pantaleoni D. On endoscopic examination of the cavity of the womb. *Med Press* 1869;8:26
5. Edstrom A, Fernstrom I. The diagnostic possibilities of modified hysteroscopic technique. *Acta Obstet Gynecol Scand* 1970;49:327–30
6. Lindemann H. Transuterine tubal sterilization by hysteroscopy. *J Reprod Med* 1974;13:21–2
7. Rubin I. Uterine endoscopy, endometroscopy with the aid of uterine insufflation. *Am J Gynecol* 1925;10:313
8. Zipper J, Stacheti E, Medel M. Human fertility control by transvaginal application of quinacrine on the fallopian tube. *Fertil Steril* 1970;21:581
9. Quinones R, Alvarado A, Ley E. Hysteroscopic sterilization. *Int J Obstet Gynecol* 1976;14:27–34
10. Kang X, Wan H, Wang P. Effectiveness of phenol-atabrine paste (PAP) instillation for female sterilization. *Int J Obstet Gynecol* 1990;33:49
11. Zaneveld L, Goldsmith A. Lack of tubal occlusion by intrauterine quinacrine and tetracycline in the primate. *Contraception* 1984;30:161
12. Richart R, Neuwirth R, Goldsmith A, Edelman D. Intrauterine administration of methyl cyanoacrylate as an outpatient method of permanent female sterilization. *Am J Obstet Gynecol* 1987;156: 981–7
13. Craft I. Utero-tubal ceramic plugs. In Sciarra J, Droegemueller W, Speidel J, eds. *Advances in Female Sterilization Techniques.* Hagerstown, MD: Harper and Row, 1976
14. Brundin J. Transcervical sterilization in the human female by hysteroscopic application of hydrogelic occlusive devices into the intramural parts of the Fallopian tubes: 10 years experience of the P-block. *Eur J Obstet Gynecol Reprod Biol* 1991;39:41–9
15. Hamou J, Gasparri F, Cittadini E. Hysteroscopic placement of nylon intratubal devices for potentially reversible sterilisation. In Siegler A, Ansari AH, eds. *The Fallopian Tube: Basic Studies and Clinical Considerations.* New York: Futura, 1986
16. Sciarra J, Keith L. Hysteroscopic sterilization. *Obstet Gynecol Clin N Am* 1995;22:581–9
17. Hosseinian A, Lucero S, Kim M. Hysteroscopic implantation of uterotubal junction blocking devices. In Sciarra J, Droegemueller W, Speidel J, eds. *Advances in Female Sterilization Techniques.* Hagerstown: Harper and Row, 1976:169
18. Sugimoto O. Sterilization by electrocoagulation. In Sciarra J, Butler J, Speidell J, eds. *Hysteroscopic Sterilization.* New York: Intercontinental Medical Books, 1974
19. Hart R, Magos A. Development of a novel method of female sterilization. I. The development of a novel method of hysteroscopic sterilization. *J Laparoendosc Adv Surg Tech* 2002; 12:365–70
20. Corfman P, Taylor H. An instrument for transcervical treatment of the oviduct and uterine cornua. *Obstet Gynecol* 1966;27:880
21. Reed T, Erb R. Hysteroscopic tubal occlusion with silicone rubber. *Obstet Gynecol* 1983;61: 388–92
22. Loffer F. Hysteroscopic sterilization with the use of formed-in-place silicone plugs. *Am J Obstet Gynecol* 1984;149:261–70
23. Cooper J. Hysteroscopic sterilization. *Clin Obstet Gynecol* 1992;35:282–97
24. Dickinson R. Simple sterilization of women by cautery stricture at the intrauterine tubal openings compared with other methods. *Surg Gynecol Obstet* 1916;23:203
25. Hyams N. Sterilization of the female by coagulation of the uterine cornu. *Am J Obstet Gynecol* 1934;28:96
26. De Vilbiss L. Preliminary report on sterilization of women by intrauterine coagulation of tubal orifices. *Am J Obstet Gynecol* 1935;29:563
27. Neuwirth R, Levine R, Richart R. Hysteroscopic tubal sterilization. *Am J Obstet Gynecol* 1973;116: 82–5
28. Darabi K, Richart R. Collaborative study on hysteroscopic sterilization procedures. *Obstet Gynecol* 1977;49:48–54
29. March C, Israel R. A critical appraisal of hysteroscopic tubal fulguration for sterilization. *Contraception* 1974;11:261–8
30. Brumstead J, Shirk G, Soderling M, Reed T. Attempted transcervical occlusion of the fallopian tube with the ND:YAG laser. *Obstet Gynecol* 1991;77:327–8
31. Donnez J, Malvaux V, Nisolle M, Casanas F. Hysteroscopic sterilization with the Nd:YAG laser. *J Gynecol Surg* 1990;6:149–53
32. Valle RF, Carignan M, Wright T. Tissue response to the STOP microcoil transcervical permanent contraceptive device: results from a

pre-hysterectomy study. *Am Soc Reprod Med* 2001; 75:974–80

33. Valle RF, Cooper J, Kerin J. Hysteroscopic tubal sterilization with the Essure nonincisional permanent contraception. *Obstet Gynecol* 2002;99 (Suppl 4):11s

34. Kerin J, Carignan C, Cher D. The safety and effectiveness of a new hysteroscopic method for permanent birth control: results of the first Essure pbc clinical study. *Aust NZ J Obstet Gynecol* 2001;41:364–70

35. Cooper J. Clinical experience with Essure permanent birth control in 745 women. *Presented at Congress of Gynaecological Endoscopy and Innovative Surgery*, Berlin, Germany, April 25–28, 2002

36. Houck R, Cooper J, Rigberg S. Hysteroscopic tubal occlusion with formed in place silicone plugs: a clinical review. *Obstet Gynecol* 1983; 62:587–91

12

Applied electrophysics in endometrial ablation

R. M. Soderstrom

INTRODUCTION

When electrical energy is used to accomplish the task of endometrial ablation, an array of variables will dictate the outcome, some being in the control of the surgeon and others controlled by physiology, tissue response and anatomical variation. All methods of endometrial ablation require the delivery of enough energy to kill tissue below the basal layer of the endometrium; however, the uterus, rich with blood vessels, acts as an efficient radiator removing any intracellular heat rapidly. Also, the contour and size of the endometrial cavity will vary from one patient to another.

Either or both the resectoscope loop and rollerball are used to destroy enough tissue to reduce or eliminate the ability for endometrial regeneration. A roller bar or barrel is also available. Experience with a thick loop used for coagulation has been effective and it is easier to keep clean of coagulated debris. Since the endometrial lining, owing to its own thickness and natural resistance to the flow of electrical energy, can hinder the transfer of sufficient energy to destroy the basal layers, medications which reduce the thickness of the endometrium, e.g. gonadotropin releasing hormone agonists, may be given to the patient several weeks prior to the ablation procedure[1,2]. When the clinical situation does not allow for such endometrial preparation, many will use the resecting loop to 'shave' off the endometrium down to or including the basal layer.

There are more theories about which approach gives the best results than there are

good outcome statistics[3,4]. Regarding the questions about the best approach to deliver electrosurgical energy in ablation procedures, the basics of electricity and its variables that must come together to create heat must be appreciated. In the past, surgeons learned to use electrosurgical techniques without any understanding of what was happening during the surgery or the tissue effect after the injury had occurred. To use the visual endpoint of electrosurgery is far from accurate as to the final outcome; thus the principles of electrophysics as they are applied to endometrial ablation must be understood by the contemporary gynecologist.

BASIC ELECTRICITY

Electrons are particles of energy that, when pushed (or passed) through human tissue, create heat and sometimes destruction. Voltage is the pressure force required to push electrons. The standard unit of measurement of this 'electrical' pressure is 1 volt. Thus, if we draw the analogy of electricity to water, an electron would be analogous to a molecule of water and voltage would be analogous to water pressure.

Whereas volume of water may be measured in cubic centimeters, the volume of electrons is measured in coulombs. If we push a volume of water through a conduit at a given pressure over a specific period, we create current. In electricity, current is measured in amperes (coulombs per second), meaning the passage of a quantity of electrons through an area over a given period. With either water or electricity, as resistance increases, the flow of current decreases (given constant pressure or voltage). The difficulty of pushing the electrons through tissue or other material, defined as resistance, is measured in ohms.

As a last definition, electrical power (watts) is the energy produced. The electrical power may be defined as pressure × current, or volts × current, or volts × electron flow per second. The total energy consumed over a period of time is measured in joules (Table 1).

FUNDAMENTALS OF ELECTROSURGERY

Manipulating electrons through living tissue with sufficient current concentration to create heat and, if desired, tissue destruction, is electrosurgery. Electrogenerators or electro-surgical units are machines that produce an alternating current of electricity at a frequency that will not stimulate muscle activity (500 000 to 3 million cycles/s). Whereas direct current flows in one direction only, alternating current flows to and fro, first increasing to a maximum in one direction and then increasing to a maximum in the other direction. This 'sinusoidal waveform' can be interrupted or varied, resulting in different surgical effects.

The waveform of alternating current has a negative and a positive excursion or peak. The measurement from zero polarity to positive or negative polarity is called the peak voltage of the waveform (the relationship is the same for peak current). The measurement from plus peak to negative peak, which is twice peak voltage, is called peak-to-peak voltage. A pure cutting waveform is a simple sinusoidal, undamped or non-modulated waveform and is generally produced by continuous energy (Figure 1). An output waveform that is interrupted or varied (modulated or damped) is called a coagulating waveform (Figure 2).

Because of this continuous flow, the peak voltage need not be as high as with the damped waveform to create the same wattage. At the same level, however, when a coagulation effect must be enhanced, the damped waveform is preferable; bursts of damped waveforms are pushed through the tissue. For an instant, with the damped waveform, high voltage may be present within the electrical circuit. A combination of undamped and damped waveforms is called a blended current (Figure 3).

As electrons, pushed with a given voltage, are concentrated in one specific location, heat within the tissue increases rapidly. This concentration phenomenon is defined as current density. The diathermy generator, an example of equipment using this principle, is familiar to most physicians. Here, electrons are passed through the body by applying two large metal conductors or plates on opposite sides of the body part to be heated. The electrons are pushed through the plate called the active electrode. Electrons are received on the other plate, the return electrode or ground plate, after they leave the body. Once the electrons enter the body (conductor) they are dispersed through the tissue toward the pathway of least resistance to the return electrode. Because current is dispersed over the entire surface area of both plates, the heat generated is of low intensity. If either plate is markedly reduced in size, however, current density (and thus heat) is increased accordingly.

Table 1 Electrophysics definitions equated to a hydraulic analog

Electrical concept	Electrical unit	Equation	Hydraulic analog
Energy	joule	–	energy
Charge	coulomb (6.3×10^{18} electrons)	–	volume (mass)
Power	watt	joules/second	power
Voltage	volt	joules/coulomb	pressure difference
Current	ampere	coulombs/second	flow
Impedence	ohm	volts/ampere	resistance

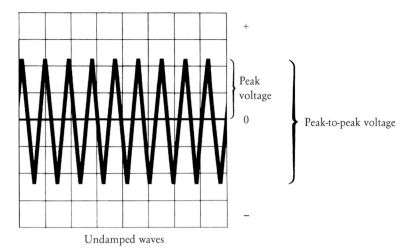

Undamped waves

Figure 1 The CUT/desiccation waveform (undamped) showing peak voltage and peak-to-peak voltage

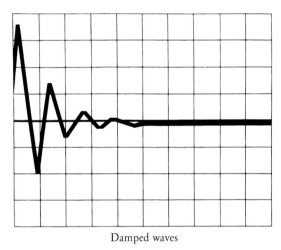

Damped waves

Figure 2 The fulguration (COAG) waveform is damped or turned off during the 'duty' cycle

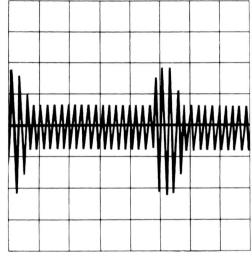

Figure 3 A blend of desiccation and fulguration waveforms

Thus, a small active electrode can create a burn where the electrons enter the body. Also, the electrons that leave the body through a small return electrode can produce another burn.

Electrons flow through the path of least resistance. If tissue resistance is high but the corresponding voltage pressure low, the current may cease to flow or may search out alternate pathways with lower resistance. When the voltage is increased, the electrons have more 'push' to find an alternate pathway. Such alternate pathways could be through a vital structure where the current might be condensed or where it might lead to an alternate return electrode, i.e. cardiac monitor electrode. Therefore, one should use the lowest voltage necessary to accomplish a given job and be sure that the dispersive electrode is in good contact with the patient and broad enough to reduce current density far below the level of tissue destruction. Isolated ground circuitry systems are desirable, as is a return electrode sentinel system, should an ineffective or incomplete return path be present.

Because operative endoscopy is remote control surgery, it is important that unexpected movements of the electrode do not occur. By reducing peak voltage, the chance of electrons jumping or sparking to nearby structures is reduced. An 8000-V pressure can push electrons 3 mm through room air under certain atmospheric conditions. Though many modern generators have a maximum peak voltage of 6000 V, most of the time they are used in the 1000–3000 V range.

BIOLOGICAL BEHAVIOR OF ELECTROSURGERY

As mentioned, at the end of an electrode, the performance depends on the shape and size of the electrode, the frequency and wave modulation, the peak voltage and the current coupled against output impedance. The tissue may be cut in a smooth, deliberate fashion without arcing, or it can be burned and charred. This great variation of tissue effects is frequently ignored or misunderstood, which is why some surgeons claim that the laser provides better control of the energy needs and provides better wound healing.

Electrocoagulation may be carried out in many different forms: from slow, delicate contact coagulation (desiccation) to the charring effects of the spray coagulation mode (fulguration), at times leading to carbonization. The temperature differences may vary between 100°C and over 500°C.

The essential characteristic of CUT waveforms is that they are continuous sine waves. That is, if the voltage output of the generator is plotted over time, a pure CUT waveform is a continuous sine wave alternating from positive to negative at the operating frequency of the generator, 500–3000 kHz.

The COAG waveform consists of short bursts of radiofrequency sine waves. With the sine wave frequency of 500 kHz, the COAG bursts occur 31 250 times/s. The important feature of the COAG waveform is the pause between each burst. If a COAG waveform had the same peak voltage as a CUT waveform, the average power delivered (heat per second) would be less because the COAG is turned off most of the time (Figure 4).

Now if the COAG waveform had the same average voltage (root mean square (RMS) voltage) as the CUT waveform and thus could deliver the same heat per second, because the COAG is turned off most of the time, it could only produce the same RMS voltage as the CUT by having large peak voltages and currents during the periods when the generator is on (Figure 5).

A good COAG waveform can spark to tissue without significant cutting effect because the

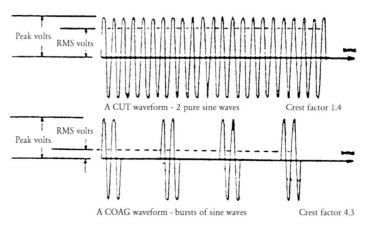

Figure 4 The peak voltage is the same in both of these waveforms, but the power is about one-third in the COAG waveform. RMS, root mean square (average) voltage

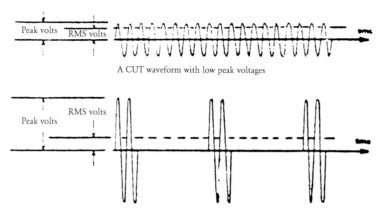

Peak volts   RMS volts

A CUT waveform with low peak voltages

RMS volts
Peak volts

Figure 5 A COAG waveform with equal power (energy per second) to the above waveform. Note that the COAG peak voltage is about three times higher in this example. Note also that the root mean square (RMS) or average voltages are equal

heat is more widely dispersed by the long sparks and because the heating effect is intermittent. The temperature of the water in the cells does not get high enough to flash into steam. In this way the cells are dehydrated slowly but are not torn apart to form an incision. Because the high peak voltage is a quality of the COAG waveform, it can drive a current through high resistances. In this way it is possible to fulgurate long after the water is driven out of the tissue and actually char it to carbon. 'Coagulation' is a general term which includes both desiccation and fulguration.

Fulguration can be contrasted with desiccation in several ways. First, sparking to tissue with any practical fulguration generator always produces necrosis anywhere the sparks land. This is not surprising when you consider that each cycle of voltage produces a new spark and each spark has an extremely high current density. In desiccation, the current is no more concentrated than the area of contact between the electrode and the tissue (Figure 6).

As a result, desiccation may or may not produce necrosis, depending on the current density. For a given level of current flow, fulguration is always more efficient at producing necrosis. However, the depth of tissue injury is quite superficial compared to contact desiccation because with fulguration the sparks jump from one spot to another in a random fashion and thus the energy is 'sprayed' rather

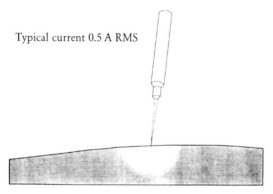

Typical current 0.5 A RMS

Figure 6 In desiccation, the electrode touches the tissue after which the energy is applied creating a deep penetration of heat destruction. RMS, root mean square (or average) voltage

than concentrated (Figure 7). In general, fulguration requires only one-fifth the average current flow of desiccation. For example, if a roller ball electrode is pressed against moist tissue, the electrode will begin in the desiccation mode, regardless of the waveform. The initial tissue resistance is quite low and the resulting current will be high, typically 0.5–0.8 A RMS. As the tissues dries out, its resistance rises until the electrical contact is broken. Since moist tissue is no longer touching the electrode, sparks will jump to the nearest areas of moist tissue in the fulguration mode, as long as the voltage is high enough to make a spark. Eventually, the resistance of desiccated tissue will stop the flow of electrons, limiting the depth of coagulation.

Electrosurgical electrodes can be sculptured to perform certain tasks. A microneedle, a knife, a wire loop or even a scissor can be shaped and sized to a specific duty. When the waveform variable is added, 'cutters' can be made to coagulate and 'coagulators' can be made to cut. The faster an electrode passes over or through tissue, the less the coagulation effect, leading to more cutting (Figure 8). The more broad the electrode, the less cutting and more coagulation effect (Figure 9). Interwoven into these acts are the output intensity and output impedance characteristics of the different electrosurgical generators.

ELECTROPHYSICS APPLIED TO OPERATIVE HYSTEROSCOPY

With endometrial ablation, either or both the resectoscope loop and rollerball are used; a rollerbar or barrel is also available. Some will shave the endometrial lining with the loop electrode; others will desiccate the endometrial lining with the rollerball or bar. A few surgeons shave first and then 'paint' the shaved myometrium with the roller electrode. Unfortunately, studies on the tissue effects of different techniques, electrodes and waveforms are few in number. Even the pressure applied to the endometrial surface will change the current (power) density; the more the pressure, the broader will be the contact surface of the electrode, creating a decreased current density. Since the speed of passage of the electrode unique to each surgeon is another variable, only the outcome statistics can be evaluated with any reasonable scrutiny. Some use a coagulation-only waveform at a low wattage of 30; other report success with a pure cutting waveform at 100 W.

My personal preference is to shave the endo-metrium first. I use a pure undamped waveform and drag the wire cutting loop in a slow, deliberate motion to 4 mm deep through the tissue so there is some coagulation effect in addition to its cutting properties. By using the cutting

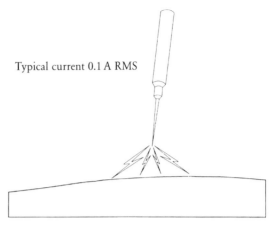

Typical current 0.1 A RMS

Figure 7 To fulgurate, the electrode is held off the surface of the tissue and sparks are allowed to strike the surface of the tissue at random, which results in a surface coagulum that impedes deep penetration. RMS, root mean square (or average) voltage

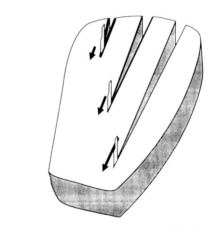

Figure 8 Influence of the speed of incision on the degree of coagulation

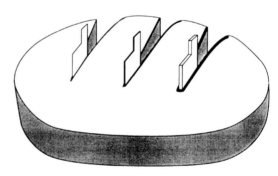

Figure 9 Influence of the shape of the electrode on the degree of coagulation

waveform, bubble formation on the anterior surface of the endometrial cavity is less than in the coagulation mode. I do not shave the cavity's lateral sulcus near the uterine vessels.

During the 'rolling' phase, I continue to use an undamped waveform with direct contact of the roller electrode set at 100 W. If the roller electrode is a bar or barrel, I will either slow up the rolling motion or increase the power output because the electrode current density is lower. At the end of the ablation procedure, I will switch to a coagulation waveform at 75 W. Here, I use a light 'painting' of the desiccated surface. Because of the increased peak voltage of this waveform, skipped areas will be 'sought out' by the electrons under higher pressure, assuring complete surface coagulation. My recent experience with the thick coagulation loop has been excellent; its self-cleaning property when compared to a roller electrode helps to speed up the process. In seven patients, histological studies performed several months after an ablation procedure demonstrated a complete absence of the endometrial lining, replaced by cuboidal cells, and a coagulation depth into the myometrium of 3–5 mm.

Outcome data

During the mid-1990s, several Food and Drug Administration (FDA)-approved studies used the resectoscope ablation procedure as a control arm to assess the success of newly developed non-hysteroscopic, endometrial ablation devices. When one collates all of these studies, the control arms have over 400 patients subjected to hysteroscopic resectoscope ablation followed in prospective fashion by the FDA. The outcome statistics of these control arms were essentially the same without statistical difference. A summary of the findings is as follows. The total amenorrhea rate using this technique was in the range of 30%, another 45% of the patients had oligomenorrhea, and 20% had eumenorrhea with the failure rate being 5%. These statistics do not differ from previous reports using lower power settings, one

electrode and either blended or coagulation waveforms[5–9]. It was found that 90% of the patients had a 90% reduction in flow and the majority of patients had a reduction or elimination of dysmenorrhea. All of the patient satisfaction surveys reported better than a 95% satisfaction rate[10–12].

HAZARDS

Two-thirds of electrical accidents during operative hysteroscopy occur at the return electrode site. As with all surgical procedures where electrosurgical generators are used, the operating-room staff need to possess the proper techniques for return electrode application. With the same magnitude required when using lasers, both the staff and surgeon should have some familiarity with the instruction manual supplied with the generators.

To date, true electrical injuries within the uterus have been few and have been associated with inadvertent perforation, partial or incomplete. Though some have worried about sparking or arcing through the uterine wall to adjacent structures, the physics of fulguration make this theory unlikely. Because a non-electrolytic solution is used for distention, water overload has occurred. A bipolar cutting loop system which allows saline to be used eliminates the risk of water intoxication but introduces the problems of possible fluid overload.

SUMMARY

Although electrosurgery has been with us for decades, few surgeons have received formal training in its proper uses. The erroneous belief that electrosurgery techniques increase scar formation or impair healing processes has led surgeons to other methods to deliver energy to the living cell. At the cellular level, a watt, is a watt, is a watt; knowing how to calculate and administer that energy is the challenge. Laser technology has forced the bioelectrical engineers to develop improved electro-generators and accessories that are easier to understand and control. The use of digital reader boards, displayed in watts rather than an arbitrary dial setting, is one example. A good electrosurgical system, with proper accessory electrodes, once mastered, can have more power and finesse than any available laser. For successful resectoscopic ablation procedures, a thorough knowledge and appreciation of the physics of electrosurgery is a basic requirement.

References

1. Brooks PG, Serden SP, Davos I. Hormonal inhibition of the endometrium for resectoscopic endometrial ablation. *Am J Obstet Gynecol* 1991; 164:1601–8
2. Brooks PG, Serden SP. Preparation of endometrium for ablation with a single dose of leuprolide acetate depot. *J Reprod Med* 1991;36: 477–82
3. Indman P, Soderstrom R. Depth of endometrial coagulation with the urologic resectoscope. *J Reprod Med* 1990;35:633–5
4. Indman P, Brown W. Uterine surface changes caused by electrosurgical endometrial coagulation. *J Reprod Med* 1992;37:667–70
5. Vancaillie TG. Electrocoagulation of the endometrium with the ball-end resectoscope ('rollerball'). *Obstet Gynecol* 1990;76:425–7
6. Townsend DE, Richart RM, Paskowitz PA, *et al.* 'Rollerball' coagulation of the endometrium. *Obstet Gynecol* 1989;74:310–13
7. DeCherney AH, Diamond MD, Lavy G, *et al.* Endometrial ablation for intractable uterine bleeding: hysteroscopic resection. *Obstet Gynecol* 1987;70:668–70
8. Letterie GS, Hibbert ML, Britton BA. Endometrial histology after electrocoagulation using different power settings. *Fertil Steril* 1993;60: 647–51
9. Onbargi LC, Hayden R, Valle RF, *et al.* Effects of power and electrical current density variations in an *in vitro* endometrial ablation model. *Obstet Gynecol* 1993;82:912–18
10. Meyer WR, Walsh BW, Grainger DA, *et al.* Thermal balloon and rollerball ablation to treat menorrhagia: a multicenter comparison. *Obstet Gynecol* 1998;92:98–103
11. Corson SL, Brill AI, Brooks PG, *et al.* One year results of the vesta system for endometrial ablation. *J Am Assoc Gynecol Laprosc* 2000;7:489–97
12. Corson SL. A multicenter evaluation of endometrial ablation by Hydro ThermAblator and rollerball for treatment of menorrhagia. *J Am Assoc Gynecol Laprosc* 2001;8:359–67

GLOSSARY

Active electrode monitoring is a technique of placing a sleeve around the electrode to detect stray energy and carry the induced energy to ground. Stray energy generally occurs due to breaks in insulation or to capacitive coupling.

Ampere is the quantity of electrons that move through a conductor over time (coulombs/second).

Bipolar refers to an electrode or electrical delivery system where the active and passive electrode are of similar size and thus similar current densities. The bipolar generators are usually calibrated against a $100 \, \Omega$ load of resistance.

BLEND is the term used when the electrical current is interrupted between 20% and 50% of the time.

Capacitance or *Capacitive coupling* is the ability of two conductors to transmit or receive electrical flow although separated by an insulator; one conductor carried the active current and induces a separate current in the nearby conductor. In general, it occurs in monopolar circuits consisting of two metal plates or tubes separated by air or another insulator. It does not occur during bipolar electrosurgery.

COAG is the term used to describe an interrupted electrical current. In some generators the period of interruption of current flow can be adjusted from 10% 'on' to 50% 'on'. At the same power settings, the voltage of the waveform is always higher than with CUT.

Coulomb is a measure of a quantity of electrons.

Current (Power) density is the surface area of an electrode in contact with tissue during electrical flow. The smaller the spot of contact, the greater the heat effect for the same amount of time, increasing by the square root of the area of contact.

Current rate (amperes) is the flow rate of a quantity (coulombs) of electrons.

CUT is the term used when referring to a continuous or undamped electrical current. At the same power settings, the voltage of the waveform is always lower than with COAG or BLEND.

Desiccation is the act of coagulating tissue after making contact with an active electrode. Either CUT or COAG may be used, but CUT is preferable. Intracellular temperature stays below 100°C, which leads to cell shrinkage and dehydration.

Direct coupling occus when two conductive materials in the same circuit touch during electrical activation or are in close enough proximity that arcing can occur. A break in the insulation of an electrode which allows sparking to tissue is an example of direct coupling.

Edge density is the affinity of electrons to concentrate at the edges of flat or irregular-shaped electrodes as they exit the electrode. This feature enhances the cutting ability of blade-shaped electrodes.

Electricity is movement of electrons between two oppositely charged poles, positive and negative.

Electrocautery refers to transfer of energy by heat, such as a hot wire. Electrons do not move into the affected tissue; only heat (molecular motion) is transferred.

Electrosurgery is the transfer of energy from an electrosurgical generator to tissue by means of energy packets (electrons).

Energy (joules) is a quantity of work produced over time. Energy (J) = work (W) × time (s).

Faradic effect is the electrical stimulation of muscle responding to a frequency of electrical current that is below 100 000 cycles/s.

Fulguration is the intentional application of sparks to tissue surface to coagulate surface bleeding. The COAG waveform is preferable.

Heat (thermal energy) is produced as electrons move from the low resistance of an electrosurgical probe to the high resistance of tissue. This energy may boil (vaporize) or denature (coagulate) tissue, depending on the extent and rapidity with which heat is generated.

A *hybrid laparoscopic trocar sleeve* is a conductive trocar sleeve covered by an outer nonconductive locking sleeve.

Impedance (ohm) is resistance to flow of electrons through a non-uniform conductor. Although resistance refers to direct current through a uniform wire, such as copper, it is generally substituted for impedance. Impedance is correctly applied with changes in voltage (alternating or fluctuating), frequency (modulating, demodulating), or tissue type (lipid membranes, soft tissue, fibrous tissue, fat, muscle, bone, artificial appliances). It can measure the combination of tissue resistance and capacitance. Impedance in human tissue is generally 100–1000 Ω and in the Fallopian tube it is 400–500 Ω.

Isolation ground circuitry is a safety feature using transformers that are not in contact with the parent generator such that the induced electrical flow 'floats' its own separate circuit. Should a break in the 'floating' circuit occur, all energy within that circuit stops and does not seek ground.

Monopolar refers to an electrode or electrical system where the active electrode is small (high current density) and the passive electrode is large (low current density). Most monopolar generators are calibrated against a 500 Ω load of resistance.

An *open circuit* is a state where a generator is activated before the active electrode touches tissue. This promotes higher voltage, especially in the COAG mode, than activating the generator after touching the tissue. Open circuitry is used to start fulguration.

The *patient return electrode* (grounding pad) is a large pad (low current density) placed on the patient to complete an electrosurgical pathway.

Return electrode monitoring is a dual-padded patient return electrode system designed to monitor irregular separation of the ground pad.

Sparking (arcing, fulguration) is the result of electrical flow through gas (air, argon).

To *vaporize* is rapidly to raise the cellular temperature above 100°C, which causes cell rupture releasing steam.

Voltage (volts) is the force (pressure) driving current.

Watts (work) is the amount of work produced by electron flow (current). Work (W) = force (V) × current rate (A).

Waveform is the oscillation characteristic of an alternating electrical current from positive to negative.

Waveform frequency is the number of oscillations of an alternating electrical current, usually between 350 000 cycles/s and 4 million cycles/s in electrosurgery.

13

Control of menorrhagia by electrodesiccation

J. A. Abbott and T. G. Vancaillie

Destruction of the endometrium by any method of energy transfer is commonly called ablation. Ablation can be understood as destruction as well as removal of tissue. The term resection applies when the electrical loop is used actually to resect the endometrium. Ablation has been perceived as being opposite to resection; it is not. Ablation could be said to entail the possibility of resection.

To avoid confusion, the term ablation will be avoided and replaced with electro-desiccation when relating to a method involving the resectoscope with a large electrode. Ablation will only be used as a generic term encompassing any method of *in vivo* destruction or removal of the endometrium.

Surgical treatment (other than hysterectomy) for excessive uterine bleeding has not been part of medical textbooks. However, attempts at conservative surgical treatment of menorrhagia are not new at all. In fact, in our modern literature, we can trace such reports back to the first two decades of the 20th century[1].

Without going into detailed philosophical discussions of why alternative methods of treating abnormal uterine bleeding are more or less widespread, it may be said that the current impetus for uterus-sparing surgical treatment is due to greater involvement of the patient in making medical decisions.

INDICATIONS

Abnormal uterine bleeding, caused by a benign condition, is a generic term for the indications for endometrial ablation. However, the true indication for this procedure is menorrhagia resulting from dysfunctional uterine bleeding and it is not recommended in women who have pathology such as fibroids or endometrial polyps. Specific treatment of these pathologies is recommended by the appropriate technique.

The objective of the procedure is cytoreduction of the endometrium, which will reduce the amount of blood flow but not influence the timing.

Currently, there is insufficient knowledge about the uterine microanatomy and the effect that this has on the type of surgery to be performed. Can the surgeon visually recognize such conditions as adenomyosis? Is it preferable to desiccate or resect the adenomyotic tissue? These questions remain unanswered.

Endometrial ablation has beneficial side-effects. Along with the reduction in menstrual flow, there seems to be a reduction in dysmenorrhea and even premenstrual syndrome (PMS)[2] symptomatology. A randomized trial comparing electrodesiccation with balloon ablation reported a 75% improvement in dysmenorrhea and a 62% improvement in PMS at 1 year[3]. Neither of these conditions, however, can be considered an indication for endometrial ablation. It also seems important to mention that if a patient complains of pelvic pain, an effort should be made to characterize the pain more precisely. One cannot just assume that the pain will be improved after the procedure. In some cases, *de novo* pelvic pain presents a new challenge to the treating physician.

Patients with known endometriosis, for example, will more than likely not be satisfied. There is no reason to believe that endometrial ablation will affect the pathophysiological process of pelvic pain related to endometriosis. The question of whether a combination of laparoscopic resection of endometriosis and endometrial ablation is an acceptable alternative to hysterectomy is out of the realm of this chapter. This approach is technically feasible, and is an acceptable alternative in well-informed patients who desire to conserve their reproductive organs – and who take responsibility for this decision.

Sterility is another potential side-effect of endometrial ablation. However, endometrial ablation cannot be considered a method of sterilization because endometrial tissue may remain, and pregnancies have been reported. The pregnancy rate after endometrial ablation is about 1%, with nearly 40 pregnancies being reported. Complications occur in over 50% of pregnancies following endometrial ablation[4].

One aspect of endometrial ablation with regard to sterilization should be emphasized: endometrial ablation might be the only method of female sterilization with a physiological indicator of success, namely amenorrhea.

METHODS

Electrodesiccation of the endometrium is achieved using large monopolar electrodes. Originally, a 2-mm ball electrode was inserted into the uterus blindly and activated while the surgeon moved the probe within the uterine cavity[1]. This rather crude technique was successful in arresting menorrhagia in an emergency room set-up in the majority of cases.

Currently, the resectoscope is the method of choice for electrodesiccation of the endometrium. The decisions to be made are which electrode to choose and what settings on the electrosurgical unit are ideal.

The electrodes available are spherical or variations thereof. The objectives to be achieved are good contact with the tissue at varying angles and large contact area to lower the power density. A low power density is required to obtain desiccation and not fulguration. Sharp edges or uninsulated branches are to be avoided. These edges are sites that can easily lead to sparking between the electrode and the tissue. When sparking occurs, there are two detrimental coexisting effects. The first one is that the power density of electrical current at other sites of the electrode will be reduced to a level ineffective in producing desiccation. The second effect is that sparking will cause carbonization of the tissue hit by the spark. The impedance of that tissue will greatly increase and, thereby, prevent destruction by electrodesiccation of the deeper layers.

In summary, the choice of electrode should be dictated by the following factors (Figure 1):

(1) Spherical, ellipsoid shape or any variation thereof;

(2) Smooth conductive surface, non-corroded, i.e. unused;

(3) No edges or sharp angles;

(4) Intact insulation;

(5) Approximately 3 mm in diameter; a larger contact area may require a high-output electrosurgical unit.

The discussion on what type of current and what settings to use on the electrosurgical unit is found in the section on 'Surgical Technique'.

PREOPERATIVE MANAGEMENT

A thorough history and physical examination are obvious prerequisites. It should be made clear that, although an endometrial ablation is a

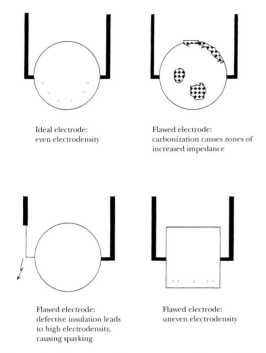

Ideal electrode:
even electrodensity

Flawed electrode:
carbonization causes zones of
increased impedance

Flawed electrode:
defective insulation leads
to high electrodensity,
causing sparking

Flawed electrode:
uneven electrodensity

Figure 1 Diagrammatic representation of the ideal electrode and the possible defects

uterus-sparing procedure, there should be no further desire for pregnancy.

Laboratory values of serum electrolytes should be considered in advance so that possible abnormalities can be dealt with prior to surgery. This is especially important in patients with systemic disorders affecting the electrolyte balance, such as liver and kidney diseases. Patients receiving diuretics should be given potassium replacement if they do not use it already. Careful evaluation of the coagulation parameters is obtained in patients with a thromboembolic disorder or on anticoagulant therapy. Abnormal values are not necessarily a contraindication for endometrial ablation, but they will require a personalized approach to management of intra- and postoperative risk of bleeding.

Histology of the endometrium is obtained in every patient either at the time of the procedure or in advance. Patients at risk for adenocarcinoma of the endometrium should undergo an endometrial biopsy or hysteroscopy and biopsy prior to scheduling of the ablation. The

patient at risk for developing endometrial cancer, such as the diabetic patient and the patient with polycystic ovary disease, should be counselled very carefully. An effort should be made to explain the risk–benefit ratio of vaginal hysterectomy versus ablation.

The objective of preoperative hormonal manipulation is to perform surgery at a time when the endometrium is reduced to the basal layer. This occurs naturally during menses or in the early postpartum. However, to ensure that a patient will indeed present with an atrophic endometrium, the use of gonadotropin releasing hormone analog (such as Lupron depot, TAP Pharmaceutical, Deerfield, IL, USA) is recommended. There are a number of studies that have examined the effect of endometrial thinning agents on outcome, and all report a shorter operative time, reduced fluid absorption rate and a higher amenorrhea rate[5]. There are no data reporting if these results are maintained for greater than 12 months. There does not appear to be an increase in the complication rate, such as perforation, when pretreatment is used[6].

Endometrial thinning is critical when ablation is performed using an electrodesiccation technique as opposed to resection. When resecting, the surgeon can visually assure that the entire endometrial lining is removed. When desiccating, there is no such visual endpoint. The latter method will, therefore, be effective only when the endometrium is thin. This can be achieved reliably only with medication, such as Lupron depot.

Patients in whom a desiccation technique is definitively preferred over resection are the individuals with coagulopathies, endogenic or iatrogenic, and in whom fluid overload is to be avoided at all cost because of reduced renal function. Some patients without systemic condition may also benefit from preparation with Lupron. They are the patients in whom ultrasonography has indicated the presence of a highly grown endometrium. In such cases, desiccation is not feasible, and resection may be quite tedious. Preoperative reduction of the bulk of the endometrial tissue will facilitate the procedure and, therefore, also increase the chances of success. The indications for hormonal suppression of the endometrium should be set liberally early in someone's experience because the use of these agents greatly facilitates the procedure.

SURGICAL TECHNIQUE

The patient is positioned in lithotomy with legs in stirrups. Use of candycane-type stirrups is indicated because of the increased mobility provided to the surgeon with regard to manipulation of the endoscope.

Local anesthesia in the form of a paracervical block combined with systemic analgesia is adequate for almost every modality of operative hysteroscopy. Conduction anesthesia or general endotracheal anesthesia are excellent alternatives. Application of a paracervical block may be used even if the patient is under general anesthesia since the block will also suppress postoperative pain. This is even more pronounced when long-lasting anesthetics, such as bupivacaine, are used.

Admixture of Pitressin® to the local anesthetic has the additional benefit of reducing blood flow during the procedure. This is advantageous when performing a resection technique. When only desiccation is used, there may not be any benefit. The impact of Pitressin on fluid absorption is unclear.

Cervical dilatation is performed using any of the established techniques. The use of KY gel appears to smooth the dilatation process. In addition, waiting until the paracervical block is well established seems to have a beneficial effect on the cervical dilatation process. Cervical lacerations are a real problem because fluid absorption through these lacerations can take dramatic proportions very quickly. When a cervical laceration is noted, the surgeon should take extra precautions in obtaining accurate estimates of the fluid deficit.

The cervix is dilated to Hegar 10. This will allow smooth maneuverability of the endoscope during the procedure. Indeed, it is important that insertion and extraction of the endoscope through the endocervical canal do not require force. This would lead to jerky movements and inaccuracy of the surgical manipulation. Over-dilatation had been advocated by some to increase the flow of distention medium. Continuous-flow resectoscopes have channels that are quite sufficient in diameter to carry the medium in and out. Smooth maneuverability of the endoscope is the first priority.

Some surgeons perform suction and evacuation of the uterus prior to electrodesiccation of the endometrium, even in cases where the endometrium was hormonally suppressed. They do this in order to ensure that there is a histological specimen.

The fully assembled resectoscope is then introduced into the uterine cavity. This can be performed under direct vision or with an obturator. Direct vision is preferred by these authors because this is the only time early in the procedure where the operator has a chance visually to inspect the cervical canal and detect lacerations, a cause for concern. In addition, blind and forceful insertion of the resectoscope, using the obturator, may lead to uterine perforation.

The irrigation system is set in place. A pump-driven system with a pressure measurement device can be used. Simple gravity with large-bore tubing used in transurethral resection of the prostate (TURP) is equally adequate. The latter is the system we favor. No matter what type of fluid is being used for distention, it is essential that a fluid monitoring system be utilized to monitor fluid deficit. This may be automated[7] or manual; however, the automated system is much less labor-intensive and may give a continuous readout of the amount of fluid intravasated.

The uterine cavity is then carefully inspected. In particular, the surgeon identifies the tubal ostia, detects and characterizes intrauterine lesions, and looks for scars left by Cesarean section and other uterine surgery. Unless the anatomy is carefully assessed, the procedure should not commence. At this time, the surgeon selects the type of electrode best suited for the particular procedure to be performed. For novices, it is recommended to start with the large ball or barrel-type electrodes. The choice of electrode will primarily depend on the pathology present. An intrauterine tumor, such as a fibroid, has to be resected with a loop-type electrode. The surgeon may elect to proceed with resection of the remaining endometrium rather than electrodesiccation. However, it is certainly not wrong to perform the electrodesiccation first and to resect the fibroid later. It is our experience that marking the fundus and ostial areas with the ball electrode helps in subsequent orientation.

Systematic is the buzz word in electrodesiccation of the endometrium. Each and every surgeon has to determine the sequence in which the endometrial surface will be desiccated. The authors begin at the fundus, drawing a line between both ostia. Then, the electrode is rolled over the anterior wall first and progressed clockwise. Some fine tuning may be required at the level of the ostia and the internal cervical os. A second pass is not required.

Choice and application of electrical current could be the subject of a book on its own. There is appreciable variation among the different electrosurgical units available in the operating room. Making recommendations is, therefore, somewhat hazardous. As surgeons, we choose the settings on the unit according to clinically observable results. These visual endpoints are typical and reproducible. The settings on particular electrosurgical units will be widely variable for identical clinical results. Therefore recommendations will not be expressed for a particular unit nor the brand name of any equipment.

The electrodesiccation process can be divided into two steps (Figure 2): the initiation phase and dynamic phase. During the initiation phase, the electrode is brought in contact with the surface of the endometrial cavity. Contact is firmly achieved before current is established. Following contact, the surgeon keys the pedal, thereby activating the electrode. Optimal current settings will result in immediate blanching of the tissue in contact with the electrode. This area of blanching slowly spreads circumferentially around the electrode. Small gas vacuoles ('bubbles') are seen arising from the tissues around the blanched area. Larger

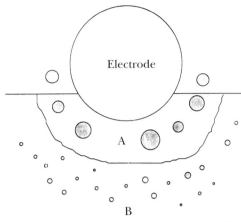

Figure 2 Diagrammatic representation of the visual control of the electrodesiccation process. A, tissue damage zone with visible blanching and large vacuoles; B, tissue damage zone with small vacuoles

vacuoles form within the blanched tissue. If sparking or tissue disintegration is observed, the settings are too high. A continuous sinusoidal (cutting) waveform is better than a damped (coagulation) waveform, provided that sufficient voltage is available to drive the current through a highly impeding tissue, such as partly desiccated endometrium. During the dynamic phase of the procedure, the electrode is painstakingly slowly rolled or dragged over the surface of the uterine cavity. The pressure on the electrode is firmly maintained while moving the instrument. The desiccation artefacts described earlier will remain visible. Vacuolization and blanching of tissue have to be observed in front of the electrode. These phenomena are the only clinical data available to the surgeon to use in estimating the adequacy of electrodesiccation. Depth of tissue destruction is not visible *per se*. However, when tissue is seen blanching in front of the electrode, one may safely assume that tissue underneath the electrode will also be affected.

Carbonization of either the tissue or the electrode has to be avoided. A new electrode should be used for each procedure because the metal will be affected by usage and carry current less effectively. A carbonized electrode requires increasing the power setting and will, therefore, likely cause sparking between the electrode and the tissue in an effort to bridge the gap created by the carbon deposit on the surface of the electrode. This sparking will, in turn, dry out the surface of the tissue too rapidly, thereby preventing desiccation of the deeper layers. Carbonization of the tissue has a similar negative effect on the depth of tissue destruction. The most likely cause of carbonization is the use of excessive electrical power.

In summary, the lowest effective power setting is the ideal setting. A low power will require slow motion of the electrode, which will lead to deep desiccation of the endomyometrial tissue. It is recommended that the surgeon use the same generator for these procedures to develop expertise with that particular unit. This, in turn, increases the likelihood of positive outcome.

Slow and systematic electrodesiccation of all endometrial surfaces is recommended. Repeat passages of the electrode over the surface do not replace the efficiency of a single slow and systematic approach. Partially desiccated tissue, resulting from a rapid pass with the electrode, will present increased impedance to the electrode during the next pass. This increased impedance may prevent all further heat generation in the tissue. Adequate ablation may not be obtained.

Lesions, such as fibroids within the cavity, represent a challenge. The rigid equipment commonly used for operative hysteroscopy limits the accessibility of areas within the cavity that are masked by the intrauterine mass. Either the surgeon accepts that the ablative procedure will be incomplete, or the mass is resected at least partially to allow the ablative procedure to be completed. The surgeon who engages in operative hysteroscopy should be well versed in the use of all different electrodes and attachments that are available. An effort should be made to resect the intrauterine mass in addition to the electrodesiccation of the endometrium. Ideally, ultrasonography has been performed prior to the ablation in order to avoid embarrassing moments for the surgeon.

When desiccating the endomyometrial surface, the endometrium has a tendency to detach from the underlying myometrium. This should be of no concern to the operator. In some instances, the strips of tissue detaching are of varying thickness and the exposed myometrial surface is irregular. This shows that the endometrium–myometrium interface is irregular. This clinical observation most likely correlates with adenomyosis. It is, as yet, unclear whether this finding should lead to alteration in surgical technique or patient management.

RISKS

The MISTELTOE study, a prospective audit of over 10 000 endometrial ablation procedures, reported that the complication rate following electrodesiccation is the lowest of any first-generation endometrial ablation technique[6]. Complication rate for hemorrhage is reported as 0.97% with perforation occurring in 0.64% of cases. The emergency hysterectomy rate is reported as 0.16% and the overall emergency surgery rate 1.11%. There were no reported visceral burns in this series and the overall complication rate was reported as 2.1%. Other risks associated with operative hysteroscopy are fluid overload, bleeding and infection.

Fluid overload is of primary concern. Careful measurement of inflow and outflow, either by automated or manual calculation, is essential when performing operative hysteroscopy. This allows the surgeon, at any time, to be aware of fluid deficit.

The choice of irrigation fluid is determined by electrical conductivity and osmolality. Nonconductive fluids are to be used with electrosurgery. This is not because the presence of electrolytes would burn the patient but because the electrolytes diffuse the current and thereby drastically reduce the power density. As a result, very little heat is generated in the tissues to be destroyed.

The osmolality of fluid is determined by the number of particles in the fluid[8]. The effects of fluids on distribution of water in the body are dependent on the permeability of cell and capillary membranes for the various particles present in the fluid.

The commonly used irrigation fluids are composed of water with particles that readily diffuse through the capillary membrane but not through the cell membrane. Therefore, infusion of these fluids will cause water redistribution in the entire extracellular compartment (EC). The intracellular compartment (IC) will be indirectly affected by the dilutional effects on the concentration of solutes (principally Na^+) in the EC. The IC will maintain the transmembranous gradient of concentrations of Na^+ and K^+ through active pumping. This process will result in intracellular low K^+ concentration and swelling due to absorption of water in the cell. Clinically, this water intoxication manifests itself by cerebral edema (confusion, drowsiness, coma and death). Acute dilutional hyponatremia is synonymous with water intoxication.

Total body fluid represents one half of body weight. Extracellular (intravascular and interstitial) fluid equals 45% of total body fluid. Table 1 demonstrates the effect that 1 liter of overload is sufficient to bring a normonatremic patient into the abnormal range! Table 2 shows the same example when there is a 3 liter

Table 1 The effects of 1 liter fluid overload

80-kg patient
Total body water = 40 l
EC = 40 × 0.45 = 18 l
Total Na^+ = 18 × 140 mEq/l = 2520 mEq
Fluid overload of 1 l of electrolyte-free solution
New EC = 19 l
New $[Na^+]$ = 2520/19 = 132.6 mEq/l

EC, extracellular compartment

Table 2 The effects of 3 liter fluid overload

80-kg patient
Fluid overload of 3 l of electrolyte-free solution
New EC = 21 l
New $[Na^+]$ = 2520/21 = 120 mEq/l

EC, extracellular compartment

overload. This will decrease the patient's sodium to 120 mEq/l, which is the level at which symptoms of cerebral edema may appear. In addition, the symptoms of cerebral edema will be masked by general anesthesia. Management of fluid overload is discussed in Chapter 6.

Bleeding is a rare complication of electrodesiccation of the endometrium. Generally, it will be due to either cervical laceration or uterine perforation. Hemorrhagic complications are more likely to occur with the loop electrode during myoma or endometrial resection of a fibroid or of the endometrium. Management of hemorrhagic complications will depend on the location of the source of bleeding and the severity of the condition. Uterine bleeding, when visualized under hysteroscopic view, can be stopped using the ball-end electrode. The electrode is firmly applied to the bleeding area. A low wattage continuous ('cutting') current is then applied for 1–2 min. This will lead to coaptation of the bleeding source and control of the hemorrhage. Diffuse bleeding from the cavity can be controlled with insertion of a balloon (Foley catheter with 30-ml bulb). The balloon is inflated with 10–20 ml of fluid until firm resistance is perceived. Methergine can be given intravenously to stimulate myometrial contractions, thereby increasing the tamponading force. The balloon is gradually deflated, e.g. 50% of its volume every 2 h, until it can be removed by gentle traction. Leaving the balloon in the uterine cavity for more than 24 h is not recommended. Antibiotic coverage is added to the treatment for the duration of the tamponade, and the patient is kept under observation for at least 23 h.

Infectious complications were the only complications initially reported in 1937 by surgeons performing endometrial electrodesiccation[1]. The incidence of endomyometritis and subsequent pelvic abscess was 3%. Some of these patients went on to develop fistulas between the uterus and small bowel! Therefore, the threat of serious infectious complications is real. The clinical manifestations of postoperative endomyometritis are hemorrhage, pain and fever. None of these symptoms needs to be dramatic to raise the suspicion of infection. When a patient presents with increasingly heavier vaginal bleeding in the early days after the procedure, treatment for endomyometritis should be initiated even in the absence of fever. Treatment consists of high-dose broad-spectrum antibiotics, which can be given on an outpatient basis. Hospitalization is required only in severe cases. Patients unresponsive to antibiotic treatment should undergo hysterectomy. A prolonged 'wait and see' attitude may be detrimental to the patient because endomyometritis may quickly degenerate into a fulminating sepsis and subsequent demise of the patient. Fortunately, infection rarely occurs[9].

Pregnancy is not a true complication of the procedure but should be discussed with the patient. The incidence of pregnancy after endometrial ablation is, in fact, unknown. A compilation of a large number of procedures demonstrated a 1% incidence of pregnancy, mostly intrauterine, after endometrial ablation[4]. Patients at risk for pregnancy after ablation should be advised to use some method of contraception or deal with the prospect of possibly undergoing a pregnancy interruption.

POSTOPERATIVE MANAGEMENT

The immediate postoperative management consists of monitoring of vital signs at regular intervals. Vaginal bleeding should not exceed the amount that can be expected after procedures such as a dilatation and curettage.

Pain, in the form of cramping, is common. When a paracervical block has been used, this pain is minimal. Otherwise, the uterine cramping during the first 2 h following the procedure can be severe and require sedation with drugs such as morphine or meperidine (Demerol). Pain requiring sedation that persists for several hours should alert the physician that a complication has occurred, related to inadvertent heat damage to neighboring organs.

Postoperative hormonal treatment has been shown to increase the proportion of patients with amenorrhea[10]. However, the combined incidence of amenorrhea and hypomenorrhea remains unchanged. Depo-Provera® is the drug most commonly used because it is conveniently administered only once, in the immediate postoperative period.

Prophylactic antibiotics are given by some. It has not been demonstrated that this reduces the incidence of infectious complications. The first postoperative visit is scheduled approximately 1 week after the procedure. The blood-tinged vaginal discharge has by that time usually ceased. On physical examination, the uterus should feel firm. Persistent or increasing blood-tinged discharge and/or uterine tenderness to palpation is a sign of endomyometritis. Immediate treatment with broad-spectrum antibiotics is recommended. Obtaining a sample from the endocervix for culture and sensitivity may be considered.

Delayed complications due to thermal damage to adjacent organs, such as the bladder and the bowel, may not become apparent until several weeks after surgery. A second postoperative visit is, therefore, scheduled within 6 weeks after surgery. The timing is individually assessed. The symptoms looked for are those of peritonitis, localized or generalized. Further visits are planned at approximately 3–4 months after surgery and then on an annual basis. During this time, the cervical canal can be evaluated for patency.

For women who have not had a sterilization performed at the time of surgery, and are not using a reliable form of contraception, pregnancy should be considered as a possible cause of amenorrhea in the postoperative setting. This is especially the case when amenorrhea occurs after regular menstrual bleeding. Pregnancy may also occur in women rendered amenorrheic following electrodesiccation and should be excluded by appropriate investigation if clinical symptoms such as breast tenderness or nausea and vomiting occur without other apparent causation.

RESULTS

Results can be looked at in two different ways. One can define success as no further need for treatment of the menorrhagia. The great majority of patients could then be considered 'cured'. If amenorrhea is considered the endpoint of the procedure, then one could say that the results are rather poor, since possibly as few as one-third of the patients will remain amenorrheic more than 1 year after surgery. When comparing results published in the literature[3,11–18] (Table 3), the rates of success and failure appear to be independent of the method of ablation used.

It is recognized that persisting and *de novo* dysmenorrhea are problems requiring our attention. In our experience, dysmenorrhea has been a reason for further surgical treatment in only a few patients. However, it has spurred more caution in selecting candidates for the procedure.

The impact of electrodesiccation of the endometrium on premenstrual symptoms (PMS) is a subject of heated debate. One fallacy of this discussion is that patients undergoing endometrial ablation, who happen to have PMS, also have excessive bleeding. In addition,

the clinical entity 'PMS' is ill-defined, to say the least. Notwithstanding the above, empirical observations confirm that reducing the bulk of the endometrial tissue has more consequences than simple reduction of menstrual flow.

Lefler and Lefler[2] performed interesting studies evaluating the impact of endometrial ablation on PMS symptoms. There was a statistically significant reduction in the severity of symptoms after endometrial ablation. This is reported to continue up to 2 years after surgery[18]. Although these beneficial side-effects of endometrial ablation are welcomed by the patients, it should be emphasized that PMS is not an indication to perform endometrial ablation. The main reason for this cautionary statement is that the currently available data have been obtained in women with menorrhagia as the primary complaint. It is unknown whether women with normal menogram would benefit in a similar fashion. The difficulty of defining 'abnormal uterine bleeding' in objective numbers will certainly add to the confusion in designing and interpreting results of studies performed on women with apparently normal menses complaining of PMS symptoms.

Table 3 Outcomes following first-generation endometrial ablation procedures

Study	No. of patients	Class of evidence*	Follow-up (years)	Amenorrhea (%)	Satisfaction (%)	Further surgery (%)	Hysterectomy (%)
Bhattacharya et al., 1997[11]	372 (Comb)	A	1	47	90	18	10
Chullaparam et al., 1996[12]	142 (ED)	B	4.2	28	84	15	8.5
Crosignani et al., 1997[13]	38 (TCRE)	A	2	23	87	NR	10
Dutton et al., 2001[14]	240 (ED)	B	5	NR	81	NR	29
Meyer et al., 1998[3]	117 (ED)	A	1	27	87	NR	2
O'Connor and Magos, 1996[15]	525 (TCRE)	B	5	32	80	20	9
Phillips et al., 1998[16]	746 (ELA)	B	6.5	37	80	NR	21
Vancaillie, 1991[†]	90 (ED)	B	2	84**	84	NR	2
Vilos et al., 1996[17]	800 (Comb)	C	1	60	NR	6	2

*Class A, randomized, controlled trials; B, prospective, cohort studies; C, retrospective, cohort studies; **combined amenorrhea and hypomenorrhea rate (spotting); †personal communication; Comb, combination of procedures; ED, electrodesiccation; TCRE, transcervical resection of the endometrium; ELA, endometrial laser ablation; NR, not reported

CONCURRENT PROCEDURES

Laparoscopy is indicated in patients in whom pelvic pathology, such as endometriosis, is suspected. This is especially valuable if the patient is complaining of pelvic pain with or without dysmenorrhea. The presence of endometriosis is not a contraindication to endometrial ablation. If pelvic pain is a major complaint of the patient besides heavy menstrual bleeding, it is recommended to evaluate the pain with care because the persistence of pain may represent a serious challenge in the further management of the patient.

Laparoscopy to monitor the procedure is not recommended because this additional procedure will not prevent the occurrence of complications, such as perforation. The objective of a laparoscopy is to assess the damage that was caused by such a complication. This surgical management decision can be taken at the time of occurrence. Systematic scheduling of laparoscopy is not warranted.

References

1. Bardenheuer FH. Elektrokoagulation der Uterusschleimhaut zur Behandlung klimakterischer Blutungen. *Zentralblatt Gynaekologie* 1937;59:209–16

2. Lefler HT, Lefler CF. Improvement in PMS related to decrease in bleeding. *J Reprod Med* 1992;37:596–8

3. Meyer W, Walsh B, Grainger D, *et al.* Thermal balloon and rollerball ablation to treat menorrhagia: a multicentre comparison. *Obstet Gynecol* 1998;92:98–103

4. Pugh C, Crane J, Hogan T. Successful intra-uterine pregnancy after endometrial ablation. *J Am Assoc Gynecol Laparosc* 2000;7:391–4

5. Sowter M, Singla A, Lethaby A. Pre-operative thinning agents before hysteroscopic surgery for heavy mentrual bleeding. *The Cochrane Library* 2000; Issue 3

6. Overton C, Hargreaves J, Maresh M. A national survey of the complications of endometrial destruction for menstrual disorders: the MISTLETOE study. *Br J Obstet Gynaecol* 1997; 104:1351–9

7. Hawe JA, Chen P, Phillips AG, *et al.* The validity of continuous automated fluid monitoring during intra-uterine surgery, luxury or necessity. *Br J Obstet Gynaecol* 1998;105:797–801

8. Rose BD. Renal function and disorders of water and sodium balance. In Rubenstein E, Federman D, eds. *Medicine.* New York: Scientific American, 1994;10:9–13

9. Loffer F. Endometrial ablation – where do we stand? *Gynecol Endosc* 1992;1:175–9

10. Goldrath MH. Use of danazol in hysteroscopic surgery for menorrhagia. *J Reprod Med* 1990; 35:91–6

11. Bhattacharya S, Cameron I, Parkin D, *et al.* A pragmatic randomised comparison of trans-cervical resection of the endometrium with endometrial laser ablation for the treatment of menorrhagia. *Br J Obstet Gynaecol* 1997;104:601–7

12. Chullapram T, Song J, Fraser I. Medium term follow-up of women treated by rollerball endometrial ablation. *Obstet Gynecol* 1996;8:71–6

13. Crosignani P, Vercellini P, Apolone G, *et al.* Endometrial resection versus vaginal hysterectomy for menorrhagia: long-term clinical and quality-of-life outcomes. *Am J Obstet Gynecol* 1997;177:95–101

14. Dutton C, Ackerson L, Phelps-Sandall B. Outcomes after rollerball endometrial ablation for menorrhagia. *Obstet Gynecol* 2001;98:35–9

15. O'Connor H, Magos A. Endometrial resection for the treatment of menorrhagia. *N Engl J Med* 1996;335:151–6

16. Phillips A, Chien P, Gary R. Risk of hysterectomy after 1000 consecutive endometrial ablations. *Br J Obstet Gynaecol* 1998;105:897–903

17. Vilos G, Vilos E, King J. Experience with 800 hysteroscopic endometrial ablations. *J Am Assoc Gynecol Laparosc* 1996;4:33–8

18. Grainger D, Tjaden B, Rowland C, *et al.* Thermal balloon and rollerball ablation to treat menorrhagia: two-year results of a multicenter, prospective, randomised clinical trial. *J Am Assoc Gynecol Laparosc* 2000;7:175–9

14

Control of menorrhagia by endometrial resection

A. Taylor and A. Magos

A BRIEF HISTORY OF ENDOMETRIAL RESECTION

It is somewhat surprising that the first hysteroscopic endometrial ablations were performed using laser energy rather than electrosurgery, bearing in mind the relatively short history of the former and the long one of the latter in the field of medicine. Nonetheless, the original series of Nd:YAG laser ablations, published by Goldrath and associates[1] in 1981, was followed only 2 years later by a report from DeCherney and Polan's group in Yale, when, for the first time, the resectoscope was used to control intractable uterine hemorrhage by electrocautery of the endometrium[2]. Neuwirth, the pioneer of hysteroscopic resection of submucous fibroids as far back as 1978[3], also wrote about the possibility of treating menorrhagia by resecting the endometrium in 1983, but did not include any cases in his review article[4]. Indeed, the second-ever paper in the English-speaking literature was also from Yale, when in 1987 DeCherney and colleagues wrote an update of their earlier work and first referred to actual resection of the endometrium rather than to solely cautery in a total of 21 patients[5]. In contrast, by 1987 there were already a number of published series of laser ablations by authors such as Lomano[6] and Loffer[7] involving over 300 patients, with many more publications to come in the ensuing few years.

Initial developments in the use of the resectoscope as a means of treating menorrhagia as an alternative to hysterectomy took place in the USA. The instrumentation, in general, consisted of a single-flow urological resectoscope combined with dextran 70 (Hyskon®) as the uterine distention medium. The next phase in the evolution of the technique of endometrial resection, as well as wider application of this mode of treatment for the management of dysfunctional uterine bleeding, took place in Europe.

Although the precise historical details and timings are unclear, two important modifications of the procedures as described by DeCherney and co-workers[2,5] were made by two gynecologists from Paris. First, Hamou popularized the use of electrolyte-free low-viscosity fluids for uterine distention, instead of dextran 70, thus allowing uterine irrigation as well as distention during surgery[8]. Second, Hallez designed a continuous-flow resectoscope for intrauterine surgery, using this instrument to perform hysteroscopic myomectomy[9]. The combination of non-viscous irrigant with a continuous-flow sheathing system meant that the operative environment could be easily controlled to produce optimum conditions for safe intrauterine surgery. From this emerged the treatment of 'partial endometrial resection' described by Hamou, involving excision of the endometrium and the underlying 2–3 mm of myometrium over the upper uterine cavity.

Hamou used sterile 1.5% glycine solution as the distention medium and a standard 26 Fr continuous-flow urological resectoscope fitted with a 4-mm 30° foroblique telescope (in contrast to the Hallez myoma resectoscope which only measured 21 Fr in diameter and utilized a 2.7-mm 0° endoscope).

With minor modifications, Hamou's instrumentation and technique have become the standard for endometrial resection as practised by most gynecologists today. In 1988, at a gynecological endoscopy meeting held in Oxford in the UK, Hamou demonstrated partial transcervical resection of the endometrium (partial TCRE) to a small but enthralled audience. From this encounter came two further developments to his original technique, that of resecting the entire endometrial surface down to the upper endocervical canal (total TCRE)[10,11], and that of performing surgery under local rather than general anesthesia as an outpatient procedure[12,13].

Not unexpectedly, a procedure which offered a genuine alternative to hysterectomy with advantages in terms of lower cost, shorter operating time, reduced hospitalization and faster recovery was quickly seized upon by both public and gynecologists alike. Within 2 years of its introduction into the UK almost half the acute hospitals were offering endometrial resection as a treatment for menorrhagia, in contrast to under 10% who were performing laser ablation[14].

INDICATIONS AND CONTRAINDICATIONS

Although endometrial ablation was first pioneered in 1981[1], it has only been in the last few years that prognostic factors for successful ablation have emerged from randomized controlled trials and large audit studies[15-17]. For instance, women with excessively heavy periods (defined as > 80 ml) report lower subjective failure rates than those women who undergo ablation for a normal menstrual loss, 9% compared with 18%[18]. Patient age also appears to be important, with older women having higher satisfaction rates than younger women. The Scottish Audit of Hysteroscopic Surgery showed that satisfaction rates for women over 40 years were 88%, compared to 79% for women under 40 years[15].

Currently, the criteria we have developed in our clinic (listed in Table 1) are based on the observations that TCRE:

Table 1 Indications and contraindications for endometrial resection

Indications	Contraindications
Menstrual problems justifying hysterectomy	mild menstrual symptoms
Symptoms resistant to medical therapy	not tried medical therapy
No desire for further pregnancies	wish for further pregnancies
Regular, relatively short heavy periods	irregular, prolonged periods
Satisfied with reduction in menstrual flow	wants amenorrhea
No other gynecological problems indicating hysterectomy	other gynecological problems indicating hysterectomy (e.g. uterovaginal prolapse, congestive dysmenorrhea, chronic pelvic inflammatory disease, endometriosis, pelvic mass, cervical atypia
Benign endometrial histology	malignant or premalignant endometrial histology (e.g. atypical hyperplasia)
Uterine size smaller than the equivalent of 12-week pregnancy (or uterine cavity length < 10 cm)	large uterus greater than the equivalent of 12-week pregnancy (or uterine cavity length > 10 cm)
Submucous fibroids < 5 cm in diameter	submucous fibroids > 5 cm diameter
Careful counselling (e.g. nature of treatment, recovery, likely menstrual result, fertility implications, unknown long-term consequences)	not able to be counselled adequately (e.g. communication or language problems)

(1) Is a surgical procedure with potentially major complications;

(2) Cannot guarantee amenorrhea;

(3) Is less successful when there is gross pelvic pathology;

(4) Inhibits or adversely affects future pregnancies;

(5) Is too new for us to know its long-term consequences.

When identifying a potentially suitable patient, the first matter to establish is the severity of her symptoms. This is more difficult than might be thought as menstrual history is a relatively poor indicator of genuine menorrhagia as judged by menstrual blood-loss studies[19]. Unfortunately, objective measurement of menstrual bleeding is not widely available in ordinary clinical practice; however, daily pictorial charting of menstruation has been shown to be a reasonable alternative and should be more widely administered[20]. Where women are found to have a menstrual blood loss within normal limits it should be remembered that their subjective satisfaction rates are lower following ablation than those of women with proven menorrhagia. They do, however, respond well to reassurance, explanation and counselling and often require no further treatment[21]. Dysmenorrhea and irregular periods were thought to predict a poorer outcome following ablation. However, data from a randomized controlled trial comparing TCRE with endometrial laser ablation (ELA) suggested no difference in satisfaction rates when these symptoms were present preoperatively[16].

The second decision that has to be made is whether surgery or medical treatment should be tried in the first instance. Guidelines from the Royal College of Obstetricians and Gynaecologists on the management of menorrhagia in secondary care acknowledge that 'drugs such as danazol, gestrinone and gonadotrophin releasing hormones are effective in reducing heavy menstrual blood loss but side effects limit their long term use'. They instead recommend that a progesterone-releasing intrauterine system (IUS) 'should be considered as an alternative to surgical treatment'[22]. However, although the IUS is effective in managing menorrhagia[23], where it has been compared to endometrial resection in randomized trials, it has been shown to be less effective[24,25]. In addition there is evidence that delaying surgery reduces surgical satisfaction rates and, therefore, if a woman does not want medical therapy it is reasonable to offer endometrial ablation in the first instance[26]. Our own, current view is that TCRE is an alternative to hysterectomy rather than to non-surgical treatment, with the implication that conservative pharmacological therapy should always be the first choice, and surgery should only be offered if this proves unsuccessful or is not tolerated because of side-effects. The same considerations apply to women wishing to retain their fertility for whom only medical therapy is suitable.

For those women who want to achieve complete amenorrhea and for whom nothing less will suffice, TCRE or any of the other ablative techniques are contraindicated. For them hysterectomy, preferably by the vaginal route, is the ideal and only guaranteed solution. Hysterectomy may well also be indicated in the presence of obvious pelvic pathology such as uterovaginal prolapse or a pelvic mass, in women affected by severe premenstrual congestive-type of dysmenorrhea suggestive of endometriosis or chronic pelvic inflammatory disease, and in those with a history of cervical dysplasia.

The rationale of hysterectomy must be applied even more strictly to women found to have endometrial malignancy. There can be no doubt that frank endometrial carcinoma should be treated in part by hysterectomy. For those women with atypical endometrial hyperplasia the risk of progression to adenocarcinoma is between 8.3% and 100%, but the rate of progress is variable depending on degree of hyperplasia[27]. They should also be offered hysterectomy, for the simple reason that the endometrium is rarely, if ever, excised completely at TCRE and therefore it is not possible to guarantee against persistence or recurrence of the endometrial abnormality. Simple, non-atypical hyperplasia is not thought to be premalignant, and therefore can be managed by ablation in menorrhagic women[28].

Once it has been decided that, in principle at least, TCRE is an appropriate mode of management for a particular patient, then the practicalities of the procedure should be considered. Account has to be taken, above all, of uterine size as surgery becomes progressively more difficult, more time-consuming and more hazardous with increasing size of the uterine cavity. Enlarged uteri are generally associated with the presence of myoma, and relatively large fibroids, relative that is to the size of the instruments used for TCRE, are difficult to excise completely hysteroscopically. We therefore tend to adhere to the limits of uterine and fibroid size listed in Table 1. Although these are only guidelines, and women with uteri outside these limits have been treated, there seems little doubt that surgery in these cases is often complicated, by fluid absorption and incomplete resection leading ultimately to a failure to relieve symptoms. Even with conservative estimates, it is thought that almost 60% of women with menorrhagia who currently undergo hysterectomy could be treated by TCRE[29].

The final component of the assessment process is as important as the rest, and involves careful counselling of the patient so that she understands fully the nature of her treatment and the likely menstrual outcome. Although there remain concerns about the long-term malignant risk of the procedure, there are published 5-year[30] and unpublished 10-year follow-up data (A. Magos, unpublished data)[27] that suggest it is safe. Our current policy is to discuss this potential risk, noting, however, that the chance of this complication developing in years to come may be reduced by procedures such as TCRE simply because most of the endometrium is removed during the surgery. We openly admit that we do not as yet know the malignant risk of the procedure.

PREOPERATIVE ASSESSMENT

Prior to surgery the woman should have a full blood count, blood grouping and blood saving. A clotting screen may be appropriate in some instances. The woman should be up to date with her smears and have had a normal one within the last 3 years. Initially, the uterine cavity should be investigated using transvaginal ultrasound[22]. A scan of the pelvis will not only detect any uterine fibroids and quantify their size, but may also suggest the presence of polyps and, importantly, allows assessment of the adnexa. Any adnexal mass should then be further investigated.

A diagnostic hysteroscopy and target biopsy is the optimum investigation for detecting small intrauterine lesions, and is also the best technique for assessing the position and number of submucous fibroids and for deciding on their 'resectability'; briefly, small myomas which are predominantly in the uterine cavity are the most suitable for simultaneous resection, while large ones which are deeply embedded in the myometrium are likely to be impossible to excise completely. If submucous fibroids are found, then hysteroscopic myomectomy alone should be considered as an alternative mode of management to endometrial ablation. While myomectomy cannot offer the chance of amenorrhea, the menstrual benefits can still be considerable with the added advantage of leaving the uterine cavity intact[31]. Conversely, the presence of relatively large intramural fibroids which would impossible to treat concurrently, but which would tend to make the resection more difficult, should act as a warning and rollerball coagulation[32], laser ablation possibly combined with myolysis[33], or even hysterectomy should be offered to such patients.

Dilatation and curettage is no longer indicated either as a diagnostic check or as a therapeutic intervention in menorrhagic patients. It is not as sensitive or specific as hysteroscopy in terms of detecting intrauterine lesions[34], and its beneficial effect on menstrual blood loss is short lived, generally no more than 1–2 cycles[35].

ENDOMETRIAL PREPARATION

The aim of all forms of endometrial ablation is to destroy or excise the full thickness of the endometrium; its success depends on it. However, the thickness of the endometrium varies depending on the time in the cycle. In the immediate postmenstrual phase it is 1 mm, increasing to 10 mm in the late secretory phase[36]. The radius of a standard electrosurgery loop used for resection is about 4 mm and the depth of tissue destruction with Nd:YAG laser or rollerball is 4–6 mm[37]. It would therefore seem sensible to schedule surgery for the early proliferative phase. Clearly, in most instances, this is impractical and therefore research has focused on the use of medical agents that 'thin' the endometrium in preparation for surgery.

The Cochrane Library published an excellent review of preoperative endometrial thinning agents in 1999 and what follows is a summary of that report[38]. The reviewers first looked at the evidence for gonadotropin releasing hormone (GnRH) analogs, danazol and progestogens versus no pretreatment. They found that GnRH analogs significantly reduced the endometrial thickness, led to shorter operating times and resulted in less distention medium absorption when compared with placebo. Of the postoperative outcome measures more women achieved amenorrhea in the short term in the GnRH group than in the placebo group, although interestingly the patient satisfaction rates were the same for both groups. Next they looked at danazol and progestogens. Unfortunately, as yet there are no published randomized trials of any significant size comparing danazol with placebo or progestogens with placebo and their value can only be determined by looking at the comparative trials with GnRH analogs. These reveal that the clinical differences between GnRH analogs and danazol are small with a tendency to favor GnRH analogs. What may be more important are issues of compliance and cost. Danazol is taken orally 400–800 mg daily for 4–8 weeks, whereas the GnRH analog goserelin is a 3.6 mg subcutaneous injection every 28 days for 1–2 months. Both cause side-effects, although whilst danazol can be discontinued immediately goserelin cannot. Progestogens are significantly cheaper than both GnRH analogs and danazol, and, in theory, could be an attractive alternative. However, the evidence surrounding their use is scarce. The Cochrane review found only one small randomized controlled trial that reported no effect on endometrial thickness[39].

At the time of writing, there are still some unanswered questions surrounding preoperative endometrial preparation. It remains unknown if the duration of pretreatment should be 1 or 2 months and if the latter, is it significant enough to outweigh the increased cost and possible side-effects to the woman? In addition, whilst there are intra-operative advantages and short-term postoperative advantages in using endometrial thinning agents, what impact do these agents have on long-term success rates? In our experience they may have very little effect on the long-term outcome (Figure 6c). Whatever the ultimate advantages and disadvantages of preoperative endometrial thinning, there can be little doubt that endometrial resection is easier to perform in women who have been prepared, and this is to be highly recommended for the resectionist in-training.

ANTIBIOTICS

There are no firm recommendations regarding the use of prophylactic antibiotics during endometrial resection. However, in some respects hysteroscopic surgery is comparable to vaginal surgery where antibiotics are widely used at hysterectomy and have been shown to reduce peri-operative morbidity. Although the vaginal vault is not opened as at hysterectomy, about 20% of the uterine irrigant which is absorbed during surgery escapes into the peritoneal cavity via the Fallopian tubes[40]. Of even more concern is the fact that the remaining 80% enters the circulation directly via the myometrial vasculature, and although the distention media used are sterile preparations, they are not intended for intravenous use. For all these reasons, we give our patients prophylactic antibiotics as a single dose, currently a combination of metronidazole (1 g, 1 h before surgery) and a third-generation cephalosporin (cefotaxime 750 mg intravenously at the time of surgery).

TYPE OF RESECTOSCOPE

Resectoscopic instrumentation is discussed in detail in Chapter 2. Resectoscopes used for hysteroscopic surgery share a common origin in the form of the urological resectoscope, and there is little difference between the various manufacturers' designs. Nonetheless, there are various combinations of size, sheathing system, handle mechanism and optic that are available, and our current choice is described in Table 2. As can be seen, we favor a medium-sized instrument fitted with an angled endoscope. As we use a non-viscous distention medium (1.5% glycine solution), a continuous-flow system with in- and outflow sheaths is ideal for easy control of uterine distention and irrigation. Most importantly from a safety aspect, we favor a passive type of handle mechanism whereby

Table 2 Basic equipment and settings for endometrial resection

	Settings
Resectoscope	26 Fr gauge continuous-flow sheath, 24 Fr cutting loop, passive handle mechanism, 4-mm 30° foroblique telescope
Irrigation system	sterile 1.5% glycine solution, HAMOU hysteromat set at: 100–125 mmHg irrigation pressure, –50 mmHg suction pressure, 300 ml/min maximum flow rate
Electrosurgical generator	e.g. Valleylab Force 2 set at: 100–125 W cutting power, blend 1–3, 50 W coagulating power
Illumination and video	high-intensity cold light source (at least 250 W), wide light cable, video camera, high-resolution color monitor

the cutting loop sits protected inside the inflow sheath at rest and is only pushed out immediately prior to a cut being made; this arrangement makes accidental trauma to the uterus unlikely as inadvertent activation of the electrode cannot have any tissue effect under normal circumstances.

Almost as important as the characteristics of the resectoscope itself is the coupling of the optic to a high-resolution color monitor via a small chip video camera. The advantages are considerable in terms of operator comfort, particularly with patients with an acutely anteverted uterus in whom the non-video alternative would be to operate kneeling on the floor, and for the teaching and supervision of beginners. An indirect benefit is the possibility for patients who have their surgery under local or regional anesthesia to watch their procedure 'live', something which a surprisingly large proportion of our patients opt for[11].

IRRIGATION SYSTEM

A discussion about irrigation fluids and systems used for hysteroscopic surgery is given in Chapter 6. Briefly, the first hysteroscopic myomectomies and endometrial ablations were carried out using dextran 70 as the distention medium, but most ablations are now performed using isotonic (or near isotonic) low-viscosity fluids such as normal saline or Ringer's lactate if using laser, and 1.5% glycine, or 3% or 5% sorbitol for electrosurgical procedures such as TCRE. As only electrolyte-free solutions can be used with electrosurgery, absorption of these fluids can be associated with the development of electrolyte disturbances, of which hyponatremia is clinically the most important.

The uterine cavity being a potential space has to be distended under pressure to allow a good-enough panoramic view for surgery, which in practice means a clear view of the uterine fundus. Uterine compliance seems to be highly variable, perhaps influenced by uterine size, the presence of fibroids and endometrial thickness, but typically pressures of 80–120 mmHg have to be reached for adequate distention of the cavity.

Uterine distention of this magnitude can be achieved in a number of ways, including gravity-feed systems, by the use of pressure cuffs, or with dedicated pumps of which the HAMOU Hysteromat® (manufactured by Karl Storz GmbH, Germany) is the most popular example. This unit not only gives convenient control over uterine distention, in terms of maximum intrauterine pressure and flow rate of the irrigant, but also is combined with a suction pump to complete the continuous-flow circuit. In principle, the system is adjusted to deliver the minimum distention pressure which gives an adequate view of the uterine fundus and cornual areas (to reduce fluid absorption), and the minimum suction pressure which keeps the uterine cavity clear of debris (to reduce the volume of fluid infused into the uterus). When faced with problems of insufficient distention or a cloudy view, it is important to realise that it is the irrigation pressure which controls the former and the suction pressure which regulates the latter under normal circumstances.

Whatever distention/irrigation system is used for TCRE, it is essential to monitor fluid balance throughout the procedure to avoid fluid overload by the simple measure of stopping surgery before dangerous volumes are absorbed. This is even more important with TCRE than with other ablative techniques for two reasons: first, electrolyte-free solutions are used for uterine distention with the risk of hyponatremia which is proportional to the volume of fluid absorbed[40], and, second, as surgery involves resecting across blood vessels, intravasation of the irrigant is more likely than with rollerball or laser ablation where the endometrium is coagulated.

ELECTROSURGICAL GENERATOR

The resectoscope is an electrosurgical instrument which uses monopolar current for its tissue effect of cutting or coagulation, and it is important for the surgeon to understand the theory of electrosurgery outlined in Chapter 3. Modern solid-state electrosurgical generators should be used as these tend to have an increas-ing number of safety features built into them and provide accurate control of power output. Two principles must be remembered to minimize the risk of electrosurgical burns to patients: there must be no malfunction or break in the electrical circuit, and the lowest power setting should be used that produces the desired tissue effect. The latter will vary depending on the make and model of the generator and resectoscope, so it is only possible to give approximate guidelines as to the power settings (Table 2). Basically, the uterine tissue should cut with ease with little or no drag on the cutting loop during resection. This can be achieved by using a pure cutting current; however, we prefer to utilize a blended current to provide additional hemostasis, possibly reduce the volume of fluid absorbed by intravasation as a result, and increase the depth of thermal damage to the underlying myometrium and thereby, at least in theory, lead to coagulation of any unresected islands of endometrium[37,41]. The penalty for operating with a mixed cutting/coagulating current is that higher powers have to be employed, there is a tendency for charring of the tissues which may make identification of the myometrial fibers more difficult, and the resected chips are more likely to stick to the cutting loop.

ANESTHESIA

Either general and regional anesthetic techniques can be used for endometrial resection[42]. Endometrial ablation is, however, potentially not only a day-case procedure, but also one which can be performed using a local anesthesia, intravenous sedation (or more correctly 'anxiolysis') and supplementary intravenous analgesia, a combination which has advantages in terms of medical manpower, turnaround time and patient recovery[12,42]. Local anesthesia is sufficient because the sensory nerve supply to the uterus is relatively insensitive to noxious stimuli such as cutting and heating, two of the modalities used in resection, although it is more sensitive to distention. This fact, combined with the well-known efficacy of what is often referred to as 'sedo-analgesia' (sedation with analgesia) in many other branches of medicine for endo-scopic and other invasive procedures, led us to develop this approach to the operation.

Briefly, patients now receive a premedication cocktail of temazepam 20 mg orally for sedation and a rectal suppository of diclofenac 100 mg 1 h before surgery. In the anesthetic room (or operating theater or endoscopy suite), baseline readings of heart rate, electrocardiogram, oxygen saturation and blood pressure are taken and continue to be monitored during surgery. A small intravenous dose of an opiate analgesic (e.g. fentanyl 50 μg) is then given, followed 5 min later by an anxiolytic (e.g. midazolam 2.5 mg); the dose of the anxiolytic is subse-quently titrated in 1 mg increments until the patient is relaxed (but not asleep). We routinely give facial oxygen as both fentanyl and mid-azolam are potent respiratory depressants.

When comfortable and relaxed, the patient is placed in lithotomy position and prepared for surgery in the usual manner. The cervix is grasped with a tenaculum and 10 ml of 1% lignocaine containing 1 : 200 000 adrenaline is injected into the paracervical nerve plexus (2.5 ml at 3, 5, 7 and 9 o'clock behind the cervix), and a similar volume into the substance of the cervix. While the local anesthetic takes effect, the resectoscope is assembled with an injection cannula rather than a cutting electrode, and connected to the irrigation system, electrosurgical generator, light source and video camera ready for surgery. The position of the patient, surgeon and equip-ment is shown in Figure 1.

By the time the anesthetic has taken effect, the uterine cavity can be sounded and the cervix dilated without discomfort to the patient. The resectoscope is then introduced into the uterine cavity and a further 20 ml of the lignocaine/adrenaline mixture is injected at 10–15 points into the myometrium to a depth of 1 cm. Most of the injections are made around the uterine fundus and cornua, the areas which are the least anesthetized by the paracervical block. Surgery can then commence as under general anesthesia, addi-tional small doses of fentanyl or midazolam being administered if further analgesia or anxiolysis is required; on average, 75–100 μg of fentanyl together with 5–7.5 mg of midazolam is ultimately given.

The choice of anesthesia must, of course, be up to the patient in most cases. However, there are high-risk patients who are unsuitable for general anesthesia for whom TCRE under local anesthesia offers the chance of surgery[13]. Conversely, it must not be thought that surgery under local anesthesia and sedation is an 'office' procedure. There has to be a dedicated member of the medical staff, not necessarily an anes-thetist, who is responsible for sedation and monitoring of the patient. Close and continu-ous monitoring of respiratory function and other vital signs is mandatory, and facilities for resuscitation, intubation and laparotomy must

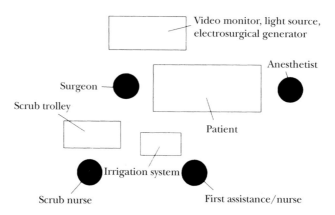

Figure 1 Position of the patient, surgeon and equipment during endometrial resection

be available. Finally, the operator should be someone experienced who can complete the required surgery quickly, efficiently and safely.

SURGICAL TECHNIQUE

There are many similarities between TCRE and the other hysteroscopic techniques of endometrial ablation. The patient is positioned and prepared as for a dilatation and curettage, and there is no need to catheterize the bladder unless it is full and making uterine palpation difficult. The operating table is tilted slightly head-down to encourage the bowel to fall away from the uterus and thereby make bowel trauma less likely should the uterus be perforated during surgery. There is a danger of air embolization in this position should air enter the uterine irrigation circuit[43]; however, this is unlikely particularly when gravity is used to pressurize the uterus. As an alternative safety measure, introducing a hydroperitoneum to float the bowel off the uterus has been suggested, but this seems unnecessarily invasive for a risk that is so slight.

The uterus is examined bimanually, the cavity sounded and the cervix dilated to admit the resectoscope easily but prevent leakage around the outflow sheath; for instance, if using a 26 Fr gauge resectoscope, which has an outer diameter of just under 9 mm, then dilatation to Hegar 10 is adequate and will ensure that loss of irrigant between the sheath and the cervix is minimal. The resectoscope is then introduced into the endocervical canal, the irrigation system opened, and the instrument guided into the uterine cavity under direct vision rather than blindly by means of an obturator.

After inspection of the cavity and injection of local anesthesia if required, the resection begins systematically in the following order: the uterine fundus and ostial areas, the upper half of the cavity starting posteriorly and working around either clockwise or anticlockwise, a similar sequence in the lower half of the cavity, and, finally, resection of the top half of the endocervical canal in women undergoing total TCRE[44]. The fundus is treated first as it is the most difficult area to resect with the greatest risk

of uterine perforation in the thin ostial regions, and the part of the uterus that becomes obscured most quickly by the resected chippings. Similarly, as the endometrial pieces tend to sink to the bottom of the uterine cavity, it is best to resect the posterior wall early on when treating the body of the uterus.

As it is mechanically difficult to resect the fundal endometrium with a standard backward-angled or right-angled cutting loop, a forward-angled electrode is used for this part of the procedure, which is a conventional cutting loop bent forward manually to 10–15° off the perpendicular (Figure 2). Rather than bending the loops backwards and forwards during surgery, a few loops are kept at the desired angle for resecting the fundus and cornual areas, and changed for the standard backward-angled loop when the remainder of the cavity is to be treated. Even with this precaution, the endometrium has to be undercut between the two cornua in a series of small chips, taking care not to push the loop more deeply into the myometrium than is necessary. Particular care has to be taken over the two tubal ostia where the myometrium is at its thinnest, and it is best to take a series of shallow shavings until all the endometrium has been resected here rather make one large cut and risk perforation. Alternatively, the fundus and cornual regions can be coagulated using a rollerball before switching to loop resection for the rest of the procedure[45].

After the fundus, the rollerball or forward-angled loop is changed for a standard,

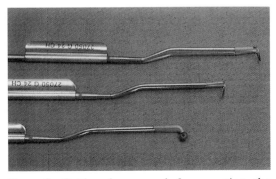

Figure 2 Cutting loops used for resecting the uterine fundus (top) and rest of the cavity (middle), and rollerball (bottom)

backward-angled loop which rests inside the insulated tip of the instrument (Figure 2). As this electrode does not protrude from the end of the irrigation sheaths, it is both safer and more efficient at cutting and should therefore be used as early as possible in the procedure. Rather than withdrawing the whole instrument from the uterus, it is easier to unlock the handle mechanism from the inflow sheath and merely remove this part of the resectoscope to change the electrode; it can then be reinserted directly into the uterine cavity via the sheathing system.

As gravity makes the resected tissue fall on to the posterior uterine wall, it makes sense to treat this part of the cavity first before it becomes obscured. Typically, therefore, surgery is started laterally by one of the tubal ostia and continued over the posterior wall to the contralateral side and then on to the anterior wall in a circular fashion, the upper cavity being treated before the lower part of the uterus. The chips of tissue, typically measuring $2.5 \times 0.7 \times 0.5$ cm as a reflection of the travel of the handle mechanism and the size of the cutting loop, are herded towards the uterine fundus with the loop, leaving the cavity relatively clear for surgery. In this way, the resection can continue uninterrupted until the whole cavity

has been treated, at which stage the pieces are removed with a flushing curette or similar instrument (Figures 3–5).

An alternative technique to the above is to cut full-length chips from the fundus towards the uterine isthmus by moving the whole instrument while cutting before finally pulling in the handle mechanism to disconnect the tissue

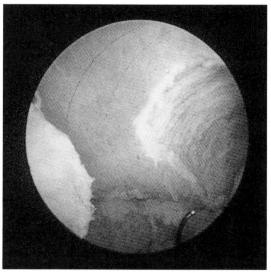

Figure 4 The endometrial/myometrial interface during surgery. See also Color Plate X

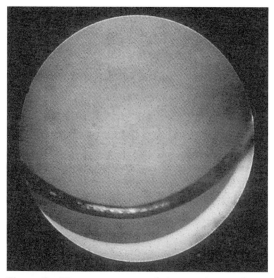

Figure 3 The appearance of the uterine cavity at the start of endometrial resection. See also Color Plate IX

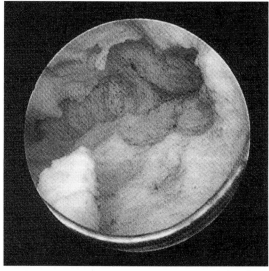

Figure 5 The appearance of the uterine cavity at the end of endometrial resection. See also Color Plate XI

from the uterus. Generally, the resected piece is then removed from the cavity immediately as the view would become obscured relatively quickly by these larger chips. Although we do not favor this approach in all cases, as it seems a less-efficient method of operating from the point of view of speed, fluid leakage via the cervix and the fact that each inflation/deflation cycle is associated with uterine bleeding which further obscures the hysteroscopic view, we do use this technique when the endometrium is very thick, during repeat resections and for removing larger submucous fibroids.

Whichever technique is used, the aim of surgery is to excise all the endometrium together with the underlying 2–3 mm of myometrium which is sufficient to remove all but the deepest extensions of the endometrium but not too deep to cut into the larger branches of the uterine artery. The circular myometrial fibers are easily visualized during resection, and once reached should only be resected further with great care as this may result in uterine perforation. If the endometrium has been prepared with an agent such as danazol or a luteinizing hormone releasing hormone (LHRH) analog, it is unusual to require more than one cut to achieve the desired depth of resection.

The lower margin of resection can be just above the uterine isthmus (partial resection) or into the upper part of the endocervical canal (total resection). Total TCRE offers the only chance of amenorrhea, although as with any of the ablative techniques, this endpoint cannot be guaranteed. Nonetheless, most women opt for total rather than partial resection, which is performed by resecting superficially into the cervical substance. Severe cervical hemorrhage necessitating hysterectomy has been recorded[46], but we have not had such complication in more than 600 procedures. As an alternative to resecting the upper endocervical canal, the rollerball can be used to ablate this area[43], although it could be argued that deep thermal damage and subsequent sloughing of the tissue could result in secondary hemorrhage.

Many patients with menorrhagia have submucous fibroids, and these can be excised easily at the time of endometrial resection provided the myomas are not numerous, are primarily intracavity in position and are < 4–5 cm in maximum diameter. Deeper fibroids are best left and only resected superficially to remove the overlying endometrium, as deep resection would promote fluid absorption, hemorrhage and risk uterine perforation. It is doubtful if menorrhagic women with multiple, deep, large fibroids are best treated by hysteroscopic surgery as opposed to hysterectomy.

At the end of surgery, once the uterus has been emptied of most of the endometrial/myometrial chips, the resectoscope is introduced back into the uterine cavity to check for any untreated areas or major bleeding points. The former are simply resected, and this demonstrates the beauty of all visual techniques, while the latter are coagulated using a loop or rollerball. Bleeding during surgery is usually minor because of the relatively high intrauterine pressure created by the irrigation system, but bleeding can be unmasked by lowering the distention pressure at the end of surgery. However, it is doubtful if it is worth spending time coagulating individual vessels or areas unless the hemorrhage is considerable.

All the collected resected tissue is sent for histological examination to exclude any unsuspected serious pathology. The availability of relatively intact tissue for such assessment is a major advantage of endometrial resection over other ablative techniques which destroy the endometrium *in situ*, and endometrial carcinoma has been uncovered in this way despite previous normal endometrial assessment[19,47].

TIPS FOR EFFECTIVE USE OF THE RESECTOSCOPE

There are four basic principles which should be adhered to for effective resectoscopic surgery.

(1) It must be remembered that it is not the cutting loop which cuts the endometrium but the arc of the cutting current passing from it; the loop must therefore be energized to make a cut, and indeed the

electrosurgical generator should be activated just before the loop comes into contact with the surface tissue to allow space for a spark of current to form[49].

(2) Cutting should only take place when moving the loop towards the resectoscope sheath, as an active loop pushed away from the sheath can easily perforate the uterus.

(3) The loop should be brought fully into the inner sheath before the generator is turned off in order to make a clean cut, otherwise a part of the resected tissue will remain attached to the uterus.

(4) The mobility of the uterus is such that a considerable pressure has to be applied between the cutting loop and the uterus

during resection to avoid skimming the surface and making a too shallow a cut; this is achieved by progressively angling the whole instrument while the loop is being pulled in, the cervix acting as the fulcrum for this movement.

TECHNICAL PROBLEMS DURING SURGERY

The most commonly encountered difficulties during and after endometrial resection are listed in Table 3 together with the likely causes and appropriate solutions. From the point of view of both safety and efficacy, it is essential that throughout surgery there is a clear view of the uterine cavity, a properly functioning

Table 3 Technical problems and solutions during endometrial resection

Problem	Cause	Solution
Poor uterine distention	low distention pressure uterine perforation cervical incompetence	increase distention pressure stop and check abdomen cervical suture or tenaculums around cervix
Slow clearance of debris/blood	insufficient suction pressure blocked outflow hole in sheath	increase suction pressure clean sheath
Inefficient cutting	cutting power too low cutting loop not in sheath at rest cutting loop broken	increase cutting power or reduce blend gently bend loop into correct position replace cutting loop
Poor view of endometrium and uterine cavity	poor uterine distention slow clearance of debris/blood resected chips restrict view bubbles on the anterior wall fibroids	see above see above remove chips before continuing with surgery increase suction pressure hysteroscopic total or partial myomectomy
Rapid fluid absorption	distention pressure too high uterine perforation	reduce distention pressure stop and check cavity
Bleeding during surgery	low distention pressure insufficient coagulation during cutting resection too deep fibroids	increase distention pressure increase coagulation blend coagulate vessel(s) and resect more shallowly coagulate vessels around pseudocapsule
Hemorrhage after surgery	resection too deep infection resected debris in cavity	uterine tamponade with balloon catheter antibiotics evacuate and give antibiotics

resectoscope, and careful monitoring of fluid balance and vital signs. If there is any concern about these aspects of the procedure, then surgery should cease immediately to be continued only if the problem has been rectified. TCRE may be a minor procedure in terms of surgical time, external trauma and recovery, but it is major surgery in terms of potential risks.

OPERATIVE COMPLICATIONS

The operative and postoperative risks of endometrial resection are listed in Table 4. These complications are unusual and TCRE is a relatively safe proceedure. This is confirmed by published data from the national survey of the complications of endometrial destruction for menstrual disorders: the MISTLETOE study[17] and the Scottish audit of hysteroscopic surgery for menorrhagia[15]. The MISTLETOE study reported on 10 686 procedures carried out by 690 doctors (1–222 cases/doctor) between 1993

and 1994. The survey investigated the complication rates for loop diathermy and rollerball when used together, loop diathermy when used alone, rollerball diathermy when used alone and laser ablation when used alone. The immediate operative complications are shown in Table 5. Overall the rates were low and ranged from 2.2% in the laser alone group to 6.4% in the loop alone group. The risk of emergency surgery following loop diathermy alone was 2.29% and for loop diathermy plus rollerball was 1.36%. This included hysterectomy, laparoscopy, laparotomy and cervical tears. In the loop alone group the results suggested that more experienced operators had fewer complications and, in particular, were less likely to perforate the uterus. Ten deaths were reported in the MISTLETOE survey, but only two appeared to be directly related to the ablation/resection procedure. Direct mortality rates in the combined procedure group were therefore 2 per 10 000 and 3 per 10 000 in the loop alone.

Table 4 Potential complications of endometrial resection

	Postoperative	
Intra-operative	*Short term*	*Long term*
Uterine perforation	infection	recurrence of symptoms
Fluid overload	hematometra	pregnancy
Primary hemorrhage	secondary hemorrhage	(uterine malignancy)
Gas embolism	cyclical pain	
	treatment failure	

Table 5 Immediate complications. Reproduced from reference 14

	Loop + ball (n = 4291)		Loop alone (n = 3776)		Laser (n = 1792)		Ball alone (n = 650)	
Complication	*n*	*%*	*n*	*%*	*n*	*%*	*n*	*%*
Hemorrhage	99	2.3	129	3.4	20	1.1	6	0.9
Perforation	52	1.2	88	2.3	11	0.6	4	0.6
Cardiovascular/respiratory	22	0.5	20	0.5	8	0.4	3	0.5
Visceral burn	3	0.07	3	0.07	0	0	0	0
Total*	171	4.2	229	6.4	46	2.7	13	2.1

Loop, loop diathermy; ball, rollerball diathermy; laser, laser ablation; *some cases had more than one complication and some complications were not specified

The current literature therefore suggests that both the morbidity and mortality associated with endometrial resection are considerably less than would be expected from hysterectomy[49,50]. It is also hoped, although it remains to be proven by continued audit, that hysteroscopic procedures such as TCRE will not be associated with the same long-term potential complications of hysterectomy such as premature ovarian failure[51], heart disease[52] and gastrointestinal dysfunction[53].

Uterine perforation is undoubtedly a major hazard of TCRE, inherently more so than with rollerball coagulation or laser ablation. If uterine perforation occurs while using the active electrode, surgery must be stopped immediately and laparotomy or laparoscopy performed depending on the experience of the operator. It is vital for the safety of the patient that serious vascular, gastrointestinal or urinary trauma is realized at once and corrective surgery performed during the same anesthetic. Provided the resection is stopped as soon as the perforation has been made, major intra-abdominal trauma is very much the exception rather than the rule; it is when the warning signs of uterine deflation with rapid fluid absorption are ignored and surgery continued that the scene is set for disaster. Conversely, we have managed several women with uterine perforation endoscopically by confirming a lack of major abdominal trauma laparoscopically, suturing the perforation laparoscopically, and then continuing with the hysteroscopic procedure once the uterus has been made 'water tight'[54].

The absorption of too much uterine irrigant is the second major potential operative complication of endometrial resection. It is difficult to compare techniques as several factors influence fluid absorption[55–57], but data from the MISTLETOE survey revealed significantly more fluid absorption in the laser ablation group than in the resection group[31]. It is probable that fluid absorption per unit time is greater with TCRE but as the operative time is faster, the total volume of irrigant absorbed is no more than with ELA. Apart from the fluid load, it must be remembered that only electrolyte-free solutions can be used with electrosurgical procedures such as endometrial resection. This means that major metabolic disturbances will accompany fluid overload, characterized by a dilutional effect on serum electrolytes, most importantly sodium[58–61]. Although hyponatremia is defined as serum Na$^+$ < 125 mmol/l, what constitutes a clinically dangerous concentration in the setting of hysteroscopic surgery in otherwise healthy, relatively young and usually fit women remains to be determined. Several authors agree that surgery should stop if the volume of fluid absorbed exceeds 1.5–2 l, and in our institution a strict protocol is followed in these situations as outlined in Table 6. Although careful monitoring of fluid balance during

Table 6   Management of fluid overload during endometrial resection

Volume absorbed (l)	Risk and action
< 1	major cardiovascular/respiratory or metabolic disturbances unlikely continue with surgery
1–2	major cardiovascular/respiratory or metabolic disturbance possible monitor vital signs closely, check serum electrolytes, treat with intravenous diuretic (e.g. 20 mg frusemide), catheterize bladder and monitor urine output complete surgery as quickly as possible
> 2	major cardiovascular/respiratory or metabolic disturbances likely actions as above if not already carried out, observe for at least 12–24 h stop surgery

surgery is paramount, labelling of the irrigant fluid with 1% ethanol has been shown to be a useful index of dilutional change[62].

Hemorrhage during or after surgery is unusual, and indeed the operative blood loss during TCRE has been shown to be only 10–20 ml when measured objectively[46]. As noted earlier, non-fatal gas embolism has been reported during endometrial resection[43], but this is preventable by ensuring that air does not enter the irrigation circuit. Postoperative complications such as endometritis, septicemia, peritonitis and pulmonary embolus have been reported but occur only in about 1% of cases[17].

POSTOPERATIVE MANAGEMENT

TCRE is day-case surgery in most cases, and potentially an outpatient procedure if performed under local anesthesia. Pain is generally slight and adequately treated by non-opiate oral analgesics. Nausea is also uncommon unless there has been a degree of fluid overload[57]. Bleeding tends to be heavy for the first 24 h or so before gradually reducing over the next 1–3 weeks to be followed by a non-offensive discharge for a short while[11]. Antibiotics are rarely given after surgery unless the uterus has been perforated. Normal activities and work can be resumed soon after surgery and the variation in recovery seen in clinical practice is more a testament to the important influences of personality and culture rather than the trauma of the operation itself. Resumption of sexual intercourse is generally advised only once the bleeding has stopped.

Women are now reviewed 3 months after surgery as it is difficult to judge the menstrual effects of TCRE before then. There are no published data regarding the use of postoperative endometrial suppression with agents such as danazol, long-acting progestogen injections or LHRH analogs as there are with laser ablation and rollerball coagulation, but there is some evidence that at least the early amenorrhea rates can be considerably increased by such a maneuver (E. Shaxted, personal communication).

RESULTS OF SURGERY

Data regarding the menstrual results of pure endometrial resection, as opposed to the other ablative techniques such as rollerball coagulation and ELA, remain limited. A distinction has also to be made between those series where the cutting loop of the resectoscope is used primarily as a coagulating tool, much like a rollerball, and where it is used to perform endometrial resection proper, the subject of this chapter. Thus, the original paper by DeCherney and Polan in 1983[2], their larger follow-up series in 1987[5], and the study by Derman and co-workers[63] with an 8-year follow-up, all essentially describe the results of endometrial coagulation with the cutting loop rather than TCRE. Other series mix techniques, even to the extent of including endometrial resection, rollerball coagulation and laser ablation on the same patients[64].

Experience regarding pure endometrial resection, with rollerball coagulation of the cornual and cervical regions in some cases, come mainly from Europe and Australia. In general, these studies come to the same conclusion, that the menstrual results of surgery are broadly comparable with the other ablative procedures, with amenorrhea occurring in about one-third of patients and failure in approximately 1 in 6[10,11,45,65,66]. Periods tend not only to become lighter but also shorter and less painful. Surgery can be effective when treating relatively enlarged uteri with simultaneous hysteroscopic myomectomy. TCRE has also been used effectively in atypical situations such as after radiotherapy for cervical carcinoma[67]. Menstrual blood-loss studies have also confirmed that TCRE is followed by a significant reduction in bleeding, by an average of 77% after total and 66% after partial resection[68,69].

How do these results compare with other methods of endometrial ablation? It is almost impossible to make a proper comparison because so many variables influence the results of surgery. The experience of the surgeon, age of the patient, presence of uterine pathology such as myomas, and the use of endometrial preparation and postoperative suppression are just a few of the factors which have to be taken into account. For instance, as the resectoscope was used initially to excise submucous fibroids, it is not surprising that women with even relatively large myomatous uteri tend to be offered hysteroscopic resection, whereas laser ablation is mainly reserved for those with dysfunctional bleeding.

An even more important consideration is the duration of follow-up of the study groups as there is now good evidence that the rate of treatment failure, as is to be expected, increases with time. Since the previous edition of this book, data on longer-term follow-up have been published. A retrospective audit of 380 women who had undergone TCRE reported 5-year results based on life-table analysis[70]. The audit revealed a hysterectomy rate of 12.4% at 1 year and 27.4% after 5 years. The rate at 5 years was higher for women under age 45 years (35%) than for those 45 and over (14.9%). Repeat TCRE was performed on 6.8% of patients, 50% of whom were then satisfied and avoided hysterectomy. Others have reported 4-year follow-up of a randomized trial of endometrial ablation versus hysterectomy. In the original trial both ELA and TCRE were performed[71], but in the follow-up paper no distinction was made between the two techniques[72]. In this follow-up series of 204 women, the probability of hysterectomy was 24% at 4 years compared with 14% at 1 year. The probability of receiving further surgery (repeat TCRE or hysterectomy) was 36%. Six women in this series had undergone two more repeat TCREs. Even at 4 years, satisfaction rates remained high at 80% compared to 89% in the hysterectomy group. We have recently conducted a 10-year follow-up survey of 525 women who underwent TCRE between 1988 and 1993 (A. Magos, unpublished data) and obtained data on 398 (75.8%) of the women. Using life-table analysis we looked at finite endpoints such as the need for repeat resection or hysterectomy. As can be seen clearly in Figure 6a, the chance of undergoing further treatment increases progressively with time, the rate depending to some extent on the nature of the initial procedure. Survival analysis showed that after 10 years the probability of hysterectomy was 28% and that of hysterectomy or repeat ablation 34%. The influence of age, endometrial preparation, presence of fibroids and uterine size on long-term hysterectomy rates are shown in Figures 6b–e. The rates of hysterectomy were greatest in those < 35 years at the time of surgery, which were twice those of women aged 45 or older at the time of surgery. The presence of fibroids or endometrial preparation appeared to have very little effect on long-term success rates. Uterine size, however, did influence the long-term probability of avoiding hysterectomy. Women with a uterine size of 10 weeks or greater at TCRE were 25% more likely to than those with a uterus less than 10 weeks in size to have undergone a hysterectomy at 10 years. Interestingly this difference between the two groups only emerged after 8 years of follow-up.

The early studies on TCRE confirmed all the expected benefits of the lesser procedure in terms of reduced operating time, shorter hospitalization, faster recovery and cost savings[73,74]. However, initially, there were doubts that the proceedure would fail in the longer term and that hysterectomy rates would be unaffected. With the emergence of longer-term follow-up data, this does not appear to be the case. For those women who undergo TCRE around 75% will avoid a hysterectomy at 4 years and its attendant morbidity and mortality; around 35% will require further surgery. Most of the failures occur in the first few years. From our unpublished data, treatment failures can occur many years later, but even at 10 years nearly 75% of women will have avoided hysterectomy. The need for these repeat surgical proceedures does have a financial implication and whilst there may be costs savings for TCRE over hysterectomy in the short term, in the longer term the difference in these savings has narrowed.

LONG-TERM COMPLICATIONS

The postoperative complications of endometrial ablation are also listed in Table 4. Apart from treatment failure (or recurrence of symptoms some time after surgery), pelvic pain, hematometra and pregnancy are the most often seen. Although menstrual pain is usually helped by surgery, in contrast to premenstrual dysmenorrhea, a small proportion of women do develop cyclical pain which is worse than preoperatively or arises *de novo*. In a certain number, the pain is related to the development

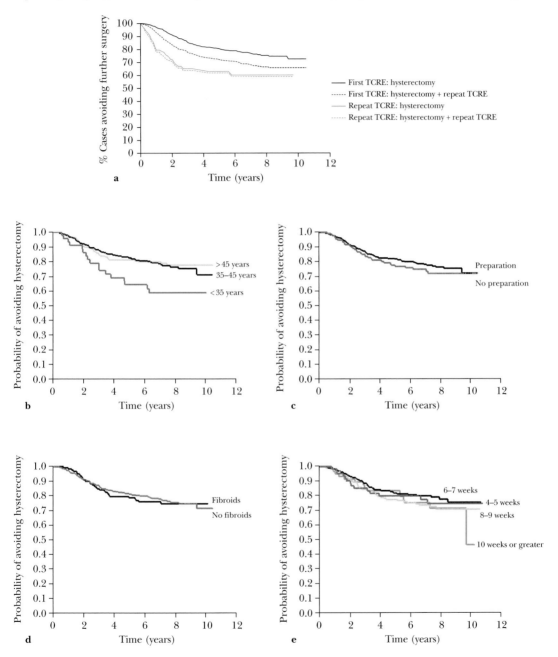

Figure 6 (a) Life-table analysis of the need for further surgery after intended total transcervical resection of the endometrium (TCRE). (b) Influence of age on the need for further surgery after intended total TCRE. (c) Influence of endometrial preparation on the need for further surgery after intended total TCRE. (d) Influence of the presence of fibroids on the need for further surgery after intended total TCRE. (e) Influence of uterine size on the need for further surgery after intended total TCRE

of a hematometra secondary to a combination of residual endometrium in the uterine cavity and cervical stenosis, a clue to the diagnosis being the absence of menstruation despite the pain[11,75]. The collection is generally fundal and presumably linked to too shallow resection in the cornual areas for fear of uterine perforation. Treatment in these cases is relatively simple and involves cervical dilatation and drainage of the hematometra followed by a repeat ablation if amenorrhea is desired; extra care has to be taken if resection is to be carried out as the myometrium has already been thinned once by the initial procedure, and rollerball coagulation would seem a safer option unless the uterine wall is known to be thick because of intramural fibroids.

Women whose pelvic pain is not associated with hematometra are more difficult to treat. Cases have been reported of granulomatous endometritis in this situation[76,77]. Interestingly, one study recently reported that endometrial ablation combined with laparoscopic treatment for pelvic endometriosis resulted in less recurrence of disease than laparoscopic treatment alone[78]. This supports the role of eutopic endometrium in the recurrence of endometriosis. Ultimately, about 25% of these patients will request a hysterectomy. The reasons for these failures are not completely understood, although increasingly adenomyosis is cited as a cause. In two studies, the histology of hysterectomies for persisting pain/bleeding following failed ablation revealed an incidence of adenomyosis between 75% and 100%[79]. Unfortunately, despite advances in imaging technology it is still not possible to identify these women accurately. In an effort to reduce these failures, some have suggested that by excluding women with dysmenorrhea and uteri > 10 cm (clinically those women with a high incidence of adenomyosis) the failure rate could be cut by 50%[80].

Endometrial resection/ablation should not be considered an absolute contraceptive, and there are now several reports in the literature of pregnancy following TCRE, rollerball ablation and ELA[81-86]. The outcomes vary from miscarriage, termination and premature labor to successful term planned pregnancy. However, there remain insufficient pregnancies to define the theoretical risks of prematurity, growth retardation and the need for abdominal delivery. A rare fetal anomaly has been reported affecting a pregnancy after endometrial ablation (single suture craniosynotosis), but this was probably coincidental[82]. Given the 0.7% frequency of pregnancy after endometrial ablation[85], it is therefore very important to offer women at risk of pregnancy either elective sterilization or advise on barrier methods of contraception.

In the very long term, the development of frank or occult endometrial carcinoma arising in islands of residual endometrium remains an unresolved risk. Even women who are amenorrheic postoperatively may have foci of inactive endometrium in the uterine cavity, and there is no reason why malignant change should not take place in some cases. This risk is the reason why women with endometrial hyperplasia showing cytological or architectural atypia should not be offered endometrial resection as they represent a high-risk group for the subsequent development of endometrial malignancy[28]. Similarly, when treated patients become menopausal and develop symptoms of the climacteric requiring estrogen replacement therapy, cyclical progestogens should be given to protect the endometrium.

CONCURRENT PROCEDURES

Hysteroscopic myomectomy is an obvious procedure to be performed during endometrial resection in women with submucous myoma, and indeed the resectoscope is most suited to the combined procedure. In contrast, deep intramyometrial fibroids should not be resected because of the risk of uterine perforation, excessive fluid absorption and probably incomplete surgery; instead, resection or rollerball ablation of the surface endometrium should suffice. It should also be remembered that hysteroscopic myomectomy on its own can be a very effective treatment for menorrhagia without the need for additional endometrial ablation[63].

Theoretically, there is no reason why TCRE should not be combined with laparoscopic pelvic surgery for endometriosis, adhesions, etc. if pelvic pain is a major component of symptomatology and there is some evidence that concurrent endometrial ablation in endometriosis reduces recurrence rates[78]. Laparoscopic sterilization, on the other hand, should be seriously considered in previously fertile women as being the most assured way to protect against unwanted pregnancy.

CONCLUSIONS

Endometrial ablative techniques have been exhaustively researched and reported in the last 10 years. There is now overwhelming evidence that they are a genuine alternative to hysterectomy[22,70,72,87] and result in high levels of patient satisfaction. Endometrial resection has a number of inherent advantages in terms of cost[88], speed of surgery, the ability to deal with fibroids, and the provision of tissue for histological assessment. However, 'pure' resection is associated with slightly higher immediate complication rates than other ablative techniques. These appear to be reduced if rollerball diathermy is used at the ostia and fundus, where the risk of perforation is probably greatest. It should be remembered that the overall morbidity and mortality of the procedure is much lower than for hysterectomy. Long-term follow-up data are now emerging that suggest that, even after 10 years, endometrial resection avoids the need for hysterectomy in 75% of women.

Finally, this chapter has focused on the first generation of endometrial ablative techniques with particular emphasis on TCRE. In the last few years there has been an explosion of new second-generation techniques[89–91]. These second-generation techniques are surgically less skill-dependent and potentially very promising. However, as yet it is too early to comment on their effectiveness and they need to be rigorously assessed against the proven first-generation techniques before any recommendations can be made about their role in the management of menorrhagia.

KEY POINTS

Endometrial resection is a fast and efficient means of removing the endometrium and submucous myoma in women with menorrhagia, that avoids hysterectomy in up to 75% of women. The ideal patient has dysfunctional uterine bleeding or a small fibroid uterus without any other pelvic pathology. The patient should understand that amenorrhea is unlikely to follow, sterility cannot be guaranteed and the long-term sequelae of surgery are as yet unknown. TCRE should only be performed by an experienced hysteroscopist with adequate training in the use of the resectoscope. The operative pitfalls of surgery should be appreciated together with the principles of appropriate corrective action. It is important to continue to monitor all patients who have undergone endometrial ablation until more is known about the long-term outcome of treatment.

References

1. Goldrath MH, Fuller TA, Segal S. Laser photovaporisation of endometrium for the retreatment of menorrhagia. *Am J Obstet Gynecol* 1981;140:14–19

2. DeCherney A, Polan ML. Hysteroscopic management of intrauterine lesions and intractable uterine bleeding. *Obstet Gynecol* 1983;61:392–7

3. Neuwirth RS. A new technique for and additional experience with hysteroscopic resection

of submucous fibroids. *Am J Obstet Gynecol* 1978; 131:91–4

4. Neuwirth RS. Hysteroscopic resection of submucous fibroids. *Obstet Gynecol* 1983;62:509–11

5. DeCherney AH, Diamnond MP, Lavy G, *et al.* Endometrial ablation for intractable uterine bleeding: hysteroscopic resection. *Obstet Gynecol* 1987;70:668–9

6. Lomano JM. Nd:YAG laser ablation of early pelvic endometriosis: a report of 61 cases. *Lasers Surg Med* 1987;7:56–60

7. Loffer FD. Hysteroscopic endometrial ablation with Nd:YAG laser using a nontouch technique. *Obstet Gynecol* 1987;69:679–82

8. Hamou JE. Hysteroscopy. *J Reprod Med* 1983; 28:359–89

9. Hallez J-P, Netter A, Cariter R. Methodical intrauterine resection. *Am J Obstet Gynecol* 1987;156: 1080–4

10. Magos AL, Baumann R, Turnbull AC. Transcervical resection of the endometrium in women with menorrhagia. *Br Med J* 1989; 298:1209–12

11. Magos AL, Baumann R, Lockwood GM, *et al.* Experience with the first 250 endometrial resections for menorrhagia. *Lancet* 1991;337: 1074–8

12. Magos AL, Baumann R, Cheung K, *et al.* Intrauterine surgery under intravenous sedation: an out-patient alternative to hysterectomy. *Lancet* 1989;2:925–6

13. Lockwood M, Magos AL, Baumann R, *et al.* Endometrial resection when hysterectomy is undesirable, dangerous or impossible. *Br J Obstet Gynaecol* 1990;97:656–8

14. Royal College of Obstetricians and Gynaecologists. *Third Bulletin of the Audit Unit*, 1991

15. Scottish Hysteroscopy Audit Group. A Scottish audit of hysteroscopic surgery for menorrhagia: complications and follow up. *Br J Obstet Gynaecol* 1995;102:249–54

16. Bhattacharya S, Cameron IM, Parkin DE, *et al.* A pragmatic randomised comparison of transcervical resection of the endometrium with endometrial laser ablation for the treatment of menorrhagia. *Br J Obstet Gynaecol* 1997;104:601–7

17. Overton C, Hargreaves H, Maresh M. A national survey of the complications of endometrial destruction for menstrual disorders: the MISTLETOE study. *Br J Obstet Gynaecol* 1997; 104:1351–9

18. Gannon MJ, Day P, Hamadich N, *et al.* A new method of measuring blood loss and its use in screening women before endometrial ablation. *Br J Obstet Gynaecol* 1996;103:1029–33

19. Chimbira TH, Anderson ABM, Turnbull AC. Relation between measured menstrual blood loss and patient's subjective assessment of loss, duration of bleeding, number of sanitary towels used, uterine weight and endometrial surface area. *Br J Obstet Gynaecol* 1980;87:603–9

20. Higham JM, O'Brien PMS, Shaw RW. Assessment of menstrual blood loss using a pictorial chart. *Br J Obstet Gynaecol* 1990;97:734–9

21. Rees MCP. Role of menstrual blood loss measurements in management of complaints of excessive menstrual bleeding. *Br J Obstet Gynaecol* 1991;98:327–8

22. Royal College of Obstetricians and Gynaecologists. *The Management of Menorrhagia in Secondary Care.* Evidence-based clinical guidelines No. 5. London: Royal College of Obstetricians and Gynaecologists, 1995

23. Andersson K, Rybo G. Levonorgestrel-releasing intrauterine device in the treatment of menorrhagia. *Br J Obstet Gynaecol* 1990;97:690–4

24. Istre O, Trolle B. Treatment of menorrhagia with the levonorgestrel intrauterine system versus endometrial resection. *Fertil Steril* 2001;76:304–9

25. Crosignani P, Vercellini P, Mosconi P, *et al.* Levonorgestrel-releasing intrauterine device versus hysteroscopic endometrial resection in the treatment of dysfunctional uterine bleeding. *Obstet Gynecol* 1997;90:257–63

26. Cooper KG, Parkin DE, Garret AM, *et al.* Two year follow-up of women randomised to medical management or transcervical resection of the endometrium for heavy menstrual loss; clinical and quality of life outcomes. *Br J Obstet Gynaecol* 1999;106:258–65

27. Creasy GW, Kafrissen ME, Upmalis D. Review of the endometrial effects of estrogens and progestins. *Obstet Gynecol Surv* 1992;47:654–78

28. Colafranceschi M, Crow J. Pathology. In Lewis VB, Magos AL, eds. *Endometrial Ablation.* Edinburgh: Churchill Livingstone, 1993:183–96

29. Rutherford AJ, Glass MR, Wells M. Patient selection for endometrial resection. *Br J Obstet Gynaecol* 1991;98:228–30

30. O'Connor H, Magos A. Endometrial resection for the treatment of menorrhagia. *N Engl J Med* 1996;335:151–6

31. Fraser IS, McCarron G, Markham R, *et al.* Measured menstrual blood loss associated with pelvic disease and coagulation disorders. *Obstet Gynecol* 1986;65:630–3

32. Vancaillie TG. Electrocoagulation of the endometrium with the ball-end resectoscope. *Obstet Gynecol* 1989;74:425–7

33. Donnez J, Gillerot S, Bourgonjon D, *et al.* Neodymium:YAG laser hysteroscopy in large submucous fibroids. *Fertil Steril* 1990;54: 999–1003

34. Loffer FD. Hysteroscopy with selective endometrial sampling compared with D&C for abnormal uterine bleeding: the value of a negative hysteroscopic view. *Obstet Gynecol* 1989; 73:16–20

35. Haynes PJ, Hodgson H, Anderson ABM, *et al.* Measurement of menstrual blood loss in patients complaining of menorrhagia. *Br J Obstet Gynaecol* 1977;84:763–8

36. Weingold AB. Gross and microscopic anatomy. In Kose NG, Weingold AD, Gershenson PM, eds. *Principles and Practice of Clinical Gynecology.* New York: Churchill Livingstone, 1990:3–32

37. Duffy S, Reid PC, Smith JHF, *et al. In vitro* studies of uterine electrosurgery. *Obstet Gynecol* 1991;78: 213–20

38. Sowter MC, Singla AA, Lethaby A. Pre-operative endometrial thinning agents before hysteroscopic surgery for heavy menstrual bleeding (Cochrane Review). *The Cochrane Library* 1999; Issue 3

39. Rich AD, Manyonda IT, Patel R, *et al.* A comparison of the efficacy of danazol, norethisterone, cyproterone acetate and medroxyprogesterone acetate in endometrial thinning prior to ablation: a pilot study. *Gynecol Endosc* 1995;4:59–61

40. Magos AL, Baumann R, Turnbull AC. Safety of transcervical endometrial resection. *Lancet* 1990;1:44

41. Duffy S, Reid PC, Sharp F. *In-vivo* studies of uterine electrosurgery. *Br J Obstet Gynaecol* 1992; 99:579–82

42. Elliott CJR, Page VJ. Anaesthesia for endometrial ablation. In Lewis VB, Magos AL, eds. *Endometrial Ablation.* Edinburgh: Churchill Livingstone, 1993:57–66

43. Wood SM, Roberts FL. Air embolism during transcervical resection of endometrium. *Br Med J* 1990;300:945

44. Magos AL. Endometrial resection: technique. In Lewis VB, Magos AL, eds. *Endometrial Ablation.* Edinburgh: Churchill Livingstone, 1993:104–15

45. Maher PJ, Hill DJ. Transcervical endometrial resection for abnormal uterine bleeding – report of 100 cases and review of the literature. *Aust NZ J Obstet Gynaecol* 1990;30:357–60

46. West JH, Robinson DA. Endometrial resection and fluid absorption. *Lancet* 1989;2:1387–8

47. Dwyer NA, Stirrat GM. Early endometrial carcinoma: an incidental finding after endometrial resection. Case report. *Br J Obstet Gynaecol* 1991; 98:733–4

48. Magos AL. Safety and hazards of endoscopic electrodiathermy. In Sutton CJG, ed. *New Surgical Techniques in Gynecology.* Carnforth, UK: Parthenon Publishing, 1993:163–71

49. Dicker RC, Greenspan JR, Strauss LT, *et al.* Complications of abdominal and vaginal hysterectomy among women of reproductive age in the United States. *Am J Obstet Gynecol* 1982;144:841–8

50. Wingo PA, Huezo CM, Rubin GL, *et al.* The mortality risk associated with hysterectomy. *Am J Obstet Gynecol* 1985;152:803–8

51. Centerwall BS. Premenopausal hysterectomy and cardiovascular disease. *Am J Obstet Gynecol* 1981;139:58–61

52. Siddle N, Sarrel P, Whitehead MI. The effect of hysterectomy on the age of ovarian failure: identification of a subgroup of women with premature loss of ovarian function and literature review. *Fertil Steril* 1987;47:94–100

53. Taylor T, Smith AN, Fulton PM. Effect of hysterectomy on bowel function. *Br Med J* 1989; 299:300–1

54. Broadbent JAM, Molnar BG, Cooper MJW, *et al.* Endoscopic management of uterine perforation occurring during endometrial resection. *Br J Obstet Gynaecol* 1992;99:1018

55. Garry R, Mooney P, Hasham F, *et al.* A uterine distension system to prevent fluid absorption during Nd-YAG laser endometrial ablation. *Gynecol Endosc* 1992;1:23–7

56. Vulgaropulos SP, Haley LC, Hulka JF. Intrauterine pressure and fluid absorption during continuous flow hysteroscopy. *Am J Obstet Gynecol* 1992;167:386–91

57. Molnar BG, Broadbent JAM, Magos AL. Fluid overload risk score for endometrial resection. *Gynecol Endosc* 1992;1:133–8

58. Baumann R, Magos AL, Kay JDS, *et al.* Absorption of glycine irrigating solution during transcervical resection of the endometrium. *Br Med J* 1990;300:304–5

59. Boubli L, Blanc M, Bautrand E, *et al.* Le risque metabolique de la chirurgie hysteroscopique. *J Gynecol Obstet Biol Reprod* 1990;19:217–22

60. Byers GF, Pinion S, Parkin DE, *et al.* Fluid absorption during transcervical resection of the endometrium. *Gynecol Endosc* 1993;2:21–3

61. Istre O, Skajaa K, Schjoensby AP, *et al.* Change in serum electrolytes after transcervical resection of endometrium and submucous fibroids with use of glycine for uterine irrigation. *Obstet Gynecol* 1992;80:218–22

62. Duffy S, Cruise M, Reilly C, *et al.* Ethanol labeling: detection of early fluid absorption in endometrial resection. *Obstet Gynecol* 1992;79: 300–4

63. Derman SG, Rehnstrom J, Neuwirth RS. The long-term effectiveness of hysteroscopic treatment of menorrhagia and leiomyomas. *Obstet Gynecol* 1991;77:591–4

64. Van Damme JP. One stage endometrial ablation: results in 200 cases. *Eur J Obstet Gynecol Reprod Biol* 1992;434:209–14

65. Hill DJ, Maher PJ. Intrauterine surgery using electrocautery. *Aust NZ J Obstet Gynaecol* 1990; 30:145–6

66. Rankin L, Steinberg LH. Transcervical resection of the endometrium: a review of 400 consecutive patients. *Br J Obstet Gynaecol* 1992;99: 911–14

67. Browning JJ, Pardey JM, Anderson RS, *et al.* Endometrial resection after radiotherapy for cervical carcinoma. *Int J Gynecol Obstet* 1991;36:243–5

68. Cooper MJW, Magos AL, Baumann R, *et al.* The effect of endometrial resection of menstrual blood loss. *Gynecol Endosc* 1992;1:195–8

69. McLure N, Mamers PM, Healy DL, *et al.* A quantitative assessment of endometrial electrocautery in the management of menorrhagia and a comparative report of argon laser endometrial ablation. *Gynecol Endosc* 1992;1:199–202

70. Pooley A, Ewen S, Sutton C. Does transcervical resection of the endometrium for menorrhagia really avoid hysterectomy? Life table analysis of a large series. *J Am Assoc Gynecol Laparosc* 1998; 5:229–35

71. Pinion SB, Parkin DE, Abramovich DR, *et al.* Randomised trial of hysterectomy, endometrial laser ablation and transcervical resection of the endometrium for dysfunctional uterine bleeding. *Br Med J* 1994;309:979–83

72. Aberdeen Endometrial Ablation Trials Group. A randomised trial of endometrial ablation versus hysterectomy for the treatment of dysfunctional uterine bleeding: outcome at four years. *Br J Obstet Gynaecol* 1999;106:360–6

73. Gannon MJ, Holt EM, Fairbank J, *et al.* A randomised trial comparing endometrial resection and abdominal hysterectomy for the treatment of menorrhagia. *Br Med J* 1991;303:1362–4

74. Dwyer N, Hutton J, Stirrat GM. Randomised controlled trial comparing endometrial resection with abdominal hysterectomy for the surgical treatment of menorrhagia. *Br J Obstet Gynaecol* 1993;100:237–43

75. Hill DJ, Maher PJ, Wood CW, *et al.* Haematometra – a complication of endometrial resection. *Aust NZ J Obstet Gynaecol* 1992;32:285–6

76. Ashworth MT, Moss CI, Kenyon WE. Granulomatous endometritis following hysteroscopic resection of the endometrium. *Histopathology* 1991;18:185–7

77. Ferryman SR, Stephens M, Gough D. Necrotising granulomatous endometritis following endometrial ablation therapy. *Br J Obstet Gynaecol* 1992;99:928–30

78. Bulletti C, DeZiegler D, Stefanetti M, *et al.* Endometriosis: absence of recurrence in patients after endometrial ablation. *Hum Reprod* 2001;16: 2676–9

79. Pagedas AC, Boe IH, Perkins HE. Review of 24 cases of uterine ablation failure. *J Am Assoc Gynecol Laparosc* 1995;2:239

80. Romer TH. Langzeitverlauf nach Endometriumsablation. Presented at *Vortrag Endoskopic-Workshop*, Rostock, 1995

81. Hill DJ, Maher PJ. Pregnancy following endometrial ablation. *Gynecol Endosc* 1992;1:47–9

82. Whitelaw NL, Garry R, Sutton CJG. Pregnancy following endometrial ablation: 2 case reports. *Gynecol Endosc* 1992;1:129–32

83. Lam AM, Al-Jumaily RY, Holt EM. Ruptured ectopic pregnancy in an amenorrhoeic woman after transcervical resection of the endometrium. *Aust NZ J Obstet Gynaecol* 1992;32:81–2

84. Edwards A, Tippett C, Lawrence, *et al.* Pregnancy outcome following endometrial ablation. *Gynaecol Endosc* 1996;5:349–51

85. Pugh CP, Crane JM, Hogan TG. Successful intrauterine pregnancy after endometrial ablation. *J Am Assoc Gynecol Laparosc* 2000;7:391–4

86. Pinette M, Katz, Drouin M, *et al.* Successful planned pregnancy following endometrial ablation with the YAG laser. *Am J Obstet Gynecol* 2001;185:242–3

87. Scottish Intercollegiate Guidelines Network. *Hysteroscopic Surgery a National Clinical Guideline.* Sign publication no. 37. Edinburgh: SIGN, 1999

88. Sculpher MJ, Bryan S, Dwyer N, *et al.* An economic evaluation of transcervical endometrial resection versus abdominal hysterectomy for the treatment of menorrhagia. *Br J Obstet Gynaecol* 1993;100:244–52

89. Hawe J, Phillips G, Chien P, *et al.* Cavaterm thermal balloon ablation for the treatment of menorrhagia. *Br J Obstet Gynaecol* 1999;106: 1143–8

90. Donnez J, Polet R, Rabinovitz R, *et al.* Endometrial laser intraterine thermotherapy: the first series of 100 patients observed for 1 year. *Fertil Steril* 2000;74:791–6

91. Hodgson D, Feldberg I, Sharp N, *et al.* Microwave endometrial ablation: development, clinical trials and outcomes at three years. *Br J Obstet Gynaecol* 1999;106:684–94

15

Endometrial ablation using heated fluids

F. D. Loffer and E. J. Bieber

INTRODUCTION

The authors, while having significant experience with resectoscopic methods of endometrial ablation such as rollerball and resection, initially like all other surgeons had limited experience with thermal ablative techniques. There was initial skepticism that balloon or other heated-fluid systems would be able to achieve the success rates seen with endometrial ablation using the resectoscope or laser. However, at this point, significant experience has been gained with a number of heated-fluid systems and early misgivings have given way to results that seem to be comparable to standard hysteroscopic techniques. The ease, simplicity, shortness of procedure and possibly decreased risk has caused many surgeons to re-evaluate incorporation of these types of techniques into the surgical armamentarium. While all patients may not be appropriate for these techniques, the majority of patients on whom we would perform a standard hysteroscopic procedure will be candidates.

The first global endometrial ablation techniques developed used heated fluid as a modality for transferring thermal energy to destroy the endometrium and superficial myometrium. Currently, four of these types of systems are commercially available. Three of the systems use a balloon to contain the fluid and the fourth allows heated fluid to circulate freely within the uterine cavity.

The three balloon methods are the Cavaterm™ (Wallsten Medical SA, Morges,

Switzerland), the MenoTreat™ system (Atos Medical AB, Horby, Sweden) and the ThermaChoice® uterine Balloon Therapy™ (Gynecare, a division of Ethicon, Inc., Somerville, NJ, USA). The free-fluid system is the Hydro ThermAblator® or HTA® system (Boston Scientific, Natick, MA, USA). While all systems are commercially available only the ThermaChoice and the HTA systems have been approved for sale in the USA. Indications and contraindications for these systems are similar to all other endometrial ablation techniques,

The balloon thermal ablation work-up and evaluation of patients is discussed in Chapter 4 and applies to all ablative techniques. In general, the authors perform hysteroscopic evaluation at the time of thermal endometrial ablation. This allows a reassessment of cavity configuration (size and shape) and rules out intracavity abnormalities such as polyps or myomata that may then be concomitantly treated. Curettage and endometrial sampling (often after dilatation) may be performed in patients, since unrecognized endometrial abnormalities have subsequently been demonstrated in what was previously reported as normal endometrium[1]. An advantage of many of the thermal ablative techniques is that it is not necessary to substantially dilate patients since most of the balloons, as well as the HTA system, are small in size. The HTA system may be used with a 3-mm, or smaller, hysteroscopic system.

ANESTHETIC CONSIDERATIONS

There was initial early enthusiasm that the limited need to dilate patients to perform these procedures would allow their placement in the clinic setting. Unfortunately, while some authors have reported on the performance of balloon endometrial ablations and the HTA system in the office, most surgeons continue to perform these procedures in the operation room[2]. Many different anesthetic techniques may be used, ranging from general anesthesia to conscious sedation. Unfortunately, few stringent data exist regarding comparison of these various techniques, or patient acceptability and outcome. In one trial, Lok and colleagues evaluated 30 patients who were undergoing endometrial ablation with the ThermaChoice balloon system and used patient-controlled sedation (propofol and alfentanil) by pump[3]. They evaluated patient pain during the catheter insertion, preheating phase, treatment cycle and end of treatment. Of interest, the pre-heating phase was the most uncomfortable for patients. However, this could be markedly reduced by having the patient pre-emptively administer a bolus of medication prior to starting this phase. In this trial, 85% of patients found the patient-controlled analgesia to be adequate and did not believe general anesthesia was required. Anecdotally, we have found that Toradol® administration prior to onset of the balloon procedure decreases pressure oscillations (probably by reducing myometrial contractions) and eases the attaining of a steady-state pressure.

THERMAL BALLOON SYSTEMS

The Cavaterm system consists of an 8-mm disposable catheter which has a distendable silastic balloon at the distal end (Figure 1). A heating element in the balloon is powered by a low-voltage battery contained in the central control unit. The fluid is circulated by a unique system in the central unit, which generates pulses through the liquid held within the catheter.

After purging the system, a syringe fills the balloon with 1.5% glycine and pressurizes it to 200 ± 20 mmHg. The low-voltage central system circulates the fluid, monitors the pressure and maintains a temperature of 75°C for the treatment time of 15 min. The catheter has a unique feature, which allows the balloon to be varied in length depending on the uterine cavity size.

Very good results are easily obtained (Table 1) with amenorrhea rates ranging between 30 and 68% and successful results (defined as eumenorrhea or better) occurring in over 90% of all patients[4–6]. In early trials, unsatisfactory results occurred when patients who were selected for treatment had submucosal myomas or septate uteri. It is now recognized that these are not good candidates for any of the balloon procedures. No major complications have been

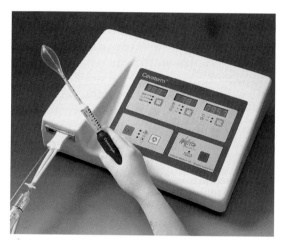

Figure 1 The Cavaterm™ system

Table 1 Results obtained in controlling menorrhagia using the Cavaterm™ system. Personal communication, Adam El-Din, Wallsten Medical S.A., Morges, Switzerland

Study	n	Follow-up (months)	Success (normal or less flow) (%)	Amenorrhea (%)
Friberg[5]	138	12–60	94	30
Hawe[6]	50	9–23	96	68
Halvorson	21	3–17	98	43
Aalailey	41	12+	97	29
Gerber	83	3–42	92	22
Frenzen	130	12+	95	44
Kleine-Gunk	42	6–15	96	42

reported with this technique. Maximum uterine length which can be treated is 10 cm.

The Menotreat system is the newest addition to balloon therapy. The instrumentation consists of an 8-mm disposable catheter with a silicone balloon. The fluid which circulates into the balloon is heated in the controller unit, which is designed to shut down with any sudden change in pressure or temperature. Treatment temperature is 85°C for 11 min with the balloon pressurized with 0.9% sterile saline to 200 mmHg. Two different disposable units are available. The standard unit is for use in cavities of 8–12 cm and a small set is for cavities measuring 6–9 cm. In a series of 51 consecutive patients evaluated at 6 months using a standardized pictorial bleeding chart, a 40% reduction of menstrual bleeding was achieved in 84.3% of the patients[7]. Five patients (10%) became amenorrheic. Quality-of-life assessments were improved and dysmenorrhea was reduced; no intraoperative complications occurred. No pretreatment endometrial thinning was used in this study.

The ThermaChoice I system consists of a disposable 5-mm catheter with a silicone balloon at the distal end. A thermistor and heating element are contained within the balloon. The balloon is pressurized with 5% dextrose and water to 180 mmHg. The central unit then monitors the pressure and temperature of the fluid. The treatment time is 8 min at 87°C. A significant drop in pressure will stop the treatment process. The ThermaChoice II differs from the ThermaChoice I in that it has an internal circulating system to mix the fluid in a silastic balloon (Figures 2 and 3). Bench studies suggest the only difference between the ThermaChoice I and the ThermaChoice II is that tissue destruction on the posterior wall is increased from 4 mm to 5 mm, respectively (Gynecare, personal communication, 1998). The ThermaChoice III system is the currently marketed device. It still has a circulating system but has been altered to give deeper penetration and better coverage in the cornual regions (Gynecare, personal communication, 2003). This may be clinically relevant since one of the technical challenges for all ablative techniques

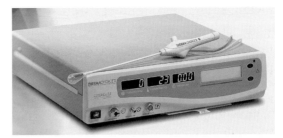

Figure 2 The Thermachoice® II system. Courtesy of Gynecare

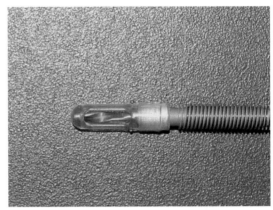

Figure 3 Thermachoice® II system – internal circulating mechanism. Courtesy of Gynecare

has been to develop technology which allows the thermal ablative effect into the cornual regions, as there are significant anatomic differences in this area from patient to patient.

Figure 4 shows the mean depth of destruction of each ThermaChoice version. Using the ThermaChoice I, a depth of destruction of 1 mm or greater in extirpated uteri was found to be 6.3 mm from the tubal ostia. With the ThermaChoice II, this distance was reduced to 4.8 mm, and to only 3.5 mm with the ThermaChoice III. In the mid-fundus, the depth of destruction was improved over the ThermaChoice I by 0.3 mm with the ThermaChoice II, and by 1.5 mm with the ThermaChoice III.

The ThermaChoice I was the first global ablation technique to be compared in a prospective 1 : 1 randomized study using traditional rollerball hysteroscopic ablation[8]. This large trial randomized 128 patients to

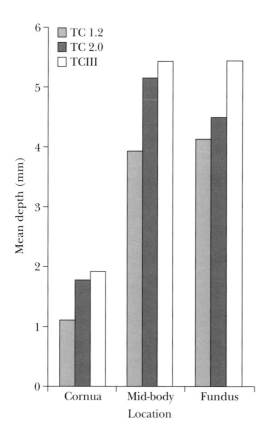

Figure 4 Mean depth of necrosis achieved by the three Thermachoice® (TC) systems, by location. Personal communication, M. Weisberg, Gynecare

thermal balloon and 117 to rollerball ablation. In this study, bleeding was measured using a standardized pictorial diary and a single brand of tampon/napkins. A score of 100 in this pictorial system had a sensitivity of 86% and a specificity of 81% for indicating menorrhagia[9]. Prior to entry into the study, patients had to have had 3 months of documented menorrhagia, which could not be treated by, or had not responded to medical therapy. Endometrial thinning was felt to be appropriate; however, at the initiation of this Food and Drug Administration (FDA) study there were no medications approved for endometrial thinning and, therefore, they could not be used to pretreat patients. As an alternative, a timed 3-min suction curettage was carried out. The maximum uterine cavity size treated was 10 cm and

patients with submucous myomas were excluded.

At 1 year, the ThermaChoice I resulted in decreased menstrual blood flow, improved quality of life and a decrease in dysmenorrhea all of which were statistically equivalent to the traditional hysteroscopic rollerball technique (Figure 5 and Table 2). While the amenorrhea rates at 12 months with ThermaChoice I were lower than with the rollerball (15.2% vs. 27.2%), it is possible that if the newer versions of ThermaChoice were used and patients were hormonally pretreated, these results could have been better[8].

The findings of this study were also reported at 2 and 3 years post-procedure and were based upon patients self-reporting their symptoms and their bleeding patterns[10,11]. Of note, there was little change in results from year 1 in the comparison between the ThermaChoice I and the rollerball technique.

Of the 255 women treated under the original protocol, 147 women were available to be interviewed 5 years postoperatively[12]. Twenty-five (17%) of these patients reported that they had had a hysterectomy, a repeat ablation or a D&C between years 3 and 5, which left 102 patients (61 in the ThermaChoice I group and 61 in the rollerball group) who were eligible for analysis. Normal bleeding (eumenorrhea or less) was reported in 95% of the ThermaChoice I and in 97% of the hysteroscopic rollerball patients. After 5 years, 42 hysterectomies had been performed on study patients, equally divided between the two arms of the study (Table 3). There were also five repeat ablations (three in the ThermaChoice I and two in the rollerball arms) and one D&C (rollerball). The amenorrhea rate of the two arms of the study had moved closer to parity, with 23% of the ThermaChoice I group and 33% of the rollerball group experiencing no bleeding (Table 4), interestingly, a higher percentage than was seen at the 12-month follow-up. These results were not biased by patients entering into menopause. The mean age at initial treatment was 40.4 years for the ThermaChoice I group and 40.9 for the rollerball group. At the 5-year contact, the mean age was 45.7 years for ThermaChoice I group

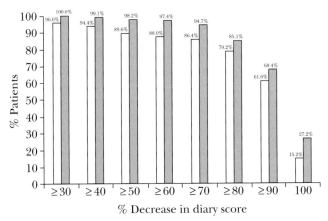

Figure 5 Decrease in diary scores of menstrual blood flow at 12 months in a study comparing uterine balloon therapy ($n = 125$; white bars) and rollerball hysteroscopic ablation ($n = 114$; shaded bars). Reproduced from reference 8 with permission. 1998 American College of Obstetricians and Gynecologists

Table 2 Quality-of-life evaluation at 12-month follow-up after uterine balloon therapy or rollerball hysteroscopic ablation. Reproduced from reference 8 with permission. 1998 American College of Obstetricians and Gynecologists

	Uterine balloon therapy (%) ($n = 114$)	*Rollerball ablation* (%) ($n = 114$)
Satisfaction		
very satisfied	85.6	86.7
satisfied	10.1	12.4
not satisfied	4.0	0.9
Dysmenorrhea		
decreased	70.4	75.4
unchanged	24.8	22.8
increased	4.8	1.8
Moderate to severe PMS (before/after procedure)	78.8/32.4	76.6/29.0
Inability to work outside home (before/after procedure)	39.8/4.0	38.5/2.7

PMS, premenstrual syndrome. Both groups before-to-after procedure, $p < 0.05$; differences between rollerball and balloon therapy, $p < 0.05$

and 46.1 for the rollerball group. In addition, a marked decrease in dysmenorrhea was noted after both treatments, which was also sustained over time (Figure 6).

Over 250 000 ThermaChoice cases have been performed throughout the world. There have been no injuries reported to date with appropriate use of the equipment. However, at least one pregnancy has been reported after thermal balloon ablation[13].

Table 3 Reasons for hysterectomy at 5-year follow-up of the comparative study of ThermaChoice® versus rollerball endometrial ablation. Adapted from reference 12

Indication for hysterectomy	*ThermaChoice*	*Rollerball*
Bleeding	9	7
Pelvic pain	3	10
Bleeding and pain	5	1
Other	4	3

Table 4 Menstrual status of patients at 3- and 5-year follow-up of balloon therapy versus rollerball ablation. Reproduced from reference 12 with permission

| | 3-year follow-up | | | | 5-year follow-up | | | |
| | Uterine balloon therapy (n = 114) | | Rollerball ablation (n = 99) | | Uterine balloon therapy (n = 61) | | Rollerball ablation (n = 61) | |
	n	%	n	%	n	%	n	%
Amenorrhea	17	14.9	26	26.3	14	23.0	20	33.0
Spotting	11	9.6	16	16.2	6	9.8	7	11.5
Hypomenorrhea	45	39.5	26	26.3	23	37.7	15	24.6
Eumenorrhea	33	29.0	25	25.2	15	24.6	17	27.9
Menorrhagia	8	7.0	6	6.0	3	4.9	2	3.3

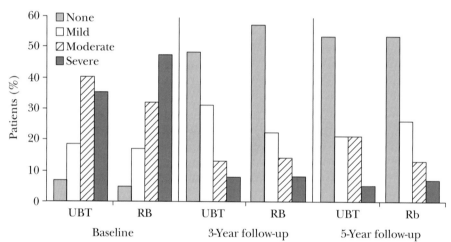

Figure 6 Dysmenorrhea at baseline and 3 and 5 years after uterine balloon therapy (UBT) or rollerball ablation (RB). Reproduced from reference 12 with permission

Bongers and colleagues prospectively evaluated 130 patients undergoing thermal ablation with the ThermaChoice device[14]. They found that 12% of their patients underwent hysterectomy in the 2 years of follow-up. Prognostic factors for poorer outcome were a retroverted uterus, pre-therapy endometrial thickness of at least 4 mm and excessive duration of menstrual flow (Figure 7). Poor outcomes were decreased with advancing age although dysmenorrhea and uterine depth were not predictive factors. It is possible that these same prognostic factors may also apply to other hot-fluid systems.

FREE-FLUID ENDOMETRIAL ABLATION

The free-fluid thermal ablation HTA system circulates heated 0.9% saline from the central monitor directly into the uterine cavity (Figure 8). The 7.8-mm insulated sheath contains a 3-mm hysteroscope, which allows the procedure to be done under direct visualization. The control unit initially cleans the cavity of debris and determines that the system is intact and leak free after which fluid is heated to 90°C for a 10-min treatment cycle. The fluid is fed by gravity into the uterine cavity with a resulting intrauterine pressure of between 50 and

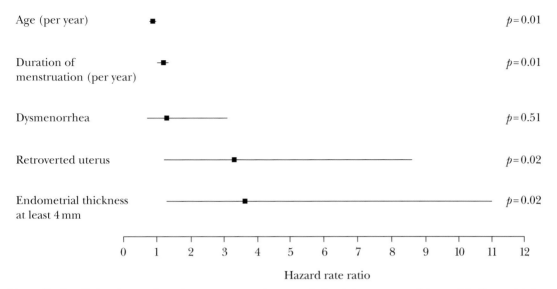

Figure 7 Predictive factors for adverse outcome in an analysis of the success of thermal balloon ablation for treatment of menorrhea ($n = 130$). Hazard rate ratio (■) and 95% confidence intervals. Data from reference 14

55 mmHg. This pressure is lower than that necessary to open the Fallopian tube. The controller pump pulls the cooler fluid from the uterine cavity back to the controller and then re-circulates it after heating.

A prospective, randomized study was undertaken with a 2 : 1 randomization of hydrothermal ablations to hysteroscopic rollerball ablations[15]. Inclusion criteria were similar to the ThermaChoice I study. Pretreatment with 7.5 mg Depo-Lupron was used in all patients. A standardized pictorial guide was used to quantitate the blood loss[16]. The ability to diminish blood loss, as well as patient satisfaction, was statistically similar between the two arms. The amenorrhea rate at 12 months was 40% in the study group and 51% in the rollerball group. Outcomes at 24 months have been consistent with those found at 1 year (S. Corson, personal communication). The only injury reported with this system was a thermal burn, which occurred when the tubing was inadvertently placed in direct contact with a patient. This problem has been solved by better insulation of the tubing.

Because the fluid is allowed to circulate freely within the uterine cavity, patients with structural abnormalities such as submucosal myomas or septum can be more easily treated than with the balloon systems. Uterine cavities up to 10.5 cm may be treated.

A preliminary study of 22 patients has shown that very good results can be obtained when treating patients with submucosal myomas[17]. The range of follow-up was 12–20 months (15.4 months average). Myomas ranged in size from 1 to 5 cm with the largest number (eight) being 3 cm. One-half of the patients had more than one myoma. The overall success rate was 91% (patients requiring no further treatment). Twelve patients reported amenorrhea (54%); two patients failed – one underwent hysterectomy and the other a repeat endometrial ablation.

PHYSIOLOGIC AND ULTRASTRUCTURAL EFFECTS OF THERMAL ENDOMETRIAL ABLATION

Prior to beginning clinical trials with each device, it was necessary to demonstrate, initially in extirpated specimens, then in patients undergoing hysterectomy, that the thermal damage was limited, yet extensive enough to produce the desired results. Several clinical trials have

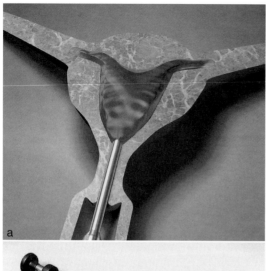

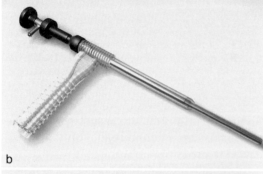

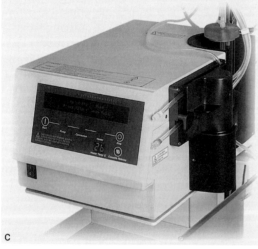

Figure 8 The Hydro ThermAblator (HTA)® system. (a) Saline is circulated into the uterine cavity; (b) insulated sheath containing hysteroscope; (c) control unit. Photographs courtesy of Boston Scientific

provided interesting results on the impact of these devices both initially and, subsequently, on the endometrium and uterus. Andersen

and colleagues used thermistors to evaluate temperatures on the serosal surface of the uterus in patients undergoing balloon endometrial ablation[18]. In the eight patients who underwent thermal balloon ablation for 8–16 min, the highest recorded temperature was only 39.1°C. Of importance, light microscopy demonstrated a maximum depth of coagulation of 11.5 mm, and election microscopy showed no effect of heat beyond 15 mm from the surface of the endometrium (Figure 9). Subsequent studies evaluated the time and pressure effect with the ThermaChoice system. Vilos and colleagues found that patients treated with balloon pressure < 150 mmHg had a statistically higher rate of persistent menorrhagia at 24-months follow-up[19]. However, increasing the time of ablation at a pressure of 150–180 mmHg from 8 min to 12–16 min did not improve success rates.

Jarvela and co-workers in Finland, prospectively evaluated and compared patients undergoing either treatment with progestins or endometrial ablation[20]. Patients underwent color Doppler imaging studies before treatment, postoperative day 1 (ablation group only) and 1 and 6 months after treatment. Surprisingly, only at 6 months were there increases in the pulsatility index noted in the uterine and spiral arteries of the endometrial ablation group. The authors suggest this may be due to the ensuing fibrosis that occurs after endometrial ablation. These same investigators also reported on ultrasonographic findings in patients after endometrial ablation[21]. They noted at 1 month after balloon ablation a 'fluid-filled clear-limited hyperechogenic zone surrounding the uterine cavity' in 60% of patients (Figure 10).

COMPARATIVE TRIALS WITH THERMAL BALLOONS

We have discussed some of the comparative trials, which have been performed to date; however, several others are worthy of discussion and many others are currently underway and will be completed in the next few years.

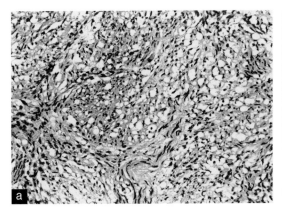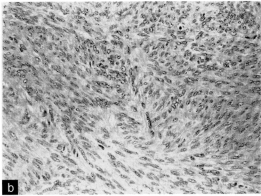

Figure 9 (a) Myometrium with nuclear shrinkage and hyperchromasia, and vacuolization in the cytoplasm; (b) normal myometrium. Original magnification ×250 (H&E). Reproduced from reference 18 with permission

Soysal and associates investigated the use of a levonorgestrel-releasing intrauterine device (IUD) versus balloon endometrial ablation in treating patients with menorrhagia[22]. At 1 year, both were noted to be effective for reducing blood loss, with ablation more effective and with fewer side-effects. Both increased hemoglobin levels similarly. This and other comparable data suggest good efficacy of the levonorgestrel IUD in diminishing bleeding in patients who may desire to retain childbearing options and thus are not candidates for endometrial ablation. The same authors also prospectively compared thermal balloon ablation to hysteroscopic rollerball ablation in patients with a myomatous uterus smaller than 12 weeks in size[23]. They found similar functional results with both techniques but noted no complications when performing thermal balloon ablations under local anesthesia, versus significantly more complications in the rollerball group.

The original ThermaChoice trial was performed without uterine preparation and included a suction curettage prior to balloon ablation. However, it is unclear if pretreatment with any of the available agents (see Chapter 5) is of value in thermal ablation patients. Lissak and colleagues performed a prospective, randomized controlled trial of immediate thermal ablation versus pretreatment with a single dose of gonadotropin releasing hormone agonist for 30 days, followed by endometrial ablation[24]. In this study of perimenopausal patients, evaluation at 6 months post-treatment demonstrated no significant difference in bleeding patterns between immediate or delayed ablation.

In another trial, two experienced hysteroscopic surgeons compared results of 73 thermal balloon ablations versus 74 endometrial resections[25]. Consistent with other data, balloon ablation took significantly less operative time. They also noted a retroverted uterus was associated with greater failure in the balloon ablation group, and age under 43 years was associated with increased failure in the hysteroscopic resection group. Overall success was comparable for both groups.

A recent report from Finland described a small trial of patients randomized to either treatment with Menotreat or Cavaterm for endometrial ablation[26]. While follow-up was short, both techniques demonstrated similar efficacy and patient acceptance.

NOVEL USES FOR THERMAL ABLATIVE TECHNIQUE

Several recent papers have suggested interesting applications for thermal balloon ablation. DeCherney and Polan reported on use of the

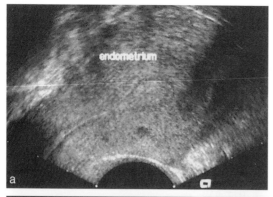

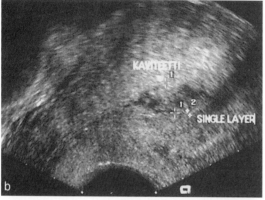

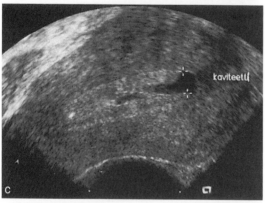

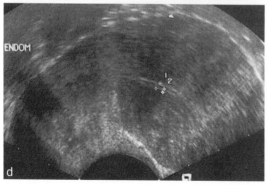

resectoscope to treat intractable bleeding in high-risk patients as an alternative to hysterectomy[27]. More recently, Nichols and Gill reported on a 44-year-old patient with liver disease, sepsis, coagulopathy, anemia and life-threatening bleeding who successfully underwent thermal balloon endometrial ablation[28]. It may be that in high-risk patients, especially those where medical therapy is ineffective or contraindicated and childbearing is not an issue, that the ease and quickness of thermal ablation makes it the procedure of choice.

Another interesting report focused on use of the thermal balloon for ablation in patients who were severely anemic and had prosthetic heart values[29]. Use of hysteroscopic techniques to perform ablation, where risk of fluid intravasation always exists, are much more difficult in this high-risk group, making thermal ablation a more optimal surgical approach.

CONCLUSION

Endometrial ablation using hot water systems appears to be safe and extremely easy to use. They afford all gynecologists the opportunity to offer their patients endometrial ablation. Although minimal training is required to use these systems, it is imperative that gynecologists understand the principles of the system they are using. Additionally, the appropriate selection of patients for endometrial ablation must be adhered to strictly.

Figure 10 Changes in the uterus following thermal balloon endometrial ablation therapy in a 42-year-old woman who suffered from hypermenorrhea (a–d). The endometrial thickness before therapy was 4.7 mm, and 6 months later it was 1.8 mm. On the first postoperative day, there were miscellaneous echoes in the uterine cavity, and the uterine tissue surrounding the cavity was more echoic than the serosal side of the myometrium (b). One month after therapy, the uterine cavity was filled with fluid, and it was surrounded by a clearly defined hyperechogenic zone, with a maximum thickness of 5.2 mm. Reproduced from Järvelä I, Tekay A, Santala M, *et al.* Ultrasonographic features following thermal balloon endometrial ablation therapy. *Gynecol Obstet Invest* 2002;54:11–16, with permission from S. Karger AG, Basel

References

1. Minassian VA, Mira JL. Balloon thermoablation in a woman with complex endometrial hyperplasia with atypia. *J Reprod Med* 2001;46:933–6
2. Fernandez H, Capella S, Avdibert F. Uterine thermal balloon therapy under local anesthesia for the treatment of menorrhagia: a pilot study. *Hum Reprod* 1997;12;2511–14
3. Lok IH, Chan M, Tam WH, *et al.* Patient-controlled sedation for outpatient thermal balloon endometrial ablation. *J Am Assoc Gynecol Laparosc* 2002;9:436–41
4. DeGrande P, El-Din A. Endometrial ablation for the treatment of dysfunctional uterine bleeding using balloon therapy. In Kochli OR, ed. *Hysteroscopy. State of the Art.* Basel: Karger, 2000:145–53
5. Friberg B, Ahlgren M. Thermal balloon endometrial destruction: the outcome of treatment of 117 women followed up for a maximum period of 4 years. *Gynaecol Endosc* 2000;9:389–95
6. Hawe JA, Phillips AG, Chien FP, *et al.* Cavaterm thermal ablation for the treatment of menorrhagia. *Br J Obstet Gynaecol* 1999;106:1143–8
7. Ulmsten J, Carstensen H, Falconer C, *et al.* The safety and efficacy of MenoTreat, a balloon device for thermal ablation. *Acta Obstet Gynecol Scand* 2001;80:52–7
8. Meyer W, Walsh B, Grainger D, *et al.* Thermal balloon and rollerball ablation to treat menorrhagia: a multicenter comparison. *Obstet Gynecol* 1998;92:98–103
9. Higham JM, O'Brien PMS, Shaw RW. Assessment of menstrual blood loss using a pictorial chart. *Br J Obstet Gynaecol* 1990;9:734–9
10. Grainger DA, Tjaden B. Thermal balloon and rollerball ablation to treat menorrhagia: two-year results from a multicenter prospective randomized clinical trial. *J Am Assoc Gynecol Laparosc* 2000;7:175–9
11. Loffer FD. Three-year results of the comparison of thermal balloon and rollerball ablation in the treatment of menorrhagia. *J Am Assoc Gynecol Laparosc* 2001;8:48–54
12. Loffer FD, Grainger D. Five-year follow up of patients participating in a randomized trial of uterine balloon therapy versus rollerball ablation for treatment of menorrhagia. *J Am Assoc Gynecol Laparosc* 2002;9:429–35
13. Cravello L, Agostini A, Roger V, *et al.* Intrauterine pregnancy after thermal balloon ablation. *Acta Obstet Gynecol Scand* 2001;80:671
14. Bongers MY, Mol BWJ, Brolmann HAM. Prognostic factors for the success of thermal balloon ablation in the treatment of menorrhagia. *Obstet Gynecol* 2002;99:1060–6
15. Corson SL. A multicenter evaluation of endometrial ablation by Hydro Thermablator and rollerball for the treatment of menorrhagia. *J Am Assoc Gynecol Laparosc* 2001;8:359–67
16. Janssen CAH, Scholten PC, Heintz APM. A simple visual assesment technique to discriminate between menorrhagia and normal menstrual blood loss. *Obstet Gynecol* 1995;85:977–82
17. Glasser MH. Beyond hysterectomy: the contemporary management of uterine fibroids. Presented at the *American Association of Gynecological Laparoscopy International Congress*, April, 2003, Scottsdale, AZ, USA
18. Andersen LF, Meinert L, Rygaard C, *et al.* Thermal balloon endometrial ablation: safety aspects evaluated by serosal temperature, light microscopy and electron microscopy. *Eur J Obstet Gynecol Reprod Biol* 1998;79:63–8
19. Vilos GA, Aletebi FA. Eskandar MA. Endometrial thermal balloon ablation with the ThermaChoice system: effect of intrauterine pressure and duration of treatment. *J Am Assoc Gynecol Laparosc* 2000;7:325–9
20. Jarvela IA, Santala M, Jouppila P. Thermal balloon endometrial ablation therapy induces a rise in uterine blood flow impedance: a randomized prospective color Doppler study. *Ultrasound Obstet Gynecol* 2001;17:65–70
21. Jarvela I, Tekay A, Santala M, *et al.* Ultrasonographic features following thermal balloon endometrial ablation therapy. *Gynecol Obstet Invest* 2002;54:11–16
22. Soysal M, Soysal S, Ozer S. A randomized controlled trial of levonorgestrel releasing IUD and thermal balloon ablation in the treatment of menorrhagia. *Zentralbl Gynakol* 2002;124:213–9
23. Soysal ME, Soysal SK, Vicdan K. Thermal balloon ablation in myoma-induced menorrhagia under local anesthesia. *Gynecol Obstet Invest* 2001;51:128–33
24. Lissak A, Fruchter O, Mashiach S, *et al.* Immediate versus delayed treatment of perimenopausal bleeding due to benign causes by balloon thermal ablation. *J Am Assoc Gynecol Laparosc* 1999;6:145–50
25. Gervaise A, Fernandez H, Capella-Allouc S, *et al.* Thermal balloon ablation versus endometrial resection for the treatment of abnormal uterine bleeding. *Hum Reprod* 1999;14:2743–7

26. Vihko K, Raitala R, Taina E. Endometrial thermoablation for treatment of menorrhagia: comparison of two methods in outpatient setting. *Acta Obstet Gynecol Scand* 2003;82:269–74

27. Decherney A, Polan MI. Hysteroscopic management of intrauterine lesions and intractable uterine bleeding. *Obstet Gynecol* 1983;61:392–6

28. Nichols CM, Gill EJ. Thermal balloon ablation for management of acute uterine hemorrhage. *Obstet Gynecol* 2002;100:1092–4

29. Soysal M, Soysal SJ. Endometrial thermal balloon ablation under local anesthesia in patients with prosthetic heart valves: a pilot study. *Zentralbl Gynakol* 2000;122:556–60

16

Endometrial cryoablation

D. E. Townsend

INTRODUCTION

Homer and Hypocrites are among the more notable who appreciated the benefits of hypothermia in treating a variety of problems. Homer used cold to reduce pain and swelling during the ancient Olympic Games. During the many battles that took place on the European continent, surgeons used cold as an anesthetic to treat wounds as well as to stem bleeding and perform amputations. However, the true potential of employing profound hypothermia was not realized until Carl Von Linde originated the present cryosurgical industry with the establishment of commercial liquefaction at the end of the 19th century. Von Linde applied the Joules–Thompson (J-T) principle that rapid expansion of gas under pressure through a narrow outlet would produce a rapid drop in temperature[1].

PATHOPHYSIOLOGY

Cryosurgery is the destruction of tissue through the application of extreme cold. The cryoprobe surface temperature is a critical determinant of tissue destruction. When a cryoprobe is applied to tissue and refrigerant is circulated, heat is withdrawn from the tissue. As heat is withdrawn from the tissue, ice formation occurs, first within the cell and then extracellularly. Death from cold occurs primarily in two ways. The first is the dehydration effect of ice crystallization, which results in destruction of enzyme systems. Second, ice crystallization, both intra- and extracellular, results in disruption of the cell membrane, which also results in cell death. Cell death begins to occur around −15°C and becomes extensive at −20°C. A freeze, partial thaw, refreeze cycle will result in greater tissue destruction.

INSTRUMENTATION

Early cryosurgical systems used liquid nitrogen, nitrous oxide, carbon dioxide gas and argon. While the liquid nitrogen systems can achieve a low surface temperature, −120 to −160°C, they are bulky, inflexible and costly. The J-T systems, which utilize nitrous oxide and carbon dioxide, are smaller and less expensive, but have a warmer surface temperature, −40 to −60°C, and higher operating pressures, 700 psi. Argon systems can achieve temperatures as low as −120°C; however, they utilize pressures in excess of 2000 psi. These high pressures raise safety concerns and limit use of these devices in some applications. Until recently, all marketed cryosurgical devices exhausted the coolant into the atmosphere and, therefore, required continual replenishment. Moreover, the operating suite must be well vented to avoid the build-up of the gases. Consequently, the convenience of these systems is reduced and the risk of exhausting the supply during a procedure is real.

In the 1990s, John Dobak and associates[2] conceived of a novel J-T cryosurgical unit that circumvents the problems noted above. This device utilizes a gas mixture to achieve a surface temperature of −115 to −125°C at pressures of 300–350 psi. The system is closed and uses an oil-free compressor to circulate the coolant. The gas mixture is non-flammable, non-toxic, non-corrosive, environmentally safe and, since it is a closed system, does not require replenishment.

HISTORY OF UTERINE CRYOSURGERY

Profound hypothermia was initially used in the uterine cavity by Cahan and Brockunier[3] in the mid-1960s. They treated three women using liquid nitrogen and then performed hysterectomies. When surgery was performed within 90 min after freezing the gross and microscopic changes were difficult to interpret. At 3 days, there was obvious necrosis of the uterine lining and at 5½ weeks, there was even more extensive destruction. They suggested that cryosurgery might be beneficial in women who have a history of abnormal uterine bleeding. Droegemueller and colleagues[4,5], in the 1970s, followed up on the study of Cahan and Brockunier and published several papers describing the effect of intense freezing on the uterus. They further emphasized the potential benefits of using cryosurgery to treat women with abnormal uterine bleeding. Freezing was well tolerated, could be performed with minimal anesthesia and was accompanied by little discomfort.

At the same time Droegemueller and colleagues were carrying out their studies on endometrial ablation, the popularity of cryosurgery for treating preinvasive cervical disease was gaining momentum[6]. In fact, the combination of colposcopy and cryosurgery has achieved a place of prominence in the management of premalignant disease of the uterine cervix. The only significant side-effect of cryosurgery of the cervix is the profuse leukorrhea that occurs after this technique. However, it can be performed in a physician's office since it is essentially painless. This analgesic property of cold is unique and is one of the major advantages of using cryosurgery.

HER OPTION™ CRYOSURGICAL UNIT

The introduction of the Her Option™ unit by Dobak was a major improvement in cryosurgical instrumentation (Figures 1 and 2). The closed system has been shown to be particularly dependable and reliable, and a recently completed multicenter study illustrated that cryosurgery was as effective as rollerball ablation in controlling abnormal uterine bleeding[7]. Moreover, the system has been shown to be effective in treating women with submucous fibroids, uterine polyps, as well as large uterine cavities. Studies are currently underway evaluating the possibility of performing laparoscopic cryomyoablation to manage women with uterine fibroids.

The multicenter study, of 279 patients, demonstrated the ease of use, safety and effectiveness of cryosurgery. Amenorrhea and spotting rates at 12 months were 44% and at 2 years were increased to 50%.

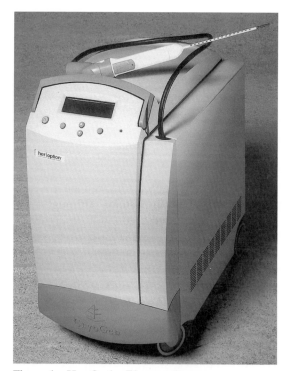

Figure 1   Her Option™ cryounit

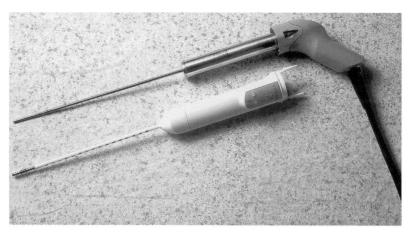

Figure 2 Cryoprobes: top, permanent unit; bottom, disposable control unit

SELECTION OF PATIENTS FOR CRYOABLATION

Prior to performing any type of endometrial ablation, proper pretreatment evaluation is necessary. Patients should have some type of investigation of the uterine cavity, by hysteroscopy, sonohysterography, ultrasonography or hysterosalpingography.

Endometrial sampling is necessary to rule out the presence of a neoplastic process. Blood studies are recommended to detect the presence of blood dyscrasias.

METHOD OF CRYOABLATION

Once a woman has been deemed to be a candidate for cryoablation, there are virtually no significant contraindications to the procedure. Women with polyps, submucous fibroids and/or large cavities can be treated with the Her Option system. Although the multicenter study used a gonadotropin releasing hormone (GnRH) agonist prior to cryo- and rollerball ablation, it is not necessary for women to have the GnRH agonist before cryosurgical ablation to achieve excellent results[7]. Therapy can be performed at any time during the menstrual cycle. It is now being performed in physician's offices with a local anesthetic as well as in an outpatient setting. Patients usually receive 10 mg of diazapam prior to treatment in the office, or when in a surgical center,

midazolam. Patients are then placed in a modified dorsolithotomy position on the operating or treatment table. Ultrasound scanning is carried out to ensure that the bladder is full. The bladder should contain at least 300–500 ml of fluid, as it will help to outline the uterus and monitor the treatment session. If the bladder is not sufficiently full, a catheter should be placed in the bladder and additional fluid added. Antibiotic coverage is recommended at the onset of therapy.

The perineum and vagina are prepped in a sterile fashion. The cervix is exposed, preferably with a weighted speculum. The anterior cervical lip should be injected with 1–2 ml of a long-acting anesthetic. A single-tooth tenaculum is then used to grasp the anterior cervical lip and a paracervical block is performed by injecting 10 ml of a long-acting anesthetic into each uterosacral area. The uterus is sounded, both in the central and cornual area. The internal os is gently dilated to 5 mm if necessary. A suction curettage is then performed of the entire cavity. This will remove excess endometrial tissue. The bleeding that follows the curettage acts as an excellent heat transfer agent. Hysteroscopy is recommended at this time if the cavity has not been well visualized prior to treatment. The cryoprobe, which measures 5 mm in diameter, is slipped into the cervix and then into the uterine cavity. Gentle traction is applied to the tenaculum in order to seat the probe into or near one of the cornua. Once positioned, as determined by ultrasound, the minus (−) button is pressed on the cryoprobe and refrigerant is circulated (Figure 3). The formation of the cryozone is observable on ultrasound. Ultrasound is performed during the course of cryoablation and the cryozone is permitted to extend to within 4–5 mm of the uterine serosa or until 6 min have elapsed, which ever occurs first (Figure 4). Timing is noted at the end of the freezing session. Treating much beyond 6 min probably does not result in a significantly greater depth of tissue destruction. It has been noted that with a 6-min freeze the depth of tissue destruction is at least 10 mm[8]. Once the probe has been warmed and loosened from the initial cryozone, it is withdrawn to the internal os and then redirected into the untreated cornual area. Again, gentle traction is applied to the tenaculum and the cryoprobe is seated as close as possible to the untreated cornua as noted by ultrasound. The second freezing session will occur more rapidly since there has been pre-cooling of the uterus. The edge of the cryozone is again permitted to extend to within 4–5 mm of the serosa or is terminated at 6 min. It is important that the second cryozone completely overlaps the first cryozone so that there is one large cryozone observable by ultrasound (Figure 5). If it appears there is not

sufficient coalescence of the two cryozones, it will be necessary to do a center freeze (Figure 6). If a center freeze is necessary, the probe is placed into the center of the uterus under ultrasound visualization, and using the same recommendations as previously outlined, i.e. permitting the cryozone to extend to within 4–5 mm of the serosa, the center of the uterus is frozen. This is seldom necessary with a normal-sized cavity.

As the last cryo session is ending, the bladder is emptied. Once the bladder has been emptied and the cryoprobe removed, the patient is sent to recovery. Recovery takes about 1 h. The patient is then permitted to go home. As a few patients will have some cramps the first day, patients are sent home with mild analgesics that will easily control the discomfort. Patients are permitted normal activity, but are urged to refrain from sexual activity or any type of heavy exercise for 2 weeks.

LARGE UTERINE CAVITIES, SUBMUCOUS FIBROIDS AND POLYPS

In women with large uterine cavities, i.e. those that are > 10 cm, more than two freeze applications will be necessary. In cases where there is a large cavity, it is best to perform a

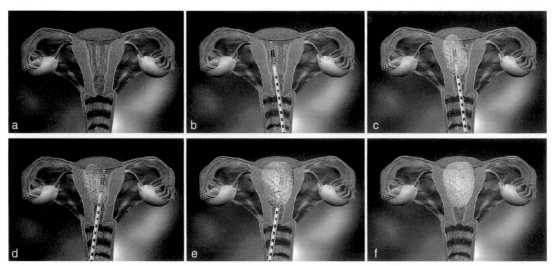

Figure 3 Stages of cryoablation: a, uterus before freezing; b, cryoprobe in right cornual area; c, end of first freeze; d, cryoprobe in left cornual area; e, end of second freeze; f, cryozone after cryoprobe removed

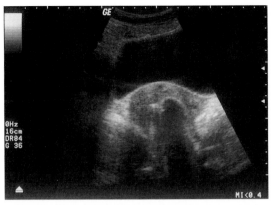

Figure 4 Transverse view. Ultrasound at 4 min. Note bladder at top (black). Oval fundus of uterus and cryozone in left side of uterus

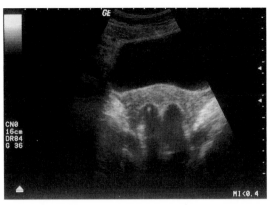

Figure 6 Transverse view. Ultrasound depicting non-overlap of cryozones. Center freeze required

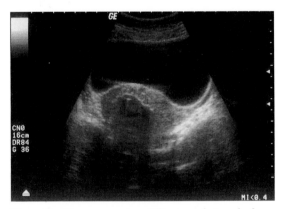

Figure 5 Transverse view. Ultrasound at end of second cryosession (6 min). Note complete overlap of both cryozones

central freeze followed by the cornua freezes. With these large cavities is may also be necessary to perform a pull-back freeze. This is necessary because the average length of the cryozone is approximately 5.5 cm. If the cavity sounds to be > 10 cm, this will mean that only 5.5 cm of a > 6 cm cavity has been frozen. In order to determine how much to pull back the cryoprobe, the length of the average cervical canal, i.e. 4 cm, should be subtracted from the depth of the uterine cavity. If the cavity is 12 cm, then the length of the fundus or endometrial cavity will be 12 – 4, or 8 cm. In these cases, it is recommended that the probe be withdrawn 4 cm and then a 4-min freeze be performed. For

this freeze it is recommended that timing be the standard of measurement for the length of the freeze. Four minutes is usually sufficient since there has been a significant amount of overlapping of the previous cryozones in the lower segment.

In women with uterine polyps, it is important to sample the polyp to rule out a neoplastic process prior to destruction. It is not necessary to remove the polyp prior to endometrial cryoablation.

In women with submucous fibroids it is suggested that if the fibroid extends < 50% into the uterine cavity, then the fibroid can be treated along with the endometrium. However, should the fibroid extend > 50% into the cavity, then the fibroid should be resected down to the level of the endometrium and then the uterine lining treated.

POSTOPERATIVE CARE

Following cryosurgery, most patients require no special care. In the multicenter study[7], few patients had discomfort and most did not have a discharge. However, timing of the freezing sessions was paramount and, generally, was of a slightly shorter duration than is recommended in this chapter. In the study, the first side was frozen for 4 min and the second side for 6 min. Despite what has come to be regarded as relatively inadequate freezing, the results were as good as rollerball ablation[7]. Through slightly more extensive freezing better results can be expected with cryoablation[9]. With longer freezes there may be a watery discharge, generally this lasts no more than 2 weeks. Pain is seldom a problem and patients have few restrictions after 2 weeks.

QUALITY OF LIFE

In the multicenter study[7], the ability to control abnormal bleeding by cryoablation was equal to that of rollerball ablation. In addition to the bleeding, quality of life was also carefully documented. Moodiness was noted to be present in 87% of women who had heavy menstrual flow. This dropped to 7% in the cryoablation group following treatment. Premenstrual syndrome (PMS) was noted to be present in over 35% of women, falling to 9% after treatment. Dysmenorrhea was noted in nearly half of the participants, dropping to 6% after treatment. At 2 years, the presence of moodiness, PMS and dysmenorrhea remained well under 10%.

PRECAUTIONS

The current recommendation is that women who have had myomectomies and classical Cesarean sections should not be treated by endometrial ablation because of the possibility of a thin uterine wall.

OTHER ISSUES

Hysteroscopic studies have been performed following cryoablation. Heppard and colleagues reported results from a group of 20 women in which no significant scarring or change of the uterine cavity occurred between 6 and 18 months after cryoablation (M. Heppard, personal communication). This was confirmed in 19 additional patients[9].

In contrast, rollerball ablation and thermal ablation have both been noted to cause extensive scarring within the endometrial cavity[9]. McCausland and McCausland[10] have recently suggested that scarring could be a

problem since it might hide areas of trapped endometrium, which could eventually turn into endometrial cancer. Since these areas of endometrium do not have access to the cervix, patients would not have vaginal bleeding and the cancer might be present for some time before it could be detected. This phenomenon has not yet been noted; however, as endometrial ablation is a relatively new procedure, most of the patients treated by heat ablation have not achieved an age when endometrial cancer occurs.

McCausland and McCausland[11], in another communication, suggested that women with deep adenomyosis should not be treated by rollerball ablation. This was based on the finding that some women had areas of adenomyosis as deep as 6 mm and that rollerball ablation destroys tissue only to a depth of 4 mm. Four millimeters is also the maximum depth of destruction noted after thermal balloon and hydrotherm ablation[12,13]. Cryosurgery, on the other hand, has been shown to destroy the myometrium to a depth of 10 mm[8].

Finally, a major advantage of cryoablation is the ability to observe the actual treatment session in real time. Of all the ablation techniques developed to date, none has the ability to predict the likely depth of tissue destruction, except cryosurgery. This is because the freezing is performed in real time and with full-thickness visualization.

SUMMARY

Cryoablation, the first technique to be suggested as an alternative to hysterectomy in women with abnormal uterine bleeding, is highly effective and extremely safe. Quality of life is dramatically improved. A unique property of cold, i.e. analgesia, permits the technique to be performed in a physician's office with little discomfort. Moreover, after treatment patients have little discomfort. It can be used effectively in women with large uterine cavities, polyps and submucous fibroids. Additional studies are underway to evaluate the effectiveness of cryosurgery in the treatment of uterine fibroids laparoscopically.

References

1. Tytus JS. Cryosurgery, its history and development. In Rand, R, Rinfret A, von Leden H, eds. *Cryosurgery*. Springfield, IL: Charles C. Thomas, 1968:3–19

2. Dobak JD, Ryba E, Kovalcheck S. A new closed-loop cryosurgical device for endometrial ablation. *J Am Assoc Gynecol Laparosc* 2000;7:245–9

3. Cahan WG, Brockunier AJ. Cryosurgery of the uterine cavity. *Am J Obstet Gynecol* 1967;1:138–53

4. Droegemueller W, Greer BE, Makowski EL. Preliminary observations of cryocoagulation of the endometrium. *Am J Obstet Gynecol* 1970;107:958–61

5. Droegemueller, Greer BA, Makowski EL, *et al.* Cryosurgery of the uterus. *Am J Obstet Gynecol* 1972;110:27–33

6. Townsend DE, Ostergard DR. Cryocauterization for preinvasive cervical neoplasia. *J Reprod Med* 1971;6:55–8

7. Duleba AJ, Heppard MC, Soderstrom RM, *et al.* A randomized study comparing endometrial cryoablation and rollerball electroablation for treatment of dysfunctional uterine bleeding. *J Am Assoc Gynecol Laparosc* 2003;10:17–26

8. Dobak JD, Willems J, Howard R, *et al.* Endometrial cryoablation with ultrasound visualization in women undergoing hysterectomy. *J Am Assoc Gynecol Laparosc* 2000;7:89–93

9. Townsend DE, Herbst S, Bush S. Comparison of thermal balloon and cryoablation for abnormal bleeding. Presented at the *50th American College of Obstetricians and Gynecologists Annual Clinical Meeting*, Los Angeles, May 4–8, 2002

10. McCausland AM, McCausland VM. Intrauterine scarring as a result of total endometrial ablation could delay the diagnosis of endometrial cancer. *Am J Obstet Gynecol* 1997;180:1598–9

11. McCausland AM, McCausland VM. Depth of endometrial penetration in adenomyosis helps determine outcome of rollerball ablation. *Am J Obstet Gynecol* 1996;174:1786–93

12. Richart RM, Botacinc GD, Nicolauo M, *et al.* Histologic studies of the effects of circulating hot saline on the uterus before hysterectomy. *J Am Assoc Gynecol Laparosc* 1999;5:2659–275

13. Meyer W, Walsh BW, Grainger DA, *et al.* Thermal balloon and rollerball ablation to treat menorrhagia, a multicenter comparison. *Obstet Gynecol* 1998;92:98–102

17

Radiofrequency endometrial ablation systems

J. Cooper and E. Skalnyi

INTRODUCTION

Traditional hysteroscopy endometrial ablation techniques require considerable experience to obtain good results. Consequently, many surgeons were unable to offer their patients this treatment for menorrhagia.

Radiofrequency (RF) energy has been successfully employed with the use of 'first-generation' (i.e. hysteroscopic) endometrial ablation systems (rollerball, rollerbar and loop resection). Both unipolar and bipolar RF energy has also found an application with the development of 'second-generation' products.

SECOND-GENERATION UNIPOLAR TECHNOLOGY

The Vesta DUB system (Valleylab Inc., Boulder, CO) consists of a single-use handset, a dedicated monopolar RF generator and a control box. The handset provides for intrauterine deployment of a balloon with 12 electrodes; six are on the anterior surface and six are on the posterior surface. Each is under individual thermistor control. After adequate cervical dilatation, an 8-mm sheath extending from the handset is inserted into the uterine cavity. The sheath is retracted to allow the balloon to be first deployed and then inflated with 12–15 ml of air. Next, a pressure test is performed to check for fundal perforations and to ensure sufficient contact between electrodes and the uterine walls.

The control box is then energized, triggering equilibration of the electrodes which usually takes about 90 s. The system has a fail-safe shut-off at 3 min if equilibration has not been achieved. The tissue impedance is monitored every 0.33 s as a means of confirming tissue contact with the electrodes. Energy delivery is controlled so as to achieve a pre-set temperature of 75°C in the main body of the uterus and 72°C in the cornual regions. The energy delivery cycle self-terminates in 4 min. Upon completion of the procedure the balloon is deflated, retracted into the sheath and removed from the uterine cavity.

Clinical results

The Vesta DUB endometrial ablation system has been evaluated in several clinical trials[1–3]. Results in the multicentered, international, randomized clinical trial show that clinical outcome is comparable to that of endometrial resection followed by rollerball ablation[3]. At 12-month follow-up, there were no statistical differences in the decrease in flow as defined by pictorial blood loss assessment chart (PBLAC) scores between the Vesta arm and the resectoscopic arm of the study. Procedure success was defined as bleeding less than eumenorrhea, noted in 86.9% of patients in the Vesta arm and 83.0% of the patients in the resectoscope arm. The amenorrhea rates were 31.1% and 34.8%, respectively. Procedure time was 23.1 ± 9.5 min. No major complications were reported.

Although the Vesta system has received conditional Food and Drug Administration (FDA) approval, the manufacturer apparently was not able to overcome several manufacturing issues and chose not to meet the conditions set by the FDA for sales and distribution. As a result, Vesta is not available in the USA and is no longer manufactured.

SECOND-GENERATION BIPOLAR TECHNOLOGY

The NovaSure™ impedance-controlled endometrial ablation system (Novacept Inc., Palo Alto, CA) is another 'global' endometrial ablation system that takes advantage of the benefits of RF technology. Unlike Vesta, NovaSure employs bipolar RF energy.

The NovaSure system consists of a disposable electrode array and a portable RF controller, connecting cord, desiccant, foot switch and power cord (Figure 1). The disposable device consists of a single-patient use, bipolar electrode array, mounted on an expandable frame intended to create a confluent lesion of the entire interior surface area of the uterine cavity. The device, 7.2-mm in outer diameter, is

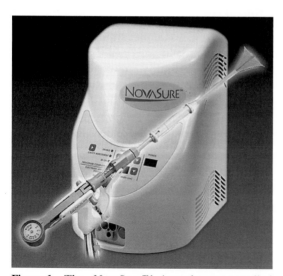

Figure 1 The NovaSure™ impedance-controlled endometrial ablation system

inserted transcervically into the uterine cavity. The protective sheath is then retracted to allow the bipolar electrode array to be deployed and conform to the uterine cavity. The electrode array consists of a gold-plated, porous fabric through which steam and moisture are continuously suctioned as tissue is desiccated[4].

The NovaSure device works in conjunction with a dedicated RF controller to perform a global endometrial ablation in an average treatment time of 90 s. There is no need for concomitant hysteroscopic visualization or endometrial pretreatment[5]. The specific configuration of the electrode array and the predetermined power (specific to the patient's uterine cavity size) delivered by the controller create a tapered depth of ablation characterized by a deeper ablation in the main body of the uterus and a more shallow ablation profile in the regions of the cornua and internal cervical os. The controller automatically calculates the required power output based on the patient's uterine cavity length and width. These figures are determined by the surgeon prior to instituting treatment. Intraoperative uterine sounding measurements allow assessment of the length of the cavity (cervix and fundus), whereas the NovaSure device measures the uterine cavity width (cornu-to-cornu distance). The operator keys these measurements into the controller. A patented moisture transport vacuum system contained within the controller creates and maintains a vacuum in the uterine cavity throughout the ablation procedure. This ensures constant apposition between the electrode array and the endometrium while simultaneously allowing for continuous removal of ablation by-products during the procedure.

A cavity integrity assessment system is an integral part of the NovaSure system. This automated safety feature was developed and implemented to assist the physician in the timely detection of uterine wall perforation, such as that caused by sounding and/or dilatation, thus preventing energy delivery. Utilizing a hysteroflator-type technology, CO_2 is delivered into the uterine cavity at a safe flow rate and pressure. When an intrauterine CO_2

pressure of 50 mmHg is reached and maintained for 4 s, thereby confirming good uterine wall integrity, the controller allows the ablation process to proceed.

During the ablation process, the flow of RF energy vaporizes and/or coagulates the endometrium regardless of its thickness. The negative intrauterine pressure created by the controller continually pulls the endometrium and myometrium towards the electrode. As the ablation process continues, the underlying superficial myometrium is also desiccated and coagulated. As tissue destruction reaches the optimal depth for a safe and effective ablation, an increase in tissue impedance to 50 Ω causes the controller to terminate power delivery, thereby providing a self-regulating process.

Clinical results

A multicenter, international 2 : 1 randomized clinical trial was conducted in support of the FDA premarket approval application and included 265 premenopausal women with excessive menstrual bleeding due to benign causes[6]. In this clinical trial the NovaSure system (175 patients) was compared to loop resection followed by a rollerball ablation (90 patients).

Twelve-month results showed that the two treatment modalities were effective in reducing excessive menstrual blood loss. A 90% or greater decrease in PBLAC scores was achieved in 84.4% of the NovaSure group and in 76.8% of the rollerball group. Normal bleeding or less (PBLAC scores ≤ 100) was reported in 90.9% of the NovaSure patients and 87.8% of the rollerball patients at 1 year post-treatment. In patients with 12-month follow-up, 41% of the NovaSure patients and 35% of the rollerball patients experienced amenorrhea. The mean procedure time (from device insertion to removal) was 4.2 min in the NovaSure Group and 24.2 min in the rollerball group. Treatment time, defined as the length of time during which RF energy is delivered, averaged 84 s in the NovaSure group.

Of the NovaSure patients 73% had the procedure performed under local and/or intravenous sedation while 82% of the rollerball patients were treated utilizing general or epidural anesthesia. Intraoperative adverse events occurred less frequently in the NovaSure group (0.6%) than in the rollerball group (6.7%) and there was a 13% occurrence rate of postoperative adverse events in the NovaSure group compared with 25.3% in the rollerball group. There was a significant decrease in premenstrual symptoms and dysmenorrhea in both treatment groups at 12 months postprocedure. Based on the results of this clinical trial, the FDA found the NovaSure system to be safe and effective and approved it for sale in the USA in 2001.

The NovaSure system has been evaluated in other clinical trials. Gallinat and colleagues conducted a clinical trial on 107 patients and found treatment was successful in 96.1% of patients[7]. The amenorrhea rate in the series at 12-month follow-up was 58%. Abbott and co-workers conducted a randomized clinical trial comparing the NovaSure with the Cavaterm™ system. Amenorrhea and satisfaction rates reported in the NovaSure arm at 12-month follow-up were 43% and 92%, respectively, compared with 11% and 83% in the Cavaterm group[8]. Fulop and associates reported a 90% amenorrhea and a 100% success rate in 75 patients at 3 years following the NovaSure procedure[9]. Laberge and colleagues conducted a clinical trial comparing intra- and postoperative pain associated with use of NovaSure and the ThermaChoice® systems. Use of the NovaSure system was associated with a statistically significantly lower intra- and postoperative pain level than that observed with the ThermaChoice system[10]. Bongers and co-workers (personal communication) conducted a randomized clinical trial comparing the NovaSure system with the ThermaChoice balloon. Amenorrhea and satisfaction rates observed in the NovaSure group of patients at 12-month follow-up were 55% and 94%, respectively, compared with 8% and 77% in the ThermaChoice group. Busund and associates, in a multicenter study, found 58% of patients reported amenorrhea and 91.5% experienced a return to normal menstrual bleeding or less at 12 months following the NovaSure procedure[11].

References

1. Dequesne JH, Gallinat A, Garza-Leal JG, *et al.* Thermoregulated radiofrequency endometrial ablation. *Int J Fertil Womens Med* 1997;42:311–18

2. Corson SL, Brill AI, Brooks PG, *et al.* Interim results of the American Vesta trial of endometrial ablation. *J Am Assoc Gynecol Laparosc* 1999;6:45–9

3. Corson SL, Brill AI, Brooks PG, *et al.* One-year results of the vesta system for endometrial ablation. *Am Assoc Gynecol Laparosc* 2000;7: 489–97

4. Laberge P. NovaSure technology overview. In: *Proceedings of the 2nd World Congress on Controversies in Obstetrics, Gynecology amd Infertility.* 2001;1:303–10

5. Cooper J, Brill A, Fullop T. Is endometrial pre-treatment necessary in NovaSure 3-D endometrial ablation. *Gynaecol Endosc* 2001;10: 179–82

6. Cooper J, Gimpelson R, Laberge P, *et al.* A randomized, multicenter trial of safety and efficacy of the NovaSure system in the treatment of menorrhagia. *J Am Assoc Gynecol Laparosc* 2002;9:418–28

7. Gallinat A, Nugent W. NovaSure impedance-controlled system for endometrial ablation. *J Am Assoc Gynecol Laparosc* 2002;9:279–85

8. Abbott J, Hawe J, Hunter D, *et al.* A double blind randomized trial comparing Cavaterm™ and the Novasure™ endometrial ablation systems for the treatment of dysfunctional uterine bleeding. *Fertil Steril* 2003; in press

9. Fulop T, Rakoczi I, Barna I. NovaSure impedance controlled endometrial ablation system. Long-term follow-up results. In *Proceedings of the 2nd World Congress on Controversies in Obstetrics, Gynecology & Infertility.* 2001;2:149–55

10. Laberge PY, Sabbah R, Fortin C, *et al.* Assessment and comparison of intraoperative and post-operative pain associated with Novasure and ThermaChoice endometrial ablation systems. *J Am Assoc Gynecol Laparosc* 2003;10:223–32

11. Busund B, Erno LE, Gronmark A, *et al.* Endometrial ablation with NovaSure GEA, a pilot study. *Acta Obstet Gynecol Scand* 2003;82: 65–8

18

A balloon endometrial ablation system

D. B. Yackel and J. R. Elliott

Thermablate™ EAS™ (MDMI Technologies Inc., Richmond, British Columbia) is a new balloon-based technology that is in the final stages of clinical validation. Because of the intrauterine temperatures achieved it may be considered to be the first of a third generation of endometrial ablation systems.

This system consists of a small, lightweight, reusable, hand-held treatment control unit (TCU) and a disposable single-use pre-filled catheter/balloon cartridge (Figure 1). Treatment time for the patient is approximately 2 min and the system is designed to be cheaper, easier to use and more effective than current therapies.

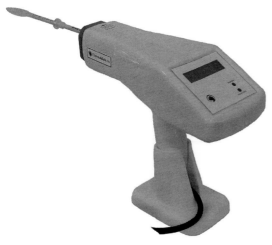

Figure 1 Thermablate™ EAS™ with LCD screen visible

DEVICE DEVELOPMENT

In reviewing the existing hot-fluid technologies, it became apparent that the target operational temperature in these systems was not necessarily the optimal treatment temperature but instead was the highest temperature that the respective systems could achieve without reaching technical limitations. Constraints on temperature, volume and pressure were clearly identified. High pressures could not be delivered in a free-circulating system for fear of tubal extravasation and temperatures could not exceed boiling points of dextrose in water or saline; therefore the only adjustments to the treatment profile in existing methods was a longer treatment time. It was felt that higher temperatures in the 'searing level range' would ultimately lead to the best treatment and a shorter treatment time.

Initial work was done by studying burn effects on raw meat to determine what combination of temperature, time and pressure would prove to be the most effective treatment. Key items learned at this stage of development were that:

(1) Time was a factor in treatment burn depth and therefore needed to be properly balanced with temperature;

(2) Re-circulation of the treatment fluid using re-circulation cycles was necessary to help promote thermal uniformity for better treatment;

(3) Uniformity at a 160–180°C 2-min cycle provided a good balance between temperature and time for the desired treatment depth.

To further enhance the development and testing of the new device, a silicone model of a uterus was created that incorporated an array of 64 thermocouples interfaced to a computer. From this, a soft-tipped catheter and pre-formed silicone balloon were designed with significant improvements in the effectiveness of circulation and thus temperature and treatment uniformity. In conjunction with the silicone model, a method of creating a uterine cavity in meat tissue was developed in which thermocouples could be placed at the balloon surface as well as at 0.5 mm and 5.0 mm distances from the balloon–meat interface.

A large number of meat model tests (Figure 2) were carried out until the optimum time, temperature and pressure profiles were ascertained. Numerous fluid solutions were also used and the one ultimately chosen is a Food and Drug Administration (FDA)-approved, biologically safe fluid that can be heated to temperatures in excess of 150°C.

An independently commissioned computer model for uterine endometrial thermal ablation provided corroborating evidence that the time, temperature and pressure parameters that had been selected by the engineers were optimal.

(1) Treatment control unit (TCU);

(2) Disposable single-use cartridge;

(3) Power supply;

(4) TCU stand.

All of which are supplied in a carrying case to facilitate transportation and handling.

The TCU, which is the size and shape of a hair dryer (Figure 3), weighs approximately 700 g (1.5 lb). The unit controls the treatment settings (time, pressure and temperature) through a computerized system that operates the electromechanical heating and pumping/draining components. The TCU has a liquid crystal display (LCD) that provides pertinent information to the user: warm-up phase, leak checks, treatment phase and completion of treatment, which are all clearly indicated on the display. The TCU is easily cleaned, is reusable, and has a planned life span of more than 600 cycles before maintenance is required.

The disposal single-use cartridge (Figure 4) is the actual treatment component of the Thermablate EAS. Twenty-eight milliliters of treatment fluid is contained inside the diaphragm of the cartridge and, after it is heated, is available for injection into the pre-shaped silicone balloon through an insulated 6-mm catheter ending with a soft tip.

DEVICE OPERATION

The Thermablate EAS shown (Figure 1) includes the following components:

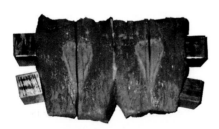

Figure 2 Example of meat model test with uniform pattern of burn demonstrated

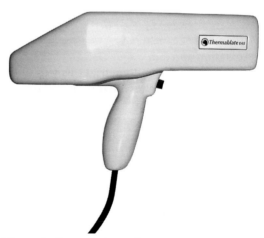

Figure 3 Lateral view of treatment control unit (TCU)

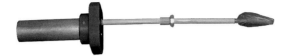

Figure 4 Disposable cartridge

The balloon conforms directly to the uterine cavity shape, contacting the endometrial tissue and performing the thermal ablation.

A power supply (not shown) converts 120–220 V alternating current to 24 V direct current for the TCU. A stand is provided to hold the TCU in a horizontal position during the system's warm-up stage and offers a sanitary rest when the unit is not in use.

Principles of operation

The ablating heat source of the Thermablate EAS is the treatment liquid, which is supplied inside the diaphragm of the disposable cartridge. This diaphragm, surrounded by an aluminum shield, is inserted into the heating chamber of the TCU and is easily locked in place with a bayonet connection. After the cartridge has been inserted and the device turned on, a warm-up phase of about 8 min is required to bring the temperature of the liquid to approximately 170°C. The temperature is visually displayed on the LCD and indicates when the device is ready for treatment. During the device warm-up phase, appropriate patient preparation is then carried out and, unless previously done, includes a diagnostic hysteroscopy as well as dilatation and curettage (D&C). The balloon is inserted into the endometrial cavity until the soft catheter tip touches the fundus and the balloon is then withdrawn 0.5–1.0 cm. Centimeter markings are clearly indicated on the catheter to compare with sounding measurements previously obtained at the time of D&C.

To initiate the treatment, the trigger is depressed and held for 5 s after which an audible beep indicates the trigger no longer needs to be held. The system then goes through a 15-s balloon leak test and other components of the device are also automatically checked.

Failure of any of these safety checks will stop the procedure and this will be indicated on the display screen.

If the safety checks are satisfactory, the treatment liquid is then forced through the catheter into the balloon by compression of the diaphragm with air pumped within the TCU heating chamber until a control set-point air pressure has been reached. The treatment liquid temperature decreases slightly as it travels through the catheter and when it enters the balloon it is approximately 150°C (302°F). Treatment temperatures measured at the endometrial lining are approximately 100°C (212°F). Thermal energy is thus transferred to the endometrial lining.

During the treatment phase, the TCU performs a series of pressurization and depressurization cycles to homogenize the temperature of the liquid in the balloon. This helps ensure a uniform endometrial remodeling to most of the uterine lining. It takes 128 s to obtain a treatment depth of 4–5 mm. At the conclusion of the treatment, the liquid is pulled back into the diaphragm and a prompt is given for the physician to withdraw the balloon.

PRE-HYSTERECTOMY CLINICAL SAFETY STUDIES

Clinical safety study at Delta Hospital

A pre-hysterectomy phase 1 safety trial using the Thermablate EAS was performed at Delta Hospital, Vancouver, British Columbia, between 10 October 2000 and 2 March 2001. All patients were scheduled for a vaginal hysterectomy for benign disease usually involving symptomatic pelvic relaxation. In all cases, the Thermablate EAS worked flawlessly and without incident. All patients had uneventful postoperative courses and no complications occurred.

Laboratory examination of the excised uterus was immediately carried out. Reviewing the thermal coagulation results in the first five cases showed that the thermal effects were less than optimal. A slight adjustment in treatment time and pump recycling was made so that the depth of thermal endometrial necrosis was increased. Because of the balloon design, treatment depth is greater at the mid-portion of the endometrial cavity and tapers toward both cornual areas as well as toward the internal os. In all cases, no thermal burn effects were observed in the endocervical canal, demonstrating the effectiveness of the insulated sheath in protecting this area (Figure 5).

Clinical safety study at Monterrey

A second pre-hysterectomy clinical safety study was carried out on 9 and 10 November 2001 by Jose Gerardo Garza-Leal at the University Hospital, Monterrey, Mexico.

This study involved thermocouple temperature monitoring within the cervical canal and on the serosal surface of the uterus during the ablation procedure. Seven procedures were performed in women scheduled for an abdominal hysterectomy. At the time of surgery, thermocouples were placed through the abdominal incision on to the outer surface of the uterus. A cervical temperature probe was placed at a measured point in the cervical canal.

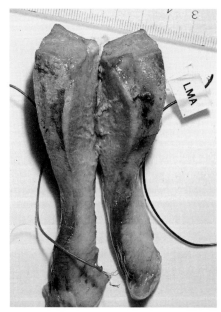

Figure 5 Hysterectomy specimen with NBT stain showing depth of tissue necrosis

Histological examination of the uterus was conducted immediately after the uterus was removed. In two patients a previous Cesarean section had been done and thermocouples were placed on the serosal surfaces of the Cesarean section scar. The device worked as intended in all cases and no adverse events were reported. The serosal and cornual temperatures were within the range of normal body temperature and there was no evidence for any thermal damage to the cervix or endocervical canal. The endometrial ablation effects were in the 3–5 mm range with uniformity of burn effect being noted in all surfaces.

INTERNATIONAL CLINICAL STUDIES

Bombay pilot study

A pilot study of 16 patients with menorrhagia was carried out by Prashant Mangeshikar in Bombay, India, in January 2001 (Figure 6)[1]. The study included an informed consent and a history of excessive uterine bleeding on a dysfunctional basis with a uterine sounding of ≥ 7 cm to ≤ 12 cm. A pre-procedure evaluation included a pelvic examination and Pap smear, a hemoglobin or hematocrit, endometrial biopsy and pelvic ultrasound. If it had not been previously obtained, hysteroscopy was performed immediately pre-treatment to assess the endometrial cavity. No gonadotropin releasing hormone analogs were used, nor were the treatments timed to the menstrual cycle. All patients had a D&C for endometrial thinning immediately pre-ablation.

Each patient was followed either by office visit or telephone interview at 2 weeks, 3 months, 6 months and 1 year. One-year results (P. Mangeshikar, personal communication) have shown eight of the 16 patients (50%) to have amenorrhea and six (38%) with spotting or hypomenorrhea. No complications occurred and all but one of the patients (94%) were satisfied or very satisfied with the results of their treatment. The single treatment failure was a 44-year-old para 4 patient with documented cystic endometrial hyperplasia who had been on cyclic medroxyprogesterone acetate for 2 years.

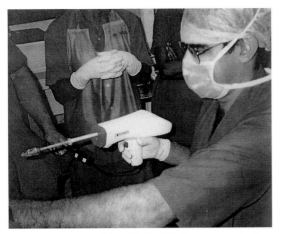

Figure 6 Thermablate™ EAS™ in use in Indian clinical trial

The high rate of amenorrhea and hypomenorrhea in this small series is not an unexpected finding. Laboratory testing in the research and development of the device had shown that a higher thermal transfer of energy for a shorter period of time combined with a pre-formed silicone balloon would give a more uniform pattern of tissue necrosis. In turn, it was felt that this would result in a predictably higher amenorrhea rate. Clinically, it appears that the anticipated result of endometrial remodeling using the Thermablate EAS has been achieved.

Guanzhou pilot study

A similar pilot study of 100 patients in Guanzhou, China, commenced in March 2002 (data on file with MDMI Technologies Inc., Richmond, British Colombia, Canada). Initial rates of amenorrhea, hypomenorrhea and patient satisfaction are similar to the Indian trial but the length of follow-up is not sufficient to draw any firm conclusions.

In both studies, it has been observed that the level of postoperative pain or discomfort is much less and of shorter duration than our experience using most other ablation methods. Because of this, additional studies to quantify dysmenorrhea are being planned for the near future.

In conclusion, the simplicity of use, low cost and portability of the Thermablate EAS are advantages when compared with other second-generation methods. The safety and ease of use of this new, compact, thermal balloon endometrial ablation instrument has been established. A high rate of amenorrhea and hypomenorrhea in international pilot studies has been observed as well as a very high level of patient satisfaction. Increased sample sizes and longer follow-up times are required but the pilot studies are extremely encouraging. FDA approval has been obtained for a randomized, prospective clinical trial at multiple sites in the USA and Canada.

Reference

1. Mangeshikar P, Kapur A, Yackel DB. Endometrial ablation with a thermal balloon system. *J Am Assoc Gynecol Laparosc* 2003;10:27–32

19

The role of repeat procedures and second-look hysteroscopes in endometrial ablation/resection

R. J. Gimpelson, E. J. Bieber and F. D. Loffer

INTRODUCTION

Second-look or repeat resectoscope procedures are indicated under three circumstances:

(1) When initial endometrial ablation (by either a roller or resection technique) fails to control menorrhagia[1];

(2) When a submucous or intramural leiomyoma is only partially resected[2,3] and is symptomatic;

(3) When a new fibroid develops[2,3].

Additionally, in higher-risk procedures such as myomectomy, where intrauterine adhesions may occur after surgery, repeat evaluation and treatment may be indicated in patients desiring fertility. In one clinical study, 95 patients underwent an operative hysteroscopic procedure followed by a second-look hysteroscope after the next menses[4]. Of interest, only one of 43 patients who underwent polypectomy or septolysis were noted to have intrauterine adhesions, whereas 10/32 (31.3%) of patients with a single myoma and 9/20 (45.5%) with multiple myoma were noted to have intra-uterine adhesions. The authors found repeat hysteroscopy to be a valuable tool in the treatment of intrauterine adhesions after hysteroscopic myomectomy.

ENDOMETRIAL ABLATION

Anatomy

When attempting a repeat endometrial ablation, one must be aware of the uterine anatomy. The cavity is usually a different shape compared to an unablated cavity. The shape is narrow and cylindrical, cornua are usually obliterated, the myometrium may be thinner and the endometrium may be sporadic, ranging from thick to non-existent in fibrosed areas. The uterus usually sounds to a shorter depth following endometrial ablation and, occasionally, the cavity is interlaced with synechiae (Figures 1 and 2).

Indications

Repeat endometrial ablation is indicated whenever there is a failure to achieve the desired results from an initial endometrial ablation and patients do not desire a hysterectomy. Patients undergoing repeat ablation fall into one of five categories[1]:

(1) Initial procedure not completed because of leiomyomas;

(2) Menstrual bleeding improved but still heavy or prolonged and impacting on quality of life;

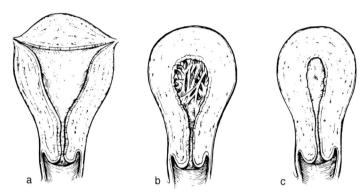

Figure 1 Drawings of uterus: (a) normal uterine cavity; (b) postablation (synechiae); (c) postablation (narrowed and cylindrical)

(3) Physical or mental disability with amenorrhea desired;

(4) Amenorrhea desired by patient despite achieving normal or light flow;

(5) Unimproved.

Most patients will fall into category 2, the 'improved but still heavy or prolonged flow' category. It is recommended that an interval of at least 6 months be observed before a repeat ablation is performed to allow for full healing of the uterus and also to allow for a recognizable and definable menstrual pattern.

Methods

Both the rollerball electrode and Nd:YAG laser have been used for repeat ablation although seemingly other methodologies could also be used[1]. Repeat ablation with the laser affords the advantage of fitting the laser fiber through a conventional 21 Fr operating hysteroscope and more easily entering the constricted uterine cavity. However, with the increased use of electrosurgical and heated-fluid techniques, increasing experience with repeat ablations has been obtained.

Surgical technique

After allowing for a recovery period of at least 6 months following initial endometrial ablation[5],

a patient can be scheduled for repeat endometrial ablation if success has not been attained. If it has been over 1 year since the initial ablation, the endometrium must be re-evaluated histologically to rule out cancer or premalignant changes. Suppression of the endometrium may be achieved either by medical suppression (Danocrine 800 mg/day for 4 weeks[6] or gonadotropin releasing hormone (GnRH) agonist for 6 weeks[7]) or by mechanical preparation (suction curettage with a 7-mm suction curette[8,9]). Mechanical preparation is carried out for 2–3 min just prior to the ablation (see Chapter 5).

The mechanical preparation of the endometrium makes repeat ablation more convenient and comfortable for the patient since surgery can be scheduled without specific time requirements or delays and the patient is free from the side-effects of endometrial suppression medications. Uterine entry is easier when a non-atrophic state is present, as is the case with mechanical preparation.

The patient is given general anesthesia, epidural anesthesia or local anesthesia with sedation. A paracervical block with 0.25% bupivacaine may make cervical dilatation easier and less uncomfortable. Pitressin® (2 units/10 ml) may be administered concurrently to reduce fluid absorption and bleeding, but it is not without risk (see Chapter 20). A paracervical block may be performed even with general and regional anesthesia to reduce postoperative discomfort.

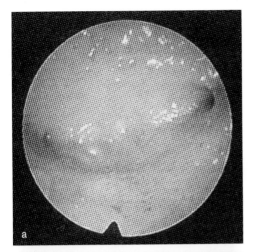

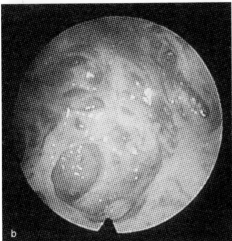

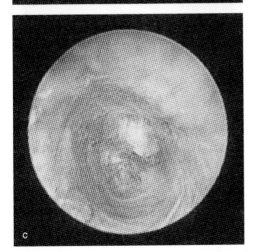

Figure 2 Photos of uterus: (a) normal cavity; (b) postablation (synechiae); (c) postablation (narrowed and cylindrical). See also Color Plates XII, XIII and XIV, respectively

Just as with other procedures using high-flow, low-viscosity liquids, the fluid inflow and outflow must be monitored very closely. Initial entry into the uterus is with a 5-mm diagnostic sheath and 4-mm telescope. Entry is usually achieved without the need for dilators. Following this initial entry, a continuous-flow operating hysteroscope (21 Fr) can be inserted 90% of the time, again without need for dilators. Use of the diagnostic sheath reduces the number of blind insertions into the uterus and reduces the risk of perforation. At this point, the suction curettage is performed if medical preparation of the endometrium has not been utilized (Figures 3 and 4). If the resectoscope is to be used, further cervical dilatation is usually performed at this time.

Usually, lactated Ringer's is used with the Nd:YAG laser. However, electrolyte-free fluids must be used with the resectoscope (see Chapter 6). The power is set at 50–55 W for the Nd:YAG laser, and a non-touch technique allows the procedure to be performed in 10–15 min. Approximately the same amount of time is used with the roller electrode set at 60 W coagulating current or 80 W cutting circuit. With either modality, the technique involves ablation from the fundus toward the internal os to enhance the success of the procedure and reduce the risk of perforation. Once the procedure is

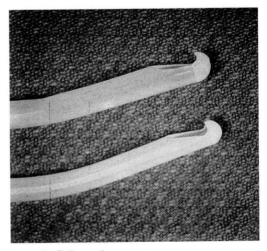

Figure 3 7 Fr suction curette

203

completed, the patient is observed and almost always discharged on the same day as surgery.

Although most ablations are now being performed with the roller electrode or loop electrode rather than the Nd:YAG laser, it is the opinion of the author (R.J.G.) that repeat ablation is more easily accomplished with the Nd:YAG laser. The reason is that a laser fiber will go through a 21 Fr hysteroscope sheath, whereas the roller or loop electrode requires a minimum 24 Fr sheath. Since the uterine cavity is usually shortened and narrowed with a cylindrical shape following endometrial ablation, a 21 Fr sheath is easier to insert than a 24 Fr sheath. However, if one prefers the roller electrode for repeat ablation, the results will probably be comparable to those from the laser. Global endometrial ablation techniques have not been described for repeat procedures. However, the Hydro ThermAblator system, which circulates hot saline in the cavity, may give the distinct advantage of being able to treat distorted cavities (see Chapter 15).

Risks

The risks of repeat endometrial ablation are the same, but increased[10], as those for initial endometrial ablation[11]: fluid overload, perforation, bleeding, infection and thermal injury to structures outside the uterus.

Fluid overload is avoided by carefully monitoring fluid inflow and outflow throughout the procedure. Many fluid monitors, which measure intake and output, are commercially available and avoid the considerable risk of inaccurate manual calculation of intake and output. If a fluid monitor is not available, a sheet for keeping track can be utilized for ease of record keeping (Figure 5). Electrolytes can be

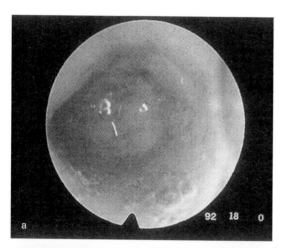

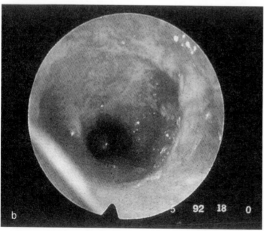

Figure 4 Uterine cavity before (a) and after (b) curettage. See also Color Plates XV and XVI

HYSTEROSCOPIC SURGERY FLUIDS INTAKE AND OUTPUT

FLOW SHEET

TIME (q 10 Min)	FLUID IN	FLUID OUT	PUMP PRESSURE	COMMENTS
TOTAL ___				

OTHER FLUIDS

IVs: _____

Urine: _____

Figure 5 Sheet for monitoring fluid use

considered prior to the procedure and absorption of fluid is limited according to published fluid monitoring guidelines[12]. However, more rigid limits are used depending on the medical condition of the patient. Usually, observation or Lasix® is used for excess fluids.

Perforation is more likely to occur with blind insertion of dilators and sounds rather than the hysteroscope or resectoscope. Such a risk may be higher in patients undergoing a secondary procedure. Theoretically, the smaller cavity may predispose patients to a perforation. If perforation occurs, with the diagnostic sheath, dilator or sound, the procedure is generally ended and observation may be all that is needed. A repeat procedure can be performed in approximately 3 months, after the perforation has sealed. If perforation occurs with the operating hysteroscope or resectoscope, laparoscopy may be utilized to assess the damage. If the laser or electrical generator is being operated when perforation occurs, then it is usually necessary to perform a laparotomy to evaluate damage to the bowel, bladder or vessels.

The most serious type of injury would be an unrecognized thermal injury to abdominal structures without perforation of the uterus. This occurrence can be minimized by avoiding powers above 55 W with the Nd:YAG laser and continually moving the tip across the uterus to avoid constant exposure in one area. The roller electrode should also be kept moving to avoid similar problems. Powers for the electrical method have not been as well studied as laser, but 60 W coagulating and 80 W cutting current have accomplished satisfactory results.

Postoperative management

Postoperative discomfort is usually easily controlled with mild analgesia, such as non-steroidal anti-inflammatory agents. Patients are given a home instruction sheet (Figure 6) and asked to return in 1 month for uterine sounding and cervical dilatation to reduce the potential for developing hematometra secondary to cervical stenosis.

Results

Early studies of endometrial ablation with the Nd:YAG laser demonstrated that repeat ablation would generally be successful in cases where ablation is a viable option, with expected good or excellent results most of the time.

Whether the Nd:YAG laser, roller electrode or loop electrode is utilized for endometrial ablation (Table 1), a small number of patients

---

Postoperative Instructions
for
Endometrial Ablation

- You should rest this evening.
- Avoid alcoholic beverages for about 48 hours.
- Avoid intercourse for about 72 hours.
- You will need to make an appointment to be seen in my office one month from the surgery for a follow-up examination, uterine sounding and hemoglobin/hematocrit.
- You should notify me if any of the following occurs:
  - Fever above 101 degrees
  - Severe pains
  - Bleeding that requires more pads than a usual period. You will expect some drainage and some bleeding that may continue for 4 to 6 weeks
- You may experience moderate to severe cramping lasting 48–72 hours that should respond to pain medication prescribed.

Figure 6   Postablation instruction sheet

Table 1 Success of endometrial ablation techniques

Author	Number of patients	Repeat procedures (success/total)	Initial technique	Repeat technique
Goldrath[13]	216	—	Nd:YAG	Nd:YAG
Loffer[14]	36	2/2	Nd:YAG	Nd:YAG
Garry et al.[15]	479	26/39	Nd:YAG	Nd:YAG
Magos et al.[16]	234	13/16	roller loop	roller loop
Leffler et al.[8]	38	2/2	Nd:YAG or roller	roller
Gimpelson et al.[1]	143	16/16	Nd:YAG or roller	Nd:YAG or roller
Rankin et al.[17]	400	28/31*	loop or roller	loop or roller
Baggish et al.[18]	568	5/8	Nd:YAG or ball electrode	
Vilos et al.[19]	800	—/32	loop or roller	

*One patient had three procedures before success

will not achieve satisfactory results with the initial procedure. However, with repeat ablation, most patients will be satisfied with the outcome and will not need further treatment[1].

Since the author's paper (R.J.G.) was published[1], an additional 69 patients have undergone initial endometrial ablation. Only two additional repeat ablations have been performed in the same time period for a total of 18 repeat ablations out of 212 patients. Amenorrhea was achieved in 12 of the 18 repeat ablations.

Only one of the patients who underwent repeat ablation had a subsequent hysterectomy and was found to have a leiomyoma and simple hyperplasia. An additional five of the 212 patients experienced a change in their menstrual pattern that occurred over 1 year following endometrial ablation and were evaluated by hysteroscopy and curettage. All findings were benign, and since flow was well within an acceptable range, no repeat ablation was performed. The uterine cavities in these patients had the same scarred and constricted appearance as the patients undergoing repeat ablation.

Three patients who had gone through menopause (documented by elevated follicle stimulating hormone and decreased estradiol) were hysteroscoped prior to estrogen replacement therapy and also had the typical post-ablation appearance of the uterine cavity.

In a large series of 568 patients undergoing endometrial ablation, the authors describe a patient who required a second endometrial ablation who had residual endometrium present in the cornua[18]. This may often be the location of residual tissue since, anatomically, this area may be the most difficult to reach with the hysteroscope. Wortman and Daggett evaluated 26 patients who had previously undergone failed hysteroscopic resection and ablation[20]. Interestingly, 81% of the patients required an endocervical resection to gain access to the endometrial cavity. Consistent with other reports on the causes for failure of endometrial ablation, 58% of these patients were noted to have adenomyosis on final pathologic evaluation. Noteworthy is the fact that 23 of the 26 patients achieved satisfactory results with sonographically guided endomyometrial resection with only three of the patients undergoing subsequent hysterectomy. We (R.J.G., E.J.B., F.L.) believe only a handful of hysteroscopists are capable of performing this type of second resection in this setting.

Although the experience with long-term results is less with thermal ablation than the YAG laser or resectoscope, a recent study suggests similar findings after surgery. Taskin and colleagues evaluated 26 patients with a second-look hysteroscopy who had previously undergone thermal ablation[21]. They noted complete atrophy, intrauterine adhesions or obliteration with endometrial fibrosis similar to the findings with other ablation methodologies.

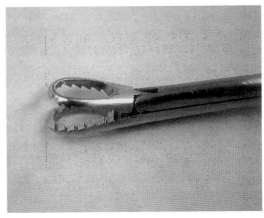

Figure 7 Corson Myoma Grasping Forceps (Karl Storz)

LEIOMYOMAS

Indications

Leiomyomas with large intramural components can often be removed by multistage operations at intervals of 1 month or more if they cannot be completely removed at the initial procedure. Infertility or continued bleeding problems are two indications that leiomyomas remain[2,3,22], thus warranting second-look resectoscopic surgery. When fertility is of concern, a final office procedure can be performed to lyse synechiae that may have developed from a resectoscopic procedure.

In a study of 51 patients undergoing resectoscopic myomectomy, Wamstecker and colleagues noted a correlation of increased intramural involvement with incomplete resection and also additional procedures[23]. It may be of value to discuss these issues with patients who have been documented by sonohysterography to have intramural involvement.

Methods

Scissors, Nd:YAG laser and unipolar or bipolar resectoscopes can all be utilized; however, the resectoscope is the quickest modality for fibroid removal. An instrument of extreme value for myomectomy is the Corson Myoma Grasping Forceps (Figure 7). Its strong jaws can tightly but gently grip a leiomyoma and completely extract it from the myometrial bed and out through the cervical canal.

Surgical procedure

When a leiomyoma with a large intramural component has been partially resected until flush with the endometrium, the next step is to remove the instruments from the uterine cavity and wait several minutes[24] (see Chapter 9). On re-examination, the leiomyoma will often rise out of the myometrium and be in a position for further resection or extraction. If the myoma does not rise out of the myometrium, one can terminate the procedure and re-evaluate the cavity using a sonohysterogram, hysterosalpingogram or office hysteroscopy several months after the procedure. If a residual myoma is seen, the patient may be brought to the operating room at that time. At this follow-up procedure, the leiomyoma has usually delivered a large portion of itself into the uterine cavity and can once more be partially or totally resected. If only partial resection is achieved, the scenario is repeated and the patient can be brought back again. This method has allowed the removal of quite large leiomyomas with ease.

In a large case series from the Netherlands, the authors report on the cases of 285 women who underwent only hysteroscopic resection of myomas with no endometrial ablations[25]. In this series, 41/285 patients underwent a repeat hysteroscopy, with 21% of these 41 patients ultimately undergoing hysterectomy. The authors suggest that resectoscopic myomectomy is best for patients with no more than two myomas with a normal uterine size, since both were independent prognosticators ($p < 0.001$ for recurrence). They also suggest the procedure may still be an acceptable alternative for other patients not meeting these criteria.

Risks

The risks for resection of leiomyomas are the same as those of any hysteroscopic procedure as described earlier in this chapter. In addition, there are certain risks that are increased with myomectomy. GnRH agonists can often be utilized to shrink leiomyomas, stop bleeding and allow for the migration of the intramural segment of the myoma into the uterine cavity as the myometrium shrinks and compresses the myoma[26]. However, the GnRH agonists have risks that must be addressed[27]. Since the uterus will shrink more than the myoma, a tumor filling half the uterine cavity prior to treatment with GnRH agonists may well fill the entire uterine cavity after a course of GnRH agonists and actually make resection of the myoma more difficult. Also, heavy uterine bleeding has been reported on occasion when GnRH agonists are used with leiomyomas[3].

Uterine perforation may occur with too vigorous a resection or attempts at extraction before the myometrium can push the leiomyoma into the uterine cavity. If visualization becomes uncorrectably poor and intrauterine pressure diminishes, one may suspect perforation, and laparotomy or laparoscopy should be considered to assess and correct the problem. Transvaginal ultrasound and sonohysterography prior to myomectomy and repeat procedures will give an estimate of myometrial thickness overlying the leiomyoma[28]. Occasionally, bleeding is encountered, but it is often limited as the uterus spontaneously contracts. If bleeding is persistent, a catheter can be inserted into the uterus and the balloon distended for several hours as a tamponade.

Fluid overload is more a concern with myomectomy than with endometrial ablation since the electrical loop used for myomectomy is more likely to expose the uterine vasculature than ablation with a roller electrode[3]. Safety measures are similar to those described with repeat endometrial ablation.

Postoperative management

Postoperative patients are usually discharged on the day of surgery and instructed to return in

---

Postoperative Instructions
for
Hysteroscopic Myomectomy

- You should rest this evening.
- Avoid alcoholic beverages for about 48 hours.
- Avoid intercourse for about 72 hours.
- You will need to make an appointment to be seen in my office in one week for a follow-up examination.
- You should notify me if any of the following occurs:
  - Fever above 101 degrees
  - Severe pains
  - Bleeding that requires more pads than a usual period.
- You may experience moderate to severe cramping lasting 48–72 hours that should respond to over the counter ibuprofen or pain mediaction that may have been prescribed.

Figure 8 Postmyomectomy instruction sheet

1 week for a follow-up visit. They are given a going-home instruction sheet for guidance (Figure 8). Antibiotics are sometimes used, and after complete myomectomy, a 3-week course of estrogen is used to stimulate endometrial growth when infertility is a concern.

The resectoscope is far superior to laser or scissors in ease of use, speed of surgery and thoroughness of removal. The author (R.J.G.) has abandoned use of the Nd:YAG laser for myomectomy, especially in combination with endometrial ablation because of the lengthy operating times and large amount of fluid absorbed[29]. Scissors are fine for small leiomyomas and for office use but are too slow compared to the resectoscope and loop electrode in the operating room.

FERTILITY

An interesting study from Israel evaluated 110 patients who had been noted to have a normal hysteroscopy and failed to conceive after three or more *in vitro* fertilization cycles[30]. In re-evaluating these patients, 20 patients (18%) were noted to have abnormalities such as polyps, hyperplasia, intrauterine adhesions, etc. This suggests that a re-evaluation may be worthwhile in patients who are not successful with *in vitro* fertilization and whose treatment regimens span a protracted period of time. A reassuring study from Canada evaluated the

risk of diagnostic hysteroscopy in causing adhesions[31]. In only one of 100 patients was any evidence of adhesions noted in patients who had previously had a normal cavity.

CLINICAL PEARLS

(1) One should not hesitate to offer repeat endometrial ablation because the outcome is usually excellent.

(2) If there is a change in postablation menstrual pattern, this should be evaluated in the same way as initial abnormal bleeding.

(3) The previous ablated cavity is smaller than the original uterine cavity.

(4) The Nd:YAG laser may be easier to use during repeat procedures, as it only requires a 21 Fr instrument.

(5) Do transvaginal ultrasound prior to myomectomy to assess the myometrium overlying the leiomyoma.

(6) If a leiomyoma is partially resected, remove all instruments, wait several minutes, and reinsert the resectoscope to see if the leiomyoma has risen out of the myometrium. If it has, finish the procedure. If it has not, discharge the patient and re-evaluate in 1 month. The leiomyoma will almost always be visible and resectable.

References

1. Gimpelson RJ, Kaigh J. Endometrial ablation repeat procedures. *J Reprod Med* 1992;37:629–35
2. Brooks PG, Loffer FD, Serden SP. Resectoscopic removal of symptomatic intrauterine lesions. *J Reprod Med* 1989;34:435–7
3. Indman PD. Hysteroscopic treatment of menorrhagia associated with uterine leiomyomas. *Obstet Gynecol* 1993;81:716–20
4. Taskin O, Sadik S, Onoglu A, *et al.* Role of endometrial suppression on the frequency of intrauterine adhesions after resectoscopic surgery. *J Am Assoc Gynecol Laparosc* 2000; 7:351-4
5. Goldrath MH, Fuller TA, Segal S. Laser photovaporization of the endometrium for the treatment of menorrhagia. *Am J Obstet Gynecol* 1981;140:14–19

6. Goldrath MH. Use of danazol in hysteroscopic surgery for menorrhagia. *J Reprod Med* 1990; 35:91–6

7. Brooks PG, Serden SP, Davos I. Hormonal inhibition of the endometrium for resectoscopic endometrial ablation. *Am J Obstet Gynecol* 1991; 164:1601–8

8. Lefler HT, Sullivan GH, Hulka JF. Modified endometrial ablation: electrocoagulation with vasopressin and suction curettage preparation. *Obstet Gynecol* 1991;77:949–53

9. Gimpelson RJ, Kaigh J. Mechanical preparation of the endometrium prior to endometrial ablation. *J Reprod Med* 1992;37:691–4

10. O'Connor H, Magos A. Endometrial resection for the treatment of menorrhagia. *N Engl J Med* 1996;335:151–6

11. Brooks PG. Complications of operative hysteroscopy: how safe is it? *Clin Obstet Gynecol* 1992;35:256–61

12. Loffer FD, Bradley LD, Brill AI, *et al.* Hysteroscopic fluid monitoring guidelines. *J Am Assoc Gynecol Laparosc* 2000;7:167–8

13. Goldrath MH. Hysteroscopic laser surgery. In Baggish MS, ed. *Basic and Advanced Laser Surgery in Gynecology*. Norwalk, CT: Appleton Century-Crofts, 1985:357–72

14. Loffer FD. Hysteroscopic endometrial ablation with the Nd:YAG laser using a nontouch technique. *Obstet Gynecol* 1987;69:679–82

15. Garry R, Erian J, Grochmal SA. A multi-centre collaborative study into the treatment of menorrhagia by Nd:YAG laser ablation of the endometrium. *Br J Obstet Gynaecol* 1991;98:357–62

16. Magos AL, Baumann R, Lockwood GM, *et al.* Experience with the first 250 endometrial resections for menorrhagia. *Lancet* 1991;337:1074–8

17. Rankin L, Steinberg LH. Transcervical resection of the endometrium: a review of 400 consecutive cases. *Br J Obstet Gynaecol* 1992;99:911–14

18. Baggish M, Sze E. Endometrial ablation: a series of 568 patients treated over an 11-year period. *Am J Obstet Gynecol* 1996;174:908–13

19. Vilos GA, Vilos EC, King JH. Experience with 800 hysteroscopic endometrial ablations. *J Am Assoc Gynecol Laparosc* 1996;4:33–8

20. Wortman M, Daggett A. Reoperative hysteroscopic surgery in the management of patients who fail endometrial ablation and resection. *J Am Assoc Gynecol Laparosc* 2001;8:272–7

21. Taskin O, Onoglu A, Inal M, *et al.* Long-term histopathologic and morphologic changes after thermal endometrial ablation. *J Am Assoc Gynecol Laparosc* 2002;9:186–90

22. Derman SG, Rehnstrom J, Neuwirth RS. The long-term effectiveness of hysteroscopic treatment of menorrhagia and leiomyomas. *Obstet Gynecol* 1991;77:591–4

23. Wamsteker K, Emanuel MH, de Kruif JH. Transcervical hysteroscopic resection of submucous fibroids for abnormal uterine bleeding: results regarding the degree of intramural extension. *Obstet Gynecol* 1993;82:736–40

24. Loffer FD. Removal of large symptomatic intrauterine growths by the hysteroscopic resectoscope. *Obstet Gynecol* 1990;76:836-40

25. Emanuel MH, Wamsteker K, Hart AA, *et al.* Long-term results of hysteroscopic myomectomy for abnormal uterine bleeding. *Obstet Gynecol* 1999;93:743–8

26. Friedman AJ, Barbieri RL. Leuprolide acetate: applications in gynecology. *Curr Probl Obstet Gynecol Fertil* 1988;11:205–36

27. Friedman AJ, Juneau-Norcross M, Rein MS. Adverse effects of leuprolide acetate depot treatment. *Fertil Steril* 1993;59:448–50

28. Batzer FR. Vaginosonographic evaluation of the nonpregnant uterus. *Am J Gynecol Health* 1992; 6:28–31

29. Gimpelson RJ. Hysteroscopic Nd:YAG laser ablation of the endometrium. *J Reprod Med* 1988;33:872–6

30. Dicker D, Ashkanazi J, Feldberg D, *et al.* The value of repeat hysteroscopic evaluation in patients with failed *in vitro* fertilization transfer cycles. *Fertil Steril* 1992; 58: 833–5

31. Fedorkow D, Pattinson HA, Taylor PJ. Is diagnostic hysteroscopy adhesiogenic? *Int J Fertil* 1991;36:21–2

20

Complications of operative hysteroscopy

E. J. Bieber and P. G. Brooks

Operative hysteroscopy generally comprises procedures that are relatively simple and safe, resulting in few complications. In a survey of its members conducted by the American Association of Gynecologic Laparoscopists, the overall complication rate for almost 14 000 hysteroscopic procedures performed by the respondents in 1988 was reported as 2%, with major complications (perforation, hemorrhage, fluid overload, bowel or urinary tract injury) occurring in less than 1% of procedures[1].

The complications seen during, or subsequent to, operative hysteroscopy are described in this chapter. They include trauma, hemorrhage, distention media-related complications, infections, risk of subsequent pregnancy, thermal injury, cervical stenosis and hematometria, and the conceptual risk of endometrial cancer. An attempt has also been made to elucidate the reasons for the complications and outline steps to avoid them, if possible, and to manage them when they occur.

TRAUMATIC COMPLICATIONS

Inserting rigid instruments through the soft cervical canal and into a hollow organ like the uterus are maneuvers that will occasionally result in traumatic lacerations or bleeding. This is especially a problem if the cervix has to be dilated enough to pass wider-caliber operating instruments. Careful placement of tenacula and gentle dilatation of the cervix minimize these risks. The use of laminaria tents is favored by

some hysteroscopists but is avoided by others because of the possibility that overdilation will occur, resulting in loss of distention medium and intrauterine pressure, in turn producing poor visualization. In addition, anecdotal cases of endometritis or purulent cervicitis have been reported subsequent to the use of laminaria, but this has not been supported scientifically.

While too low an intrauterine pressure can result in poor visualization, excessive pressures are also harmful. They will increase the risk of fluid overload due to intravascular intravasation; this is especially a problem if salt-poor distention media are used. It will also increase the risk of gas embolization, when a gaseous distention medium is used. Fortunately, this is very unlikely at flow rates routinely used for CO_2 hysteroscopy. Great care must be taken if instillation of distending media (such as high molecular weight dextran) is performed manually with syringes. The proper technique should be to infuse the medium slowly and hold the pressure steady without injecting more fluid, as long as visualization is adequate. This is where working off a video monitor with a video camera attached to the hysteroscope is especially advantageous, since both the operator and the assistant who is infusing the medium can see the view and the procedure simultaneously.

Rupture of the oviducts from excessive gas pressures with or without bilateral hydrosalpinx has been reported anecdotally. This usually results from use of the wrong equipment or excessive insufflation pressures. It is imperative that only insufflators designed exclusively for hysteroscopy be used for uterine distention. Hysteroscopic insufflators are designed to produce flow rates of only 100–200 ml/min (although flow rates of 40–60 ml/min are almost always sufficient). Most laparoscopic insufflators, even older models, deliver between 1000 and 3000 ml/min. A case was reported where, due to a lack of available equipment, a CO_2 tank was attached directly to a hysteroscope without any insufflator with governors, etc. This resulted not only in the rupture of normal oviducts but also the rupture of the patient's diaphragm, resulting in massive pneumothorax, cardiac arrest and death[2].

In addition to restricting flow rates, the hysteroscopist should also use equipment that can be set to deliver pressures under 100 mmHg. The basic physiology is that, once the intrauterine surgery opens sinuses and venous channels, gas or fluid will flow into the vascular tree when the intrauterine pressure exceeds the intravascular pressure in the vessel open to the endometrial cavity.

Perforation of the uterus is a well-documented risk of operative hysteroscopy, with most hysteroscopists encountering it at one time or another. Lomano and colleagues reported one perforation of the uterus in 61 laser endometrial ablation procedures, while Goldrath and Fuller reported it once in his first 196 laser ablations[3,4]. We reported one perforation in 216 uterine resectoscopic operations involving both resections of intrauterine growths and ablations[5], and, at the time of writing, we have still had only one in almost 500 resectoscopic procedures.

Most perforations result in little or no serious bleeding or other problems, but often require a diagnostic laparoscopy to ensure that there is no damage to adherent or adjacent structures and that there is no unsuspected laceration of large blood vessels. As such, when operative hysteroscopy is scheduled, all patients should have given prior consent for laparoscopy. More about the use of concomitant laparoscopy to avoid or manage complications of hysteroscopy will be discussed at the end of this chapter.

HEMORRHAGIC COMPLICATIONS

Intraoperative bleeding other than from lacerations due to forceful dilation or tenaculum tears, as noted above, occurs infrequently and is usually the result of inadvertent or unintentional trauma to the uterine wall. It can occur from lacerations or false passages created during either the dilatation of the cervix or the insertion of the hysteroscope and sheath through the endocervical canal.

In addition, excessive bleeding can occur after operative procedures, such as the incision of uterine septae or synechiae, especially when deep penetration into healthy myometrium occurs. This can occur whether using mechanical methods (scissors), or electrical or laser energy, although using either of the latter two is usually associated with coagulation of the smaller vessels.

Intraoperative bleeding sufficient to require intrauterine tamponade with a Foley catheter or a balloon catheter specially designed for intrauterine use by Neuwirth, was reported in nine out of 40 (22.5%) resectoscopic procedures by DeCherney and colleagues[6], one out of every three resectoscopic cases by Neuwirth (personal communication), and four of the first 216 cases in one series (1.9%)[5–7].

The technique that we use for intrauterine tamponade is to place the balloon into the uterine cavity in the operating room (often performing a paracervical block with a longer-acting anesthetic drug to minimize the cramping postoperatively) and then fill the balloon with approximately 10–15 ml of liquid (saline, water, etc.) until moderate resistance is felt. After about an hour, half of the liquid is removed. If no bleeding occurs over the next hour, the rest of the liquid is removed, but the catheter is left in the uterine cavity. If no bleeding is encountered over the next hour, the catheter is removed and the patient is usually discharged. If active bleeding recurs at any time prior to removal of the catheter, it is reinflated and left in place for a longer period, often overnight. An unusual complication of this technique was reported by Galka and Goldfarb who noted disseminated intravascular coagulation in a patient who had an intrauterine balloon placed to tamponade bleeding[8].

To minimize bleeding during operative procedures, it is possible to inject about 4–6 units of Pitressin®, diluted 10 units/20 ml of saline, directly into the cervical stroma prior to each procedure. Care must be taken to avoid intravascular injection, which can cause significant cardiovascular changes. The small amount of Pitressin decreases the likelihood of systemic reactions. In a double-blind, randomized, prospective study, Corson and colleagues showed a statistically significant reduction in blood loss and amount of intravasation of distending media (sorbitol or glycine) when Pitressin was used as contrasted with placebo[7]. In another randomized, double-blind study, Phillips and co-workers found that intracervical injection of dilute vasopressin (0.05 U/ml) into the cervical stroma, prior to dilatation or operative hysteroscopy reduced blood loss, operative time and fluid intravasation, 448 ml versus 819 ml[9].

Townsend has reported on the use of a vasopressin-soaked pack in 17 women with refractory bleeding after submucous myoma resection[10]. A 1-inch gauge pack was soaked in a solution of 20 units Pitressin and 30 ml saline solution. The pack was then placed in the uterine cavity by forceps and left for no more than 1 h. Resolution of bleeding without significant systemic side-effects was noted in all patients.

Stotz and co-workers describe a patient who underwent hysteroscopic myomectomy who became hypotensive and bradycardic with signs of dilutional hyponatremia (sodium, 125 mg) and anemia[11]. They believed this to be consistent with volume overload and treated the patient appropriately for this clinical scenario. When the patient's anemia worsened and abdominal pain increased, laparotomy revealed a tear in the right internal iliac vein and 3000 ml of blood in the abdomen with two necrotic areas in the posterior uterine wall. Unfortunately, her vascular injury was confused with a presumption of volume uptake causing the dilutional anemia and hyponatremia.

Preoperative medical therapy has been used to decrease the thickness and vascularity of the endometrium or to shrink myomata. Such therapy reduces the risk of bleeding and makes the procedure easier to perform (see Chapter 5). Of all the drugs used for this purpose, we prefer using a gonadotropin releasing hormone (GnRH) analog such as leuprolide acetate depot, for a minimum of 4 weeks prior to the procedure[12,13], although Danocrine and progestins have been used by others[14]. Our experience with the latter two drugs is that the endometrium is often fluffier, more deciduous and more vascular as confirmed histologically. On microscopic examination, after the use of GnRH analogs for at least 3–4 weeks, the endometrium is thinner, more compact, markedly devoid of intra- and extracellular fluid, and contains fewer and more inactive glands, and smaller and fewer blood vessels.

UTERINE RUPTURE

Uterine rupture after prior Cesarean section is a recognized complication, with or without labor. Recently, several cases of uterine rupture have been reported following lysis of a uterine septum, uterine perforation at dilatation and curettage (D&C) and lysis of adhesions. Generally, it has been believed that patients who previously underwent hysteroscopic septoplasty may experience labor in a routine fashion and, that since their active segment was not surgically affected, they would be at a low risk for uterine rupture. The published case reports of uterine rupture include hysteroscopic septolysis performed with scissors, electrosurgery and laser energy[15–17]. One of the cases occurred during labor induction with prostagladins[18]. Of interest, in one report, follow-up hysterosalpingography following metroplasty revealed a 'small residual septum' suggesting an incomplete resection[15]. Unfortunately, in this case, a cornua to cornua rupture during early labor allowed complete exteriorization of the fetus and placenta. In another case, a patient who probably had an unsuspected perforation during D&C for late first-trimester fetal demise was found to have a 5-cm fundal defect[19]. Gurgan and colleagues reported on a patient who had a fundal perforation during hysteroscopic lysis of adhesions who conceived with *in vitro* fertilization and later presented at 36 weeks pregnant with uterine rupture[20]. Because of the small number of case reports, it is believed that the risk to a given patient is probably small. It will take a much larger series and follow-up to ascertain the actual increase in relative risk (if any). Until this information exists, it may be prudent to view cases of prior septoplasty, lysis of significant intrauterine adhesions or patients with history of uterine perforation in a watchful fashion during pregnancy. In patients presenting with acute onset of pain or with fetal distress during labor, the clinician may consider the possibility of uterine rupture.

DISTENTION MEDIUM HAZARDS

Complications specifically related to distention media were reported to have occurred in less than 4% of cases in a retrospective survey[1].

Carbon dioxide

Embolism is the most feared complication from the use of CO_2 as a distention medium. Fortunately, when the principles of low flow and low pressure, i.e. using a hysteroflator only, are followed, the risks are very low.

Two studies, one with dogs[21] and one with sheep[22], both showed that, even with infusion of the gas directly into the femoral veins of these animals, CO_2 produces very few systemic cardiovascular problems unless the flow rates were higher than those recommended for hysteroscopy and were maintained for longer periods of time. Thus, when CO_2 is the chosen distending medium, the margin of safety is quite wide. Several reports of fatal or near fatal CO_2 embolization during diagnostic and operative hysteroscopy have appeared in the literature[23-26]. Some of these complications resulted from the inappropriate use of CO_2-cooled laser fibers with sapphire tips for intrauterine operative procedures. The problem occurred because the flow rates of CO_2 for cooling laser tips are equivalent to those of a laparoflator, or greater than 1 l/min, thus over ten times greater than

the flow rates recommended for hysteroscopy. As a result of these reports, the Food and Drug Administration (FDA) has issued a warning never to use gas-cooled laser fibers or tips for intrauterine surgery[27].

More recently it has become apparent that prior to beginning CO_2 hysteroscopy the connection tubing should be purged of air with CO_2[28]. In a study from Germany, Brandner and colleagues identified a number of patients with clinically undetectable CO_2 emboli during CO_2 hysteroscopy[29]. They found that by purging the connector tubing of room air with CO_2 prior to onset of the procedures they had no further clinical or subclinical emboli.

High molecular weight dextran (Hyskon®)

A major complication from the use of dextran 70, although very rare, is that of anaphylactic shock. No data exist regarding the frequency of this problem, and reports are sporadic and anecdotal. It is believed to be an immunological reaction and can be prevented, according to Renck[30], by the intravenous injection of a small amount of 15% dextran 2 min prior to the use of dextran 70. However, very few hysteroscopists using dextran 70 consider the risk serious enough to warrant this method of prophylaxis routinely. Multiple reports have continued to be published in the obstetric, anesthesia and pulmonary literature discussing a 'dextran syndrome' including acute hypotension, non-cardiogenic pulmonary edema, anemia and coagulopathy[31-34]. Anaphylactic shock remains one of the most catastrophic risks and is probably to attributable to the antigenicity of Hyskon (CooperSurgical, Trumbull, CT, USA)[35].

Although still uncommon, a more frequent problem resulting from the use of dextran 70 as a distention medium may occur when a substantial volume is retained in the patient, due to intravascular intravasation via open vessels or sinuses.

The potential for dextran 70 to draw in large volumes of water osmotically may result in ascites when the fluid is in the peritoneal cavity or fluid overload when excessive Hyskon enters the vascular tree. When this occurs, careful use of diuretics and electrolyte management may be required. Coagulation abnormalities may also be associated with Hyskon use (see Chapter 6). Consistent with these reports, Romero and associates published, in the anesthesia literature, on pulmonary hemorrhage in a patient, secondary to Hyskon use[33]. Prevention is most important and is accomplished by limiting the amount of dextran used during a procedure and carefully monitoring the volume retained in the patient, i.e. assessing the amount used less the amount retrieved at the end of the procedure. One note of medicolegal importance is that the package insert provided by the manufacturer of dextran 70 states that no more than 500 ml of this liquid should ever be used during operative hysteroscopy. It would be difficult to defend if more liquid was used and the patient developed a serious problem, even if it can be shown that much of the liquid ran out onto the floor or drapes.

Low-viscosity liquid complications

Low-viscosity fluids, such as sorbitol, glycine, mannitol, dextrose in water, etc. which are used primarily with intrauterine electrosurgical (resectoscopic) procedures, may result in significant hyponatremia and fluid overload when retained in the patient because they are sodium-free. These issues are extensively discussed in Chapter 6. In our experience, retention of these fluids mainly occurs from intravasation resulting from opening into large venous sinuses during the operative procedure or from lacerations or false passages produced during a difficult dilatation of the cervix. It is mandatory to monitor intake and output of these liquids during and after each procedure, with the immediate assessment of serum electrolytes if a discrepancy of 1000 ml or more occurs in the healthy patient, or 750 ml in the older patient and/or in those with a history of cardiovascular compromise (a flow sheet for fluid monitoring is found in Chapter 19).

If hyponatremia (serum sodium < 125 mg) or fluid overload occurs, it is strongly recommended that the surgeon *stop the procedure immediately* and consider completing it in the near future. The use of diuretics and restriction of intravenous fluids may be necessary. To re-emphasize prevention of this very serious problem, it is essential to monitor the inflow and outflow volumes of these liquids when they are used for distention during operative hysteroscopy.

In addition to the hyponatremia that results from excessive intravasation of low-viscosity liquids, there are scattered reports of central nervous system toxicity from glycine, mainly in the urological[36] and orthopedic[37] literature. One study found oxygen desaturation and increases in blood CO_2 in six of 46 patients undergoing operative hysteroscopy with glycine as the distention medium[38]. Four of the six had concomitant coagulopathy but only two had hyponatremia. A syndrome including encephalopathy and transient blindness has been reported after transurethral prostatectomy and after electrosurgical arthroscopic procedures associated with the use of glycine as an irrigation medium and wherein very high levels of serum glycine and its metabolic byproduct, ammonia, are detected. No such syndrome has been reported after the use of glycine for gynecologic resectoscopic procedures, but again, careful monitoring of inflow and outflow volumes is essential to prevent the retention of too much distention medium fluid in the patient's vascular tree.

GAS AND AIR EMBOLI

In recent years, significant attention has been given to the issues of air and gas embolism. While largely unrecognized until the mid 1990s as a problem in hysteroscopic surgery, multiple case reports of patient morbidity have now been published. Several different mechanisms exist whereby air or gas embolism may occur during surgical procedures. The process of entry into the endometrial cavity may be difficult with creation of false passages, endomyometrial trauma or laceration, perforation, etc. Wide cervical dilatation in and of itself presents an opportunity for room air to enter these areas, and the placement of patients into the Trendelenburg position, with the heart lower then the uterus, sets up a gradient to promote air emboli. Other factors such as incomplete purging of tubing were discussed previously. The use of electrocautery during operative hysteroscopy may also be associated with gas production and gas emboli[39]. Bloomstone and co-workers evaluated patients undergoing operative hysteroscopy with a unipolar ball or loop electrode[40]. They performed continuous echo evaluation of heart, liver and the inferior vena cava during hysteroscopic procedures. Nine of 11 patients evaluated demonstrated identifiable gas bubble entrapment in the heart. The pictorial demonstration of microbubbles filling hepatic veins from the inferior vena cava is seen in Figure 1.

Air absorbtion into the venous vascular tree is much more problematic than CO_2. Room air is composed largely of nitrogen which is much less soluble in blood than CO_2. Once air has entered the circulation and enters the right heart there is decreased blood outflow, with increased pulmonary pressure and decreased cardiac output. This results in hypotension, hypoxia, tachypnea and ultimately cardiac arrest if untreated. Other clinical findings include a sudden fall in end-tidal CO_2, dysrythmias or a precordial millwheel murmur.

Brooks previously reported on seven patients with air embolism during hysteroscopy who had some or all of these findings[41]. Unfortunately, five of the seven patients died of the complication.

It is critical in such cases to quickly recognize the problem, and for the anesthetist and the surgeon to work closely and expediently. Immediately on diagnosis, the surgical procedure should be stopped, any open channels should be occluded (i.e. cervix and vagina), and the patient placed in the left lateral decubitis position with slight Trendelenburg (Durant maneuver). Depending on the degree of physiological changes, the patient may require 100% oxygenation, use of pressors, increasing vascular volume and pulmonary artery catheter placement[42]. Another alternative is jugular vein catheterization to attempt aspiration of the air. The likely key to patient outcome is quickly recognizing the problem and reacting before

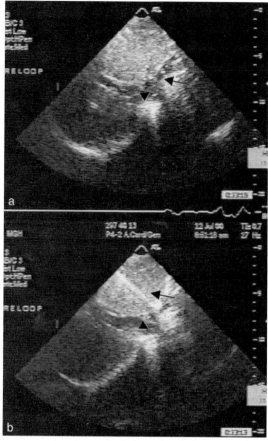

Figure 1 Ultrasound scans of the liver bed before and during hysteroscopic resection. (a) The hepatic veins (arrow) before hysteroscopic resection are not filled with microbubbles. Note scant white contrast. (b) During hysteroscopic resection, the hepatic veins fill retrograde from the inferior vena cava (arrowhead) with microbubbles and appear as white contrast. Reproduced from reference 40 with permission

there is significant cardiopulmonary compromise. Keys to prevention of this potentially catastrophic complication include:

(1) Avoid Trendelenburg position;

(2) Preform cervical dilatation and entry with care;

(3) Purge all lines prior to hysteroscopy;

(4) Do not leave a dilated cervix open to the air;

(5) Recognize the physiological changes associated with embolism, some of which may be confused with fluid overload.

A recent question has been raised regarding differences between production of gases with unipolar versus bipolar vaporizing electrodes. In an interesting *in vitro* model, Munro and colleagues evaluated rates of gas production at various generator settings[43]. Results demonstrated that the power settings impacted gas production more than use of bipolar versus unipolar. In a prior study, Munro and co-workers had evaluated the composition of gas produced with bipolar or unipolar electrodes[44]. Results demonstrated that there was little difference between monopolar or bipolar vaporizing electrodes with hydrogen, carbon monoxide and carbon dioxide, the main gaseous byproducts, all of which are highly soluble in serum.

INFECTION

Endometritis is an occasional complication following hysteroscopy, occurring in one out of 4000 cases performed by Salat-Baroux and colleagues[45] and in two of 216 patients in another series[5]. Bracco and colleagues noted development of pelvic inflammatory disease (PID) in two of 253 hysteroscopic cases using CO_2 as the distention medium[46]. Both of these patients were noted to have untreated *Chlamydia trachomatis* on cervical culture. In a large case series spanning 10 years, Agostini and associates found only 18 cases of endometritis in 2116 patients undergoing operative hysteroscopic procedures (0.85%)[47]. They did note patients undergoing intrauterine lysis of adhesions had a greater risk than other operative procedures.

When infection occurs, it is usually following longer operative procedures, especially with repeated insertion and removal of the hysteroscope through the cervical canal. Endometritis, in our experience, is usually treated with oral antibiotics and rarely requires hospitalization. To prevent it from occurring, the use of prophylactic antibiotics is recommended when long procedures are contemplated, as well as for all patients being treated for infertility.

McCausland and co-workers[48] reported that, out of 200 cases of operative hysteroscopy where no prophylactic antibiotics were used, three of the patients with a history of PID developed tubo-ovarian abscesses, whereas no cases were seen in 500 patients treated prophylactically prior to and immediately after the procedure. In addition, it may be appropriate to obtain cervical cultures prior to hysteroscopy when the patient's past history (or additional high-risk factors) suggests a possible risk for infection.

Finally, while extremely uncommon, a flareup of PID has been reported (even after diagnostic hysteroscopy), occurring in one of a series of 34 such diagnostic procedures reported by Cohen and Dmowski[49].

PREGNANCY FOLLOWING ABLATION

Pregnancies have been reported following endometrial ablation by laser, resection, rollerball and thermal balloon[50–54]. Because of known obstetric complications in patients with Asherman's syndrome, there has been appropriate concern regarding obstetric outcome. Little information exists in the literature to understand what level of risk for pregnancy is present for the unsterilized patient postablation with an unsterilized partner. Hill and Maher reported on an uneventful pregnancy following endometrial coagulation and resection[50]. Placental pathology revealed a single placental infarct with other non-specific findings.

Whitelaw and colleagues polled members of the British Society for Gynaecological Endoscopy, and ten pregnancies were reported[51]. Most of these patients chose elective termination, but two patients elected to carry to term. One patient who had undergone Nd:YAG laser ablation had an uncomplicated pregnancy. The second patient, who was 44 years old, had also undergone laser ablation. She was delivered at 39 weeks' gestation for breech, intrauterine growth restriction (IUGR) and pregnancy-induced hypertension. The infant was subsequently diagnosed with single-suture craniosynostosis (premature fusion of the cranial vault sutures). In an addendum to Whitelaw's paper, 16 additional pregnancies in a series of 985 ablations were reported[51]. Again, most patients elected for termination. Three patients of the 16 chose to continue their pregnancies. One patient was delivered by Cesarean section at 31 weeks for severe IUGR. Placenta increta was noted, for which the patient underwent three subsequent dilations and curettages. In the second patient, placenta accreta necessitated hysterectomy. In the third patient, Cesarean section was performed at 29 weeks for severe IUGR and oligohydramnios. The placenta had to be shaved off. In contrast, Pinette and colleagues recently described a patient who had a prior laser endometrial ablation who subsequently desired pregnancy[52]. Work-up and evaluation interestingly demonstrated a normal intrauterine architecture and the patient subsequently conceived a viable pregnancy.

All patients should be counselled that endometrial ablation is not a sterilization procedure. The risk of pregnancy following endometrial ablation has been estimated at 0.7%[53]. It is unclear if there are differences in risk between the different ablation methods.

While the exact risk of obstetric complications in patients who conceive after ablative procedures is unknown, patients should be counselled that, should they choose not to be sterilized or use a reliable form of contraception, their risk is increased. Frank discussion and documentation is important.

ELECTRICAL AND LASER INJURIES

Injury resulting from the use of electrical energy and its thermal effects is rarely a problem but, when it occurs, can be life-threatening. Electrical shocks to the patient or to the surgeon from the body of the resectoscope occurred with the early prototypes of the resectoscope, but improvements in design have corrected the problem.

In patients desiring future fertility, thermal injury to the walls of the uterus with resultant scarring is a potential problem that may result from electrical as well as laser energy. Although theoretical, this problem has not been reported and no sequelae appear to occur in the few studies reporting on the efficacy of using laser or electrical (resectoscopic) energy to incise septae. When possible, intrauterine surgery in the patient with intrauterine adhesions should be performed with hysteroscopic scissors to minimize the theoretical risk of excessive scarring inside the uterus due to thermal damage occurring from electrical or laser energy.

Laser or electrical injury to the adjacent bowel is almost always due to perforation of the uterus during operative procedures requiring energy. However, a study evaluating efficacy of using a hysteroscopically inserted coagulation electrode into the tubal cornu for the purpose of inducing tubal sterilization was abruptly stopped because of the significant risk of bowel injury, adjacent or adherent to this very thin part of the uterine wall, which resulted in one death and several other cases of bowel damage[55]. Caution must be taken not to apply strong electrical or laser energy to these areas for long periods of time. There have been reports of bowel thermal injury occurring during Nd:YAG laser endometrial ablation. Indman and Brown have reported a lack of significant increase in temperature occurring on the serosal surface when a resectoscopic electrode is held against the endometrial surface, using standard power settings, even when held there for up to 5 seconds[56].

Kivneck and Kanter reported on full thickness myometrial necrosis with small bowel injury in a patient undergoing endometrial coagulation ablation[57]. The patient presented on the second postoperative day, and at laparotomy was noted to have an ileal serosal burn and perforation. Interestingly, no area of uterine perforation could be documented on pathological examination of the hysterectomy specimen.

Sullivan and colleagues reported a case of uterine perforation during resectoscopic resection of a uterine myoma[58]. Laparoscopy demonstrated a midline uterine perforation but failed to identify a transmural sigmoid injury secondary to inadequate visualization. However, at laparotomy a sigmoid burn was noted and primary repair of the non-prepped sigmoid were performed with no apparent sequelae.

In a recent report, Vilos and colleagues detailed 13 cases of genital tract burns during hysteroscopic endometrial ablation[59]. Of interest, the posterolateral walls of the vagina were involved with thermal injury in all cases. In four of the 13 cases the surgeon reported equipment difficulties, eight out of 13 used reusable electrodes and in two cases there was a sense of decreased effect based on visualization. Several theories were proposed to explain the findings including: placement of the weighted speculum into the vagina when still too warm from autoclaving, patient reaction to scrub/prep solution, patient reaction to inadequate cidex removal or electrical injury. Based on the authors' *in vitro* experiments as well as cumulative clinical accumen, speculum placement and scrub or cidex solution were felt to be unlikely sources of the injury and that the most likely cause of the injuries was from 'capacitive coupled currents and/or stray currents arising from defective insulation of electrodes to the telescope and thus to the entire resectoscope'[59]. We have long concurred with Vilos and will routinely remove and destroy our electrodes prior to case completion to eliminate the possibility of reuse.

CERVICAL STENOSIS AND HEMATOMETRIA

Another undesirable result is the development of cervical stenosis and/or hematometria after endometrial ablation using any of the currently available methodologies for endometrial ablation. This problem can be avoided by being especially careful not to ablate tissue at or below the internal os. Interestingly, a recent case report documented cervical occlusion and hematometria in a patient who had a history of cervical incompetence and subsequently underwent thermal balloon endometrial ablation[60]. Leung and co-workers evaluated 22 patients after thermal ablation with second-look hysteroscopy[61]. Two of the twenty-two had complete obliteration of the cavity and six

had focal fundal adhesions. They noted an association between amount of menstrual bleeding and visual postablation appearance.

While hematometria or cervical stenosis has not occurred in all series, it has been noted in several studies of endometrial ablations in fewer than 5% of cases, particularly subsequent to the use of the Nd:YAG laser to destroy the endometrium.

Goldrath suggested that all patients should undergo office suction curettage following Nd:YAG laser ablation[62]. He noted 12 cases of postoperative hematometria during these procedures and recommended repeating curettage weekly to decrease the recurrence. It is unclear whether Nd:YAG laser ablation may have a higher incidence of hematometria than coagulation or thermal ablation.

Townsend and colleagues described a post-ablation tubal sterilization syndrome where they noted an association of pelvic pain and vaginal spotting in women who had undergone a previous tubal sterilization and more recent rollerball endometrial ablation[63]. Laparoscopy and hysteroscopy revealed dilated Fallopian tubes and scarified endometrial cavities but patent cornua that were thought to contain endometrial tissue. This may have been a subset of patients with cornual hematometria who are unable to pass endometrial tissue and secretions transtubally, secondary to the previous sterilization or, transcervically, secondary to adhesions.

Ultrasonographic evaluation in patients with symptoms of cyclical pain may help in evaluating the adnexa to rule out hydro- or hematosalpinx and in evaluating the uterine cavity for evidence of fluid collections consistent with hematometria. Goldrath suggested that hematometria are unlikely to develop remotely more than 3 months following surgery[62]. However, there is a report of a hematometria developing in a patient who was subsequently placed on estrogen replacement therapy[64].

ENDOMETRIAL CANCER

There is the concern that performing endometrial ablations may result in remaining viable endometrial glands that might later undergo malignant change and go undetected until very late. The fear of hiding a subsequent endometrial cancer by performing endometrial ablation is entirely theoretical and has no basis in fact. To begin with, the belief that the entire endometrial cavity is obliterated by scar tissue, much like what may happen in the development of Asherman's syndrome, is not true. We have performed office hysteroscopy for over 30 patients from 4 to 12 months following ablation and have noted a narrow tubular cavity with access to the vagina in every case (see Chapter 19). Goldrath reported the same using serial hysterosalpingography[65]. Furthermore, patients with recurrences of abnormal bleeding, even years after ablation, present with external bleeding not unlike patients who have not had ablations.

In addition, in the 20 or more years since the first reports of laser ablation, there have been few cases of endometrial carcinoma reported after an endometrial ablation. In one case, endometrial cancer was diagnosed in a patient with a persistent history of adenomatous hyperplasia for 8 years prior to the ablation[66]. It may be that endometrial ablation is less appropriate for patients with significant hyperplastic endometrial disease. One reason for the low frequency of later endometrial problems may be that the single layer of cuboidal epithelium we find covering the myometrium in postablation hysterectomy specimens is unresponsive to the endogenous stimuli that induce malignant change.

What is unknown is whether patients will present later in the disease course of endometrial cancer, since residual endometrium exists in a significant percent of patients. Most of the 35 000 new cases of endometrial cancer present as stage I lesions, many with abnormal bleeding. Cervical stenosis could potentially prevent vaginal bleeding and cause delayed diagnosis. This underscores the importance of a patent cervical canal following those procedures. In one case of an endometrial carcinoma presenting after endometrial ablation, abnormal bleeding through a patent canal allowed rapid diagnosis of the patient's potentially surgically curable early stage lesion[66].

It is for similar reasons that the use of a combination regimen of estrogen and progestin in postmenopausal patients who require hormone replacement therapy and have previously undergone endometrial ablation is recommended.

FAILURES AND POOR OUTCOMES

Obviously, the inability of the hysteroscopic surgery to correct the patient's presenting problem may be considered one of the most significant complications.

It is an undesirable outcome when abnormal bleeding is not controlled, the intrauterine synechiae recur or occur *de novo* following surgery, or if the procedure must be abandoned due to the development of complications, such as perforation of the uterus or fluid overload. Fortunately, these are very uncommon and, in many cases, may be avoided by care and experience.

Table 1   When to perform concomitant laparoscopy

WISE TO ALWAYS GET CONSENT FOR:
Lysis of adhesions
Always with dense adhesions or total obstruction
Rarely for isolated or focal adhesions

Septoplasty
Always (unless under ultrasound monitoring)

Ablation
Rarely necessary
Beginners (?)

Myomectomy
Rarely for pedunculated tumors
Maybe for intramural lesions

Tubal sterilization
When patient has not solved contraception
  question
Perform sterilization *AFTER* ablation or
  myomectomy is done

WITH PERFORATION
Always if perforation done with energy source
If perforation is lateral
If continued bleeding

THE ROLE OF LAPAROSCOPY IN REDUCING THE RISK OF RESECTOSCOPIC SURGERY

Since perforation of the uterus and injury of adjacent organs (bowel, bladder, blood vessels, etc.) are among the most serious complications of operative hysteroscopy, it is often very beneficial to perform concomitant laparoscopy. Although we do not schedule all patients to have laparoscopy at the time of all operative hysteroscopies, we obtain consent for it in all cases, in case it is needed (Table 1).

Laparoscopy is indicated in the following situations:

(1) *For lysis of intrauterine adhesions* Laparoscopy should be used when there are lateral dense adhesions or total uterine obstruction, to warn the hysteroscopic surgeon that he or she may be getting dangerously close to the serosal surface. For isolated or focal intrauterine adhesions, laparoscopy monitoring is rarely necessary.

(2) *For incision of uterine septae* Laparoscopy is helpful in protecting against incising too far and perforating the fundus.

(3) *For endometrial ablation* It is rarely necessary, except possibly for beginners. In our experience, after performing laparoscopy during the first 30 ablations, the lack of evidence of getting too deep into the myometrium or producing any thermal change on the serosa left the impression that concomitant laparoscopy was not cost- or risk-effective enough to perform routinely for this procedure.

(4) *For hysteroscopic myomectomy* Laparoscopy is rarely necessary for pedunculated tumors but, sometimes, may be useful for myomata with a significant intramural component. It is our recommendation that intracavitary sessile myomas be resected hysteroscopically only if more than 50% of the tumor protrudes into the endometrial cavity, and that the resection be carried down only to the level of the concavity of the uterine wall.

(5) *For tubal sterilization at the time of the hysteroscopic procedure* The tubal sterilization procedure should be performed at the conclusion of the hysteroscopy so that the intrauterine pressure necessary to achieve adequate uterine distention does not force occluded tubes open.

Laparoscopy is seldom necessary if the perforation of the uterus is in the midline and occurs with blunt instruments, such as uterine sounds or dilators. If the perforation is lateral into the parametrium or occurs with a laser fiber or an electrosurgical electrode, it is almost always necessary to evaluate for damage to adherent or adjacent organs (bowel, bladder, etc.). It is well understood that thermal injury to the bowel wall, for example, may result in a slow devitalization of the tissue and a long delay before breakdown ensues. However, it is almost always essential that the surgeon performs laparoscopy after such perforation to try to detect damage if at all possible.

LARGE POPULATION STUDIES

Recently, a number of large surveys, audits and studies have evaluated complications associated with hysteroscopic surgery. One such audit evaluated 978 cases of endometrial ablation performed at 13 hospitals in Scotland[67]. Sixty-five per cent of cases were endometrial resection, 32% laser endometrial ablation and 3% rollerball. There was a high overall complication rate of 12%: 5.2% of cases had fluid overload of 1–2 liters and in 1.0% of cases there was overload of 2 liters or more; 2.9% of patients required intrauterine catheters for excessive bleeding and 1% of patients had uterine perforations. In this audit where surgical operator experience was also tracked, the authors noted no association between complication and operator experience. They did find that laser ablation was associated with a greater risk of fluid overload.

Under the auspices of the German Society of Endoscopic Gynecology, 92 centers in Germany registered 21 676 operative hysteroscopic procedures[68]. Half of all cases were for resection of fibroids or polyps and almost three-quarters of the cases were performed by one-quarter of the participants. Operator experience was quite limited with the median surgical experience slightly less than 4 years. In this registry, the overall uterine perforation rate was only 0.12%; however, in five cases there was concomitant perforation of the bowel or bladder.

Another interesting study was performed in 82 hospitals in the Netherlands during the calendar year 1997 with a 100% response rate from the participating hospitals[69]. The overall complication rate was only 0.28% for the 13 600 hysteroscopic procedures, although only 2515 of the procedures were considered operative. Half of all complications were entry related. Although both diagnostic and operative complication rates were low, operative procedures had a seven-fold greater risk of complication versus diagnostic hysteroscopies (0.95% vs. 0.13%). Uterine perforation was the most frequently reported complication with half of these associated with difficult entry. The overall rates of complications were: adhesiolysis 4.48%, endometrial resection 0.81%, myomectomy 0.75% and polypectomy 0.38%. Complications occurred at a greater frequency with more experienced surgeons, suggesting a different case selection and mix.

Propst and colleagues evaluated 925 patients who underwent hysteroscopic surgery at Brigham and Women's Hospital in Boston during 1995 and 1996[70]. They reported a 2.7% complication rate with excessive distention media absorbtion (1 liter or more) the most frequently complication. Table 2 demonstrates the odds ratios for operative complications based on patient characteristics. Of note, patients using preoperative GnRH agonist therapy, as well as surgery performed by a reproductive endocrinologist, were both associated with increased odds ratio likely secondary to types of cases being performed. These data are consistent with the prior report. Table 3 lists the odds ratios by procedure type.

These studies are consistent in documenting the overall low incidence of complications with hysteroscopic surgery. While they vary on which procedures are associated with the greatest risk, operative procedures such as intrauterine lysis of adhesions, myomectomy or endometrial resection generally have elevated risk versus diagnostic procedures. It is interesting that unlike other surgical procedures, surgeons with the greatest experience may have greater complication rates, although this is most likely due to case selection and referral trends rather than operator experience.

Table 2 Odds of operative complications by selected patient characteristics. Reproduced from reference 70 with permission

Variable	Number of patients	Age-adjusted OR (95% CI)
Age 35–50 years*	510	0.6 (0.2,1.4)
Age > 50 years*	308	0.2 (0.1, 0.8)
Premenopausal[†]	606	2.8 (0.6, 12.9)
Preoperative GnRHa therapy	42	6.6 (2.5, 17.6)
Reproductive endocrinologist[‡]	253	2.9 (1.2, 6.8)
General gynecologist[‡]	632	0.4 (0.2, 1.0)
1 or 2 live births**	254	1.3 (0.5, 3.2)
> 2 live births**	173	1.2 (0.4, 4.0)
Weight > 200 lbs[††]	81	0.4 (0.1, 3.2)
History of Cesarean delivery	101	0.3 (0.0, 2.4)
Previous myomectomy	43	0.8 (0.1, 5.9)
Cervical stenosis	55	1.5 (0.4, 6.8)

OR, odds ratio; CI, confidence interval; GnRHa, gonadotropin releasing hormone agonist
*Relative to those ≤ 34 years, not age-adjusted; [†]relative to postmenopausal women; [‡]relative to all surgeons; **relative to nulliparity (207 of 925 patients did not have parity information); [††]relative to women ≤ 200 pounds

Table 3 Odds of complications by type of procedure. Adapted from reference 70 with permission

Procedure	Number of patients*	Complications†		
		n	%	OR (95% CI)
Myomectomy	128	13	10.2	7.4 (3.3, 16.6)
Septum resection	21	2	9.5	4.0 (0.9, 19.6)
Lysis of adhesions	20	1	5.0	1.9 (0.2, 15.0)
Hysteroscopy and/or curettage	410	7	1.7	0.5 (0.2, 1.1)
Endometrial ablation	78	1	1.3	0.4 (0.1, 3.3)
Polypectomy	270	1	0.4	0.1 (0.0, 0.7)

OR, odds ratio; CI, confidence interval
*Total number of procedures adds up to 927 because two of 925 patients had more than one primary procedure; †complications odds ratio relative to all 925 patients

CLINICAL PEARLS

(1) Complications of operative hysteroscopy are relatively infrequent and can often be prevented if the surgeon is experienced and observes due caution.

(2) Once you suspect that the patient is in even a little trouble, STOP THE PROCEDURE AND COME BACK ANOTHER TIME!

(3) Patients get into severe trouble faster than it takes to get into a little trouble!

(4) Understanding the risks inherent in the use of the instruments and media selected will minimize the chances of complication and enhance the chances of a good surgical result.

(5) The performance of concomitant laparoscopy in selected cases can help to avoid some of the more severe complications that can occur during operative hysteroscopy.

References

1. Survey of American Association of Gynecologic Laparoscopists. Office hysteroscopy, national statistics. 1988 AAGL Membership Survey. *J Reprod Med* 1990;35:590–1
2. Obstetrician connected in sterilization death is placed on probation. *Obstet Gynecol News* 1974;9:4
3. Lomano JM, Feste JR, Loffer FD, *et al.* Ablation of the endometrium with the Nd:YAG laser: a multicenter study. *Colposc Laser Surg* 1986;2:203–7
4. Goldrath MH, Fuller TA. Intrauterine laser surgery. In Keye WR, ed. *Laser Surgery in Gynecology and Obstetrics*. Boston: GK Hall Medical, 1985:93–110
5. Serden SP, Brooks PG. Treatment of abnormal uterine bleeding with the gynecologic resectoscope. *J Reprod Med* 1991;36:697–9
6. DeCherney AH, Diamond, Lavy G, *et al.* Endometrial ablation for intractable uterine bleeding: hysteroscopic resection. *Obstet Gynecol* 1987;70:668–70
7. Corson SL, Brooks, PG, Serden SP, *et al.* The effects of vasopressin administration during hysteroscopic surgery. *J Reprod Med* 1994;39:419–23
8. Galka E, Goldfarb HA. Disseminated intravascular coagulation as a complication of intrauterine balloon tamponade for posthystero-

scopic acute uterine bleeding. *J Am Assoc Gynecol Laparosc* 2000;7:573–6

9. Phillips DR, Nathanson HG, Milim SJ, *et al.* The effect of dilute vasopressin solution on blood loss during operative hysteroscopy: a randomized controlled trial. *Obstet Gynecol* 1996;88:761–6

10. Townsend DE. Vasopressin pack for treatment of bleeding after myoma resection. *Am J Obstet Gynecol* 1991;165:1405

11. Stotz M, Lampart A, Kochli OR, *et al.* Intra-abdominal bleeding masked by hemodilution after hysteroscopy. *Anesthesiology* 2000;93:569–70

12. Brooks PG, Serden SP, Davos I. Hormonal inhibition of the endometrium for resectoscopic endometrial ablation. *Am J Obstet Gynecol* 1991; 164:1601–8

13. Brooks PG, Serden SP. Preparation of the endometrium for ablation with a single dose of leuprolide acetate depot. *J Reprod Med* 1991; 36:477–8

14. Siegler AM, Valle RF, Lindemann HJ, *et al.* Endometrial ablation. In *Therapeutic Hysteroscopy, Indications, and Techniques.* St. Louis: CV Mosby, 1990:149–63

15. Angell NF, Tan Domingo J, Siddiqi N. Uterine rupture at term after complicated hysteroscopic metroplasty. *Obstet Gynecol* 2002;100:1098–9

16. Kerimis P, Zolti M, Sinwany G, *et al.* Uterine rupture after hysteroscopic resection of uterine septum. *Fertil Steril* 2002;77:618–20

17. Lobaugh ML, Bammel BM, Duke D, *et al.* Uterine rupture during pregnancy in a patient with a history of hysteroscopic metroplasty. *Obstet Gynecol* 1994;83:838–40

18. Gabriele A, Zanetta G, Pasta F, *et al.* Uterine rupture after hysteroscopic metroplasty and labor induction. A case report. *J Reprod Med* 19999;44:642–4

19. Reed WC. Large uterine defect found at cesarean section. A case report. *J Reprod Med* 2003;48:60–2

20. Gurgan T, Yarali H, Urman B, *et al.* Uterine rupture following hysteroscopic lysis of synechiae due to tuberculosis and uterine perforation. *Hum Reprod* 1996;11:291–3

21. Lindemann HJ, Mohr J, Gallinat A. Der einfluss von CO_2-Gas wahrend der hysteroskopie. *Geburtshilfe Frauendheilkd* 1976;36:153–63

22. Corson SL, Hoffman JJ. Cardiopulmonary effects of direct venous carbon dioxide insufflation. *J Reprod Med* 1988;33:440–4

23. Perry PM, Baughman VL. A complication of hysteroscopy: air embolism. *Anesthesiology* 1990; 73:546–8

24. Challener RC, Kaufman B. Fatal venous air embolism following sequential unsheathed (bare) and sheathed quartz fiber Nd:YAG laser endometrial ablation. *Anesthesiology* 1990;73: 51–2

25. Nishiyama T, Hanaoka K. Gas embolism during hysteroscopy. *Can J Anaesth* 1999;46:379–81

26. Sherlock S, Shearer WA, Buist M, *et al.* Carbon dioxide embolism following diagnostic hysteroscopy. *Anaesth Intensive Care* 1998;26: 674–6

27. Gas/air embolism associated with intrauterine laser surgery. FDA Bulletin. Washington, DC: Food and Drug Administration, May 1990:6–7

28. Anonymous. Air embolism and CO_2 insufflators: the need for pre-use purging of tubing. *Health Devices* 1996;25:214–15

29. Brandner P, Neis KJ, Ehmer C. The etiology, frequency, and prevention of gas embolism during CO_2 hysteroscopy. *J Am Assoc Gynecol Laparosc* 1999;6:421–8

30. Renck H. Prevention of dextran-induced anaphylactic reactions. *Acta Chir Scand* 1983; 149:335

31. Ellingson TL, Aboulafia DM. Dextran syndrome. Acute hypotension, noncardiogenic pulmonary edema, anemia, and coagulopathy following hysteroscopic surgery using 32% dextran 70. *Chest* 1997;111:513–18

32. Huhn AM. Anaphylactic reactions to high molecular weight dextran during hysteroscopic surgery. *CRNA* 1995;6:167–71

33. Romero RM, Kreitzer JM, Gabrielson GV. Hyskon induced pulmonary hemorrhage. *J Clin Anesth* 1995;7:323–5

34. Schinco MA, Hughes D, Santora TA. Complications of 32% dextran-70 in 10% dextrose. A case report. *J Reprod Med* 1996;41:455–8

35. Perlitz Y, Oettinger M, Karam K, *et al.* Anaphylactic shock during hysteroscopy using Hyskon solution: case report and review of adverse reactions and their treatment. *Gynecol Obstet Invest* 1996;41:67–9

36. Hoekstra PT, Kahnoski R, McCamish MA, *et al.* Transurethral prostatic resection syndrome – a new perspective: encephalopathy with associated hyperammonemia. *J Urol* 1983;130:704–7

37. Burkart SS, Barnett CR, Snyder SJ. Transient postoperative blindness as a possible effect of glycine toxicity. *Arthroscopy* 1990;6:112–14

38. Goldenberg M, Zolti M, Seidman DS, *et al.* Transient blood oxygen desaturation, hypercapnia, and coagulopathy after operative hysteroscopy with glycine used as the distending medium. *Am J Obstet Gynecol* 1994;170:25–9

39. Imasogie N, Crago R, Leyland NA, *et al.* Probable gas embolism during operative hysteroscopy caused by products of combustion. *Can J Anesth* 2002;49:1044–7

40. Bloomstone J, Chow CM, Isselbacher E, *et al.* A pilot study examining the frequency and quantity of gas embolization during operative hysteroscopy using a monopolar resectoscope. *J Am Assoc Gynecol Laparosc* 2002;9:9–14

41. Brooks PG. Venous air embolism during operative hysteroscopy. *J Am Assoc Gynecol Laparosc* 1997;4:399–402

42. Stoloff DR, Isenberg RA, Brill AI. Venous air and gas emboli in operative hysteroscopy. *J Am Assoc Gynecol Laparosc* 2001;8:181–92

43. Munro MG, Brill AI, Ryan T, *et al.* Electrosurgery induced generation of gases: comparison of *in vitro* rates of production using bipolar and monopolar electrodes. *J Am Assoc Gynecol Laparosc* 2003;10:252–9

44. Munro MG, Weisberg M, Rubinstein E. Gas and air embolization during hysteroscopic electro-surgical vaporization: comparison of gas generation using bipolar and monopolar electrodes in an experimental model. *J Am Assoc Gynecol Laparosc* 2001;8:488–94

45. Salat-Baroux J, Hamou JE, Maillard G. Complications from microhysteroscopy. In Siegler A, Lindemann JHJ, eds. *Hysteroscopy, Principles, and Practices.* Philadelphia: Lippincott, 1984:112–17

46. Bracco PL, Vassallo AM, Armentano G. Infectious complications of diagnostic hyster-oscopy. *Minerva Ginecol* 1996;48:293–8

47. Agostini A, Cravello L, Shojai R, *et al.* Post-operative infection and surgical hysteroscopy. *Fertil Steril* 2002;77:766–8

48. McCausland VM, Fields GA, McCausland AM, *et al.* Tubo-ovarian abscesses after operative hysteroscopy. *J Reprod Med* 1993;38:198–200

49. Cohen MR, Dmowski WP. Modern hysteroscopy. Diagnostic and therapeutic potential. *Fertil Steril* 1973;24:905–9

50. Hill DJ, Maher PF. Pregnancy following endometrial ablation. *Gynecol Endocrinol* 1992;1:47–8

51. Whitelaw NL, Garry R, Sutton CJG. Pregnancy following endometrial ablation: 2 case reports. *Gynecol Endocrinol* 1992;1:129–31

52. Pinette M, Katz W, Drouin M, *et al.* Successful planned pregnancy following endometrial ablation with the YAG laser. *Am J Obstet Gynecol* 2001;185:242–3

53. Pugh CP, Crane JM, Hogan TG. Successful intrauterine pregnancy after endometrial ablation. *J Am Assoc Gynecol Laparosc* 2000;7:391–4

54. Ismail MS, Torsten U, Serour GI, *et al.* Is endometrial ablation a safe contraceptive method? Pregnancy following endometrial abla-tion. *Eur J Contracept Reprod Health Care* 1998;3:99–102

55. Darabi K, Roy K, Richart RM. Collaborative studies on hysteroscopic sterilization pro-cedures: final report. In Sciarra JJ, Zatuchni GI, Speidel JJ, eds. *Risks, Benefits, and Controversies in Fertility Control.* Hagerstown, MD: Harper and Row, 1978:81–101

56. Indman PD, Brown WW. Uterine surface temperature changes caused by electrosurgical endometrial coagulation. *J Reprod Med* 1992;37:667–8

57. Kivneck S, Kanter MH. Bowel injury from rollerball ablation of the endometrium. *Obstet Gynecol* 1992;79:883–4

58. Sullivan B, Kenney P, Siebel M. Hysteroscopic resection of fibroid with thermal injury to sigmoid. *Obstet Gynecol* 1992;80:546–7

59. Vilos GA, Brown S, Graham G, *et al.* Genital tract electrical burns during hysteroscopic endo-metrial ablation: report of 13 cases in the United States and Canada. *J Am Assoc Gynecol Laparosc* 2000;7:141–7

60. Hubert SR, Marcus PS, Rothenberg JM, *et al.* Hematometra after thermal balloon endo-metrial ablation in a patient with cervical incompetence. *J Am Laparosc Adv Surg Tech* 2001;11:311–13

61. Leung PL, Tam WH, Yuen PM. Hysteroscopic appearance of the endometrial cavity following thermal balloon endometrial ablation. *Fertil Steril* 2003;79:1226–8

62. Goldrath MH. Use of danazol in hysteroscopic surgery for menorrhagia. *J Reprod Med* 1990;35:91–2

63. Townsend DE, McCausland V, McCausland A, *et al.* Postablation tubal sterilization syndrome. *Obstet Gynecol* 1993;82:422–3

64. Dwyer N, Fox R, Mills M, *et al.* Haematometra caused by hormone replacement therapy after endometrial resection. *Lancet* 1991;338:1205–6

65. Goldrath MH. Hysteroscopic laser ablation of the endometrium. *Obstet Gynecol Forum* 1990;4:2–4

66. Copperman AB, DeCherney AH, Olive DL. A case of endometrial cancer following endo-metrial ablation for dysfunctional uterine bleeding. *Obstet Gynecol* 1993;82:640–2

67. Anonymous. A Scottish audit of hysteroscopic surgery for menorrhagia: complications and follow up. Scottish Hysteroscopy Audit Group. *Br J Obstet Gynaecol* 1995;102:249–54

68. Aydeniz B, Gruber IV, Schauf B, *et al.* A multi-center survey of complications associated with 21 676 operative hysteroscopies. *Eur J Obstet Gynecol Reprod Biol* 2002;104:160–4

69. Jansen FW, Vredevoogd CB, van Ulzen K, *et al.* Complications of hysteroscopy: a prospective, multicenter study. *Obstet Gynecol* 2000;96:266–70

70. Propst AM, Liberman RF, Harlow BL, *et al.* Complications of hysteroscopic surgery: predicting patients at risk. *Obstet Gynecol* 2000;96:517–20

Index